The Research Pro

Other books of interest

Writing for Nursing and Allied Professions
D.S.F. Cormack
0 632 01129 7

Professional Discipline in Nursing, Midwifery and Health Visiting
Second Edition
R. Pyne
0 632 02975 7

The Research Process in Nursing

EDITED BY

DESMOND F.S. CORMACK

RMN, RGN, Dip Nurs, MPhil, Dip Ed, PhD
Honorary Reader in Health and Nursing,
Department of Health and Nursing,
Queen Margaret College, Clerwood Terrace, Edinburgh EH12 8TS

FOREWORD BY

BARONESS McFARLANE OF LLANDAFF

Hon DSc (Ulster), MA (Lond.), Hon MSc (Manch.),
BSc (Soc.)(Lond.), SRN, SCM, HV Tut. Cert. FRCN
Emeritus Professor
University of Manchester, Stopford Building
Oxford Road, Manchester M13 39T

and

MARJORIE SIMPSON

OBE, SRN, BA (Hons), FRCN
Formerly Principal Nursing Officer (Research)
Department of Health and Social Security London

SECOND EDITION

OXFORD

BLACKWELL SCIENTIFIC PUBLICATIONS

LONDON EDINBURGH BOSTON

MELBOURNE PARIS BERLIN VIENNA

© 1984, 1991 by
Blackwell Scientific Publications
Editorial offices:
Osney Mead, Oxford OX2 0EL
25 John Street, London WC1N 2BL
23 Ainslie Place, Edinburgh EH3 6AJ
3 Cambridge Center, Cambridge,
    Massachusetts 02142, USA
54 University Street, Carlton
    Victoria 3053, Australia

Other Editorial Offices:
Librairie Arnette SA
2, rue Casimir-Delavigne
75006 Paris
France

Blackwell Wissenschafts-Verlag
Meinekestrasse 4
D-1000 Berlin 15
Germany

Blackwell MZV
Feldgasse 13
A-1238 Wien
Austria

First Edition published 1984
Reprinted 1985, 1987, 1989
Second Edition published 1991
Reprinted 1992

Set by DP Photosetting, Aylesbury, Bucks,
    England
Printed and bound in Great Britain by
Hartnolls, Bodmin, Cornwall

DISTRIBUTORS

Marston Book Services Ltd
PO Box 87
Oxford OX2 0DT
(*Orders:* Tel: 0865 791155
        Fax: 0865 791927
        Telex: 837515)

USA
    Blackwell Scientific Publications, Inc.
    3 Cambridge Center
    Cambridge, MA 02142
    (*Orders:* Tel: 800 759-6102
                617 225-0401)

Canada
    Times Mirror Professional Publishing, Ltd
    5240 Finch Avenue East
    Scarborough, Ontario M1S 5A2
    (*Orders:* Tel: 800 268-4178
                416 298-1588)

Australia
    Blackwell Scientific Publications
    (Australia) Pty Ltd
    54 University Street
    Carlton, Victoria 3053
    (*Orders:* Tel: 03 347-0300)

British Library
Cataloguing in Publication Data

The research process in nursing.
    1. Nursing. Research
    I. Cormack, Desmond F. S.
    610.73072

    ISBN 0-632-02891-2

Contents

List of Contributors

ANNIE ALTSCHUL BA, MSc, RGN, RMN, RNT, FRCN, Emeritus Professor of Nursing, University of Edinburgh, Adam Ferguson Building, 40 George Square, Edinburgh EH8 9LL, UK

F. IAN ATKINSON BSc (Hons), PhD, RGN, RMN, Research Fellow, Nursing Research Unit, Department of Nursing Studies, University of Edinburgh, 12 Buccleuch Place, Edinburgh EH8 9JT, UK

PHILIP J. BARKER RNMH, PhD, Clinical Nurse Consultant, Royal Dundee Liff Hospital, Liff, By Dundee DD1 5NF, UK

DAVID C. BENTON RGN, RMN, BSc, MPhil, District Research Nurse, North Essex Health Authority, District Headquarters, Turner Road, Colchester, Essex CO4 5JR, UK

SENGA BOND RGN, BA, MSc, PhD, FRCN, Lecturer in Nursing Research, Centre for Health Service Research, University of Newcastle-upon-Tyne, 21 Claremont Place, Newcastle-upon-Tyne NE2 4AA, UK

DIANA E. CARTER RGN, SCM, DIPNurs, RNT, BA, MSc, Lecturer in Nursing Studies, Department of Nursing Studies, University of Glasgow, 68 Oakfield Avenue, Glasgow G12 8LS, UK

JAMES CONNECHEN RGN, RMN, RNT, RCT, BEd (Hons), Management Development Adviser, Management Development Group, Scottish Health Service Centre, Crewe Road South, Edinburgh EH4 2LF, UK

DESMOND F.S. CORMACK RMN, RGN, DipNurs, MPhil, DipEd, PhD, Honorary Reader in Health and Nursing, Department of Health and Nursing, Queen Margaret College, Clerwood Terrace, Edinburgh EH12 8TS, UK

PETER T. DONNAN DCR, BA, MSc, FRSS, Research Fellow, Medical Statistics Unit, Department of Community Medicine, Medical School, Teviot Place, Edinburgh EH8 9AG, UK

LISBETH HOCKEY OBE, RGN, SCM, HV, QNCert, RNT, FRCN, BSc (Econ), PhD, Honorary Reader in Health and Nursing, Department of Health and Nursing, Queen Margaret College, Clerwood Terrace, Edinburgh EH12 8TS, UK

MAURA HUNT RGN, SCM, HVT, MPhil, PhD, Nursing Research Liaison Officer, South East Thames Regional Health Authority, Thrift House, Collington Avenue, Bexhill-on-Sea, East Sussex TN39 3NQ

PATRICIA OSBORNE RGN, DN, CertEd (FE), Nurse Tutor, Mid Glamorgan

School of Nursing, Prince Charles Hospital, Merthyr Tydfil, Mid Glamorgan CF47 9DT, UK

LINDA C. POLLOCK BSc, RGN, RMN, Dip in ClinNur, DistNurs Cert, PhD, Director of Nursing Services, Royal Cornhill Hospital, Cornhill Road, Aberdeen AB9 2ZY, UK

ALLAN S. PRESLY MA, DipPsych, PhD, FBPsS, CPsychol, Head of Adult Psychology Services, Psychology Department, Stratheden Hospital, Cupar, Fife KY15 5RR, UK

ANNE MARIE RAFFERTY RGN, DN, BSc, MPhil, Nurse Teacher, Clinical Practice Development Team, School of Nursing, John Radcliffe Hospital, Headington, Oxford OX3 9DU, UK

PHYLLIS J. RUNCIMAN BSc, RGN, SCM, HV, MPhil, MSc, RNT, Senior Lecturer (Research Development), Department of Health and Nursing, Queen Margaret College, Clerwood Terrace, Edinburgh EH12 8TS, UK

RUTH A. SCHRÖCK MA, PhD, DNS, SRN, RMN, RNT, Professor of Nursing and Social Sciences, Fachhochschule Osnabruck, Aibrechtstrasse 30, 4500 Osnabruck, Germany

ALISON J. TIERNEY BSc (SocSc-Nurs), PhD, RGN, Director, Nursing Research Unit, Department of Nursing Studies, University of Edinburgh, 12 Buccleuch Place, Edinburgh EH8 9JT, UK

CHRISTINE WEBB BA, MSc, PhD, SRN, RSCN, RNT, Professor of Nursing, Department of Nursing, University of Manchester, Stopford Building, Oxford Road, Manchester M13 9PT, UK

JENIFER WILSON-BARNETT SRN, DipN, RNT, BA, MSc, PhD, FRCN, Professor and Head of Department, Department of Nursing Studies, King's College London, 552 Kings Road, London SW10 0AU, UK

Foreword

THE RESEARCH PROCESS IN NURSING

The Past

Change in nursing practice, organization and education is inevitable and indeed proper as new knowledge becomes available and society itself changes. Research has a place in determining the direction of change. This book throws light on the nature of the research and should be helpful to all nurse decision makers.

Historically, statistical and fact-finding exercises, as well as medical research relevant to nursing practice, were going on even in the plateau between Florence Nightingale's major work and the spate of new approaches following World War II. Nurses were not prepared for research, and work by them is sparse. Other disciplines stepped in. The nurse and organizational aspects of her life and work received attention, whilst research relating to nursing practice had mainly to wait until nurses acquired research skills.

For the emergence of nurse researchers, growing points were needed. The Royal College of Nursing Research Discussion Group, started in 1959, provided a rallying point for nurses trying to break into the research field. From 1962 the government health departments began to build a framework within which nurses could develop their research potential. Practical encouragement was given with finance for fellowships, projects, programmes and research units, underwriting of research publications, provision of a research index and research abstracts, and the setting up of such focal points as the nursing research liaison group. Concurrently, nursing education opportunities were opening up in the universities, producing graduate nurses, suitable settings for research units and the growth of independent centres for healthy research development.

With the growth of nurse participation in research, the studies of nurses and administrative problems prevalent in the 1940s and 1950s came to be accompanied by more studies of nursing practice and more sophisticated work. Theoretical underpinning of nursing research, however, has remained weak.

The breadth of this book gives an indication of the level to which research in nursing has developed. It should stimulate the researcher to improve the techniques of the craft and to produce comprehensible reports for research users.

Tierney (p. 331) comments 'Using research is a complex task; ...'. She distinguishes usefully between utilization and implementation of findings; describes the illumination research reports can bring and suggests using developed research methods as audit tools.

In Chapter 34 Connechen places responsiblility on management to provide a climate conducive to enquiry, and Osborne (Chapter 33) accepts squarely the task of education to produce a research-minded profession.

Used selectively, *The Research Process in Nursing* should enable all sections of the profession to contribute to the further advancement of research in nursing.

H. Marjorie Simpson

The Future

The growth of nursing research in the last forty years is a tribute to those who pioneered its development and brought the profession to the position where it was acknowledged that 'nursing should be a research-based profession'.

The first edition of *The Research Process in Nursing* helped many nurses to equip themselves to appreciate the process involved in research and for some who undertook research, it was a valuable textbook. This second and enlarged edition is in itself a tribute to the developments which have taken place in nursing research since the first edition was published in 1984. It deals in far greater depth with the research process including research design, but there are new and valuable additions dealing with qualitative research, grounded theory, action research, historical research, evaluation research and the differences between descriptive and experimental research. It thus becomes a valuable sourcebook for those making choices about research design and methods.

If nursing is to become a research-based profession, the implication is that the practitioners of nursing must be knowledgeable about the research relevant to their field of practice, able to critically evaluate it and use it. This means that research appreciation must become an integral part of the preparation of all practitioners and that its application is accepted as part of a 'research and development' continuum in which practitioners and researchers alike are involved.

The advent of UKCC Project 2000 has opened the door to new approaches in nursing education which should open up educational strategies and will generate research awareness. The closer links with higher education and the transfer of schools and colleges of nursing and midwifery to higher education will greatly facilitate this process as will the systems of credit accumulation and transfer and Open University courses at post registration level. Opportunities to study a wide range of research methods and to carry out research at Masters and Doctoral level continue to expand and for all of these, this book which gathers together the wisdom and experience of so many respected nurse researchers will be invaluable.

Inevitably, much of the early research in nursing has been descriptive, for a profession needs first to describe the phenomena or basic concepts operating in its field. But a profession like nursing needs to be able to prescribe nursing care that is based on sound scientific principles. For this it needs to develop 'prescriptive' theories. The dominant goal of nursing research must remain the development of theories for nursing practice which demonstrate the relationship between patient needs, nursing interventions and patient outcomes. A greater involvement of nurse practitioners in such work together with those who specialise in nursing research and those of other disciplines, may help to achieve this.

Just as the profession worked on and produced a *Strategy for Nursing* so it now recognises the need for a parallel *Strategy for Nursing Research* with targets for research and development that embrace the practice of nursing, education and management. This book which Desmond Cormack has so skillfully edited and expanded is poised to assist in these developments.

McFarlane of Llandaff

Preface

The general inspiration for this book came from the now widely accepted sense of the need for all *nurses* to become aware of, and knowledgeable about, the application of the research process to *nursing*. All these teachers, some nurses and some not, from whom I have had the privilege of learning my research skills are recognized as having sown the seeds of this work. All these teachers, some of whom have contributed to this book, have made a unique contribution to the development of nursing research.

Students to whom I have taught the subject and whose research I have supervised, have also contributed to this work. It might be argued that one of the best means of extending one's knowledge of a subject is to teach it – research is no exception.

Not all nurses will carry out research work, although the potential for all professional nurses to do so exists. Many nurses will choose to remain consumers of the research undertaken by others. A thorough understanding of the research process as outlined in this book, however, is essential to both researchers and consumers of research. Thus, *all* professional nurses should acquire an understanding of the research process in nursing; this text offers one means of doing so. It has been prepared for all professional nurses and is so designed that it can be used to introduce the subject either during or after training.

Although the title and terminology used in this text imply that it relates only to nurses and nursing, this is not so. The terms *nurse* should be taken to encompass other staff groups who are part of, or are in close relationship with, the nursing profession. Examples are midwives, health visitors, district nurses, occupational health nurses, and community psychiatric and mental handicap nurses. Indeed, because the research process is the same irrespective of the discipline being studied, other health care groups such as occupational therapists, psychologists, social workers, pharmacologists, and chiropodists may find this book of value.

Although the contribution of both men *and* women in nursing and nursing research is firmly recognized, nurses and researchers will be referred to as 'she' throughout this text. Where the subject of the research is referred to, for example the patient or client, the term 'he' will be used. Thus, the repeated use of the clumsy alternative 'he/she' or 'he or she' will be avoided.

Finally, bear in mind that those who contributed to this book have done so recognizing that no single text or experience can, of itself, provide all the answers relating to the research process in nursing or any of its parts. This book should be used as part of a planned programme of study for one of two purposes. First, by those who wish to read and understand research findings; examples of this group are all nurses in training. Second, as part of a programme of study which will enable reading and understanding of research, and which will then underpin further reading and *supervised* research being undertaken by some nurses.

Desmond F. S. Cormack
Edinburgh

Part I
Introduction to the Research Process in Nursing

The purpose of Part I is to put the subsequent discussion of the research process into context and to 'set the scene' for the more detailed material which follows. The extensive introduction is presented in the belief that a firm understanding of the place of research in nursing must precede a consideration of the detailed phases of the research process. Only with the initial more general introduction, will readers be able to optimize their understanding of research, and their potential contribution to the development of nursing as a research-based profession. Chapter 1 presents a clear description of what research is and why it is of importance to the nursing profession. Not all readers will have a prior belief in the value of research to nursing; this chapter provides a persuasive argument which will reinforce the views of the converted, and convert the sceptic.

An understanding of the research process in nursing, and any subsequent contribution to the development of it as a research-based profession must be placed within a framework of previous research development. As is the case with researching a specific subject area, when the researcher makes herself aware of previous work on the subject, she should be equally aware of how her study will contribute to the general growth of research in nursing. Chapter 2 traces the landmarks in this development and gives some pointers for the future.

Chapter 3 is intended to reduce the potential isolation which many aspiring researchers experience or fear because they are unaware of the many and varied agencies which are available to give support. Some of these agencies may be unknown; others may be known but thought of as being for the use of non-nurse researchers only.

A full consideration of moral issues pervades all aspects of research, particularly that which deals with human subjects as is often the case in nursing. Chapter 4 considers these issues and offers guidelines which will direct both those who do and those who consume research.

The use of specialist research terms may inhibit nurses' use of published research and frustrate their attempts to understand what the research process is, and how to make use of it. The selected common terms and concepts discussed in Chapter 5 are intended to introduce readers to the specialist language of research. Although over-use of technical terms or 'jargon' is to be strongly condemned, a number of terms and concepts must be understood by the reader of research reports. The purpose of this chapter is not to present a comprehensive list of such terms, rather it is intended to demonstrate the need to understand these, and the relative ease with which their meaning can be understood.

It is anticipated that this text will be used by those who wish to understand the research process, and by those who teach the subject. Chapter 6 provides a structure which might be used to help students learn about the research process. The chapter explores a range of means, both formal and informal, by which a knowledge of the nursing research process can be developed.

Finally, Chapter 7 emphasizes the sequential nature of the research process and the interrelationship of each of its phases. This general overview of the research process should be seen as an introduction to the more detailed discussion of the steps in the process which are presented in Part II.

1

Chapter 1
The Nature and Purpose of Research
Lisbeth Hockey

THE NATURE OF RESEARCH

What is research?

It might have been reasonable to assume that the question 'What is research?', addressed in the first edition of this volume (1984) is no longer relevant. By now, all nurses should have a clear idea of the nature of research. After all, many books on nursing research have appeared in the last few years on both sides of the Atlantic. However, remarkably few include a definition of the term, for example, Clark (1987), Macleod Clark and Hockey (1989). On the whole, authors of research texts seem to assume that the meaning of the term is self-evident. Treece and Treece (1982) offer the following definition:

'Research in its broadest sense is an attempt to gain solutions to problems. More precisely, it is the collection of data in a rigorously controlled situation for the purpose of prediction or explanation.'

In my view, neither part of the above version is unreservedly acceptable because neither constitutes a necessary or a sufficient characteristic of research. Not all research attempts to solve problems, and the collection of data in a rigorously controlled situation is not appropriate for all types of research.

My recent and current experience suggests that misconceptions about the nature of research remain. Even in 1990, some people, lay and professional, believe that research connotes the kind of advanced scientific activity which is only undertaken by scientists in an academic setting, probably in a laboratory. Whilst such activity is likely to be research, the interpretation is narrow and does not include many other types of endeavour which are not necessarily undertaken by academic scientists in a laboratory. For others, it means little more than common sense, which is also a misguided belief. Common sense is extremely useful but not adequate. The essential characteristic of research is its scientific nature; research is a process which has to be undertaken according to certain scientific rules, the research process.

The research process can be learned and applied by people who are not necessarily academic scientists and it need not be confined to a laboratory. The research process consists of a sequence of steps, which includes mental activities that are designed to increase the sum of what is known about certain phenomena in all types of disciplines. Thus, one might wish to increase the sum of what is known about the history of nursing, about the prevention and treatment of pressure sores, about organizational change, about the effectiveness of certain

3

educational programmes, about sleep, about patient anxieties, and so on.

The researcher must distinguish between the 'sum of what is known' and 'what I know'. To increase what I know I must read and learn; I do not need to undertake research, providing, of course, that what I want to know has already been found out and documented by somebody; in other words, that it is part of 'what is known'. I can find out what is already known by referring to libraries and other resources and this is a necessary early step in the research process. Clark (1987) explains different ways of acquiring nursing knowledge.

It will be evident that processes designed to further explore the history of nursing, the prevention and treatment of pressure sores, organizational change, the effectiveness of educational programmes, sleep, patient anxieties, and any other topics, must differ from each other. The questions being asked must determine the type and design of the research. What remains static is the logical sequence of the steps in a process which is being undertaken according to the scientific rules of the respective discipline – history, physical sciences or behavioural sciences, for example.

Defining research

It is now possible to offer a definition of research as: an attempt to increase the sum of what is known, usually referred to as 'a body of knowledge', by the discovery of new facts or relationships through a process of systematic scientific enquiry, the research process (Macleod Clark & Hockey 1989).

It is important to recognize that it is not only the discovery of new facts which adds to available knowledge, but also that of new relationships. To return to some of the above examples, basic facts about the development of nursing can be retrieved from documentary sources of the time through systematic scientific historical enquiry. Such historical research will also attempt to disentangle the events of the time, to explore primary and secondary sources in the hope of offering plausible explanations of events, and to throw new light on those events by the discovery of relationships.

The science of physiology has provided new knowledge about the relationship between skin integrity and pressure. However, it is possible that other variables, such as the action of certain drugs or mental state, may also play a part in causing sores.

In order to discover effective treatments, experimental research, that is the collection of data in rigorously controlled situations, will be appropriate. Organizational change might best be explored through action research (see Chapter 17) which deliberately rules out any control of the situation. Sleep research is another relevant example that demonstrates the importance of discovering new relationships. Sleep has been observed and described; a number of facts about sleep are known. Sleep research is likely to continue for some time because much more knowledge is needed about the relationship between sleep in its many forms and various aspects of the human body and mind. Research into sleep-inducing drugs is concerned with relationships between the drug, the characteristics of the person taking it, and the form of sleep in terms of the quality and amount that it induces. In this example, one finds oneself in the realm of experimental research which attempts to establish causal relationships. A causal relationship implies knowledge about cause and effect and experimental research can create such knowledge.

Main types of research

In the preceding brief account of the meaning of research, four main types are alluded to. Historical research, such as that related to the history of nursing, which explores documentary data sources; descriptive research, such as the study of sleep, which describes phenomena, situations and events as they are; experimental research, such as treatment research, which manipulates the situation by introducing variables, for example the application of a certain ointment in order to test its effect; action research, which carefully describes the processes leading to planned change.

Many versions and different levels of sophistication within each of the main types of research have been developed. It is not my purpose to present the intricacies of the research method but rather to introduce the topic and to convey the fundamental principle that the type of research and the design and methods used to create new knowledge, must be appropriate for the problems to be explored. The research process is a means to a desired end and not an end in itself; an inappropriate process will not lead to the desired end.

Defining nursing research

Having offered a definition of research, it remains to explain the nature of *nursing* research or research in *nursing*. What is it? Is it different from other research and, if so, in what way? Many different definitions of nursing research have been advanced and there cannot be a totally right or wrong answer to the questions about its nature. Because nursing encompasses a wide range of activities, because it is interpreted differently in different parts of the world, and because it changes over time, a definition of the term nursing research and an explanation of its nature should make provision for these variations.

Nursing research is defined here as research into those aspects of professional activity which are predominantly and appropriately the concern and responsibility of nurses. Where nurses have little or no appropriate or predominant responsibility, nursing research makes little sense. Where nurses have responsibility for nursing education, for the administration of nursing services, and for all aspects of nursing practice, nursing research encompasses all these areas. At the time when nurses were not the appropriate personnel to monitor patients' vital signs, for example, blood pressure, nursing research would not have included studies of such monitoring procedures. Similarly, where nurses are not permitted to give patients information about how they can expect to feel after certain surgical procedures, for example, research into the relationships between information giving and patient outcomes would not fall into the category of either nursing research or research in nursing. In many countries, nurses are not in control of nursing education; in those cases, research in the field of nursing education would lie outside the scope of nursing research and the same is true for nursing administration. In terms of the research process – the series of logical steps which have to be undertaken to develop further the available knowledge – nursing research is no different from any other. The same rules of the scientific method apply and, just as in any other research, the specific type, design, the method of the research must be appropriate for the problems or questions to be investigated. Nursing represents a unique mix of several disciplines and any of the disciplines underlying nursing might be appropriate for research in nursing: for example, patients' anxiety can be viewed and studied from a psychological perspective, in which case psychological knowledge will be applied and psychological measurements might be utilized. Patients' anxiety can also be viewed and studied from a physiological perspective, in which case the biological sciences will be invoked to provide the necessary scientific guidelines. In time, nursing will develop more of its own nursing perspectives and nursing measures.

Deductive and inductive research

Nursing research may set out to test theories developed in other settings: for example, organizational theories developed in industry have been tested in nursing. It may set out to test theories or models developed by other researchers in nursing. Research which is designed to test general theories in particular situations is referred to as deductive research. It is also possible to study nursing inductively. Here, the particular situation would be the starting point for study. Inductive research, which also has its own scientific rules, might result in the identification of certain patterns, eventually leading to the formulation of hypotheses or the advance of general theories which can then be tested deductively.

Quantitative and qualitative research

The distinction between quantitative and qualitative research is also important. As the terms suggest, quantitative research simply attempts to demonstrate and present its findings in terms of numbers, frequencies, amounts: quantitative research quantifies or measures. Quantitative research is dependent on numbers for its conclusions and usually employs statistical techniques. Qualitative research is more concerned with individual situations, with incidents and phenomena which either occur infrequently or which are deliberately explored in isolation.

There is no intention in qualitative research to count or quantify, the aim is rather to describe in detail with a view to explaining the object of study. The researcher will be guided by certain ideas, perspectives or hunches in the overall approach to the area to be investigated but the aim will be to allow the 'subjects' of the research, such as patients, nurses, and relatives, to provide information in a more spontaneous way.

A survey of registered nurses in the UK, in an attempt to establish age structure, educational background and marital state – and using mainly postal questionnaires to gather the information – would be an example of quantitative research. A case study of nurses in one single intensive care unit which might include observations, interviewing and other forms of information gathering, would be an example of qualitative research.

Many research projects consist of a combination of quantitative and qualitative approaches. By now, it should be clear to the reader that the nature and the purpose of research are closely interrelated. Various research designs are explained in Chapters 13 to 21.

THE PURPOSES OF NURSING RESEARCH

As suggested by the definition of research advanced, its purpose is to increase the body of knowledge, the sum of what is known. The purpose of research in nursing is, therefore, to increase the sum of what is known about the professional activity of nurses, which may be nursing education, nursing administration or nursing practice in its many forms and settings. Research in nursing is relatively new and a great deal of what nurses do and teach is based on tradition, convention, hunches, and beliefs rather than on evidence. Research in nursing attempts to change this situation and to provide the professional discipline of nursing with a base which can be defended on grounds of scientifically established knowledge.

Research in nursing begins with questions about nursing. Questions may be generated by an intelligent curiosity, by a wish to find out more about the respective activity; they may also be generated by an urgent need to identify more effective and (probably also) less costly methods of providing nursing care, of educating nurses, or of providing an effective administrative structure. There are many unanswered questions in nursing and there are even more questions which have not yet been asked.

The main purposes of nursing research may be summarized as:

(1) To establish scientifically defensible reasons for nursing activities;
(2) To provide nurses with an increased repertoire of scientifically defensible nursing intervention options;
(3) To find ways of increasing the cost-effectiveness of nursing activities;
(4) To provide a basis for standard setting and quality assurance;
(5) To provide evidence of weaknesses and strengths in nursing;
(6) To provide evidence in support of demands for resources in nursing;
(7) To satisfy the academic curiosity of thinking nurses;
(8) To facilitate inter-disciplinary collaboration in health care research;
(9) To facilitate multi-national collaboration in nursing and nursing research;
(10) To earn and defend a professional status for nursing.

All these purposes are worthy of urgent pursuit, and therefore research in nursing is not an optional extra, a luxury, or an activity reserved for an academic elite who have chosen to opt out of nursing. Although the type and level of involvement is bound to vary according to interest, aptitude, ambition, competence, motivation and opportunity, research in nursing is every nurse's business.

OFFICIAL STATEMENTS ABOUT NURSING RESEARCH

The Committee on Nursing

As early as 1972, the Committee on Nursing stressed the need to give nursing a research base. The Committee stated:

'. . . a sense of the need for research should become part of the mental equipment of every practising nurse or midwife.'

Cormack (1979) suggested that the nursing profession will be recognized as being 'research based' when the above situation is achieved *and* when research becomes an integral part of nursing practice.

United Kingdom Central Council (UKCC) for Nursing, Midwifery and Health Visiting

The Report of the Committee on Research of the UKCC was presented to Council in 1983, just a little too late for the first edition of this book. The Report provides strong support for the development of nursing research and sets out the Council's suggested strategies and recommendations.

Code of Professional Conduct (UKCC 1984)

In its second edition (1984), the UKCC sets out a concise code of professional conduct for the nurse, midwife, and health visitor.

'Each registered nurse, midwife and health visitor shall act, at all times, in such a manner as to justify public trust and confidence, to uphold and enhance the good standing and reputation of the profession, to serve the interests of society, and above all to safeguard the interests of individual patients and clients.'

'Each registered nurse, midwife and health visitor is accountable for his or her practice . . .'

Research awareness is implicit in the above document. A nurse who is oblivious of the latest available knowledge relevant to his or her area of practice, using redundant methods, cannot expect public trust and confidence and such a nurse will *not* enhance the good standing and reputation of the profession. The interests of society will *not* be served and interests of individual patients and clients will *not* be safeguarded.

The International Council of Nurses ICN

In 1985, the ICN published *Guidelines for Nursing Research Development*. The introduction states the commitment of the ICN to the development of nursing research worldwide.

'The International Council of Nurses is convinced of the importance of nursing research as a major contribution to meeting the health and welfare needs of people. The continuous and rapid scientific developments in a changing world highlight the need for research as a means of identifying new knowledge, improving professional education and practice, and effectively utilising resources.'

'ICN believes that nursing research should be socially relevant. It should look towards the future while drawing on the past and being concerned with the present.'

'Nursing research should include what relates to a total research plan and what may be undertaken independently. In nursing research, available resources of different levels of sophistication should be utilised and research should comply with accepted ethical standards. Research findings should be widely disseminated and their utilisation and implementation encouraged when appropriate.'

'ICN is aware that nursing research is at various stages of development in different countries, . . . but efforts to promote it are made everywhere.'

RESEARCH INVOLVEMENT

Because nursing research is at different stages of development, the involvement of nurses must take different forms. First, there must be a research awareness, a recognition that questions can and should be asked, that reading of research articles and research-based texts is essential, and that research findings should be assessed in terms of their usefulness, their relevance, and their potential for implementation. Research awareness must be cultivated by all nurses in all spheres of activity and at all levels. Such awareness should be inculcated early in the professional preparation of nurses and kept alive throughout it. Existing professional and academic education must continue to strengthen and refine research awareness and its application to nursing.

The systematic collection of information, in which most nurses are involved in one way or another, is another form of research involvement; for example, community nurses who keep records for their employing authority should be keenly aware of the purpose of the information they collect and record, and of its ultimate use in the formulation of policy.

Many nurses, knowingly – or, alas, sometimes unknowingly – become research assistants for their medical colleagues; they may collect specimens, for example, as part of medical research, or help in some other way. Such involvement can be helpful as a learning experience but it should be part of an official and fully understood contract. The nurse's part of the contract should be the contribution of the nursing dimension to the research in return for which she should be initiated into the scientific aspects of the research process and should be encouraged to participate as a colleague in the preparation of research papers.

An increasing number of nurses, especially those in first level administrative and teaching positions, find themselves with a research component as part of their job description. This aspect of their job should be clarified as soon as possible and jealously guarded. It is a precious jewel which gives opportunity for stimulating innovative activity. It should also provide legitimate time for thinking. Sometimes, nurses feel insecure in this research role and attempt to evade it by creating other 'more urgent' demands on their time. It is only too easy to do that but it may be a retrograde step in the long-term. There are opportunities for nurses to obtain advice and help with the research component of their role and they should strive to develop confidence in it. It is almost bound to add to job satisfaction, providing, of course, that the thinking process is deemed to be both desirable and satisfying.

The research component of nursing may take many different forms: it may consist of initiating others in facilitating the creation of a research-oriented environment, or it may consist of direct personal involvement. Finally, research may be undertaken by the nurse on a full-time basis, either as a member of a research team or as an individual. Several opportunities for such research exist and are discussed elsewhere in this book. (See Chapter 3.)

In spite of the many positive aspects of research involvement and its acknowledged defensible and urgent purposes and aims, there are still many arguments in favour of leaving research in nursing well alone. Some of these arguments stress the urgency of other nursing activities at a time of scarce resources. It is considered that research activity cannot be defended when finance and manpower are not adequate to provide the necessary care and essential professional preparation for the basic licence to practise nursing. Managers with limited budgets feel reluctant to support research, the results of which are often unpredictable, when they could use the money for other, seemingly more urgent and certainly more easily defensible, purposes. Their views and hesitations must be respected and they must not be accused out of hand of being 'unprogressive'. Research does not always come up with results which can be utilized and, therefore, the type of research to be undertaken must be carefully considered.

However, some importance must be attached to the beneficial effects of continuing research within an organization, the dynamism it ensures, and the interest it generates. A recognition of possible long-term benefits rather than immediate results may change the outlook of understandably careful managers. In the long-term, it may be possible to save either time or money or both on redundant equipment or practices by investing some of these resources in research in the short-term.

Many members of the nursing profession fail to see, or do not wish to see, the importance of research and only perseverance and demonstration of its worth can be expected to change their attitude. Sometimes their lack of interest or enthusiasm is at least partially the fault of researchers who fail to communicate appropriately with their peer groups. The communication of research is as important as the research itself.

There is also a body of opinion that holds that research in nursing should be the concern of trained researchers and that it should not infiltrate the profession as a whole. Some reasons for this view are worthy of thought; poor research by incompetent people can do a great deal of harm and so can thoughtless implementation of findings. The more urgent attention must therefore be devoted to the appropriate education of nursing personnel for different levels of research involvement. An evasion of that responsibility can be expected to reverse any progress which has been made in advancing the sum of what is known in and about nursing.

SUMMARY AND SPECULATION FOR THE FUTURE

In this chapter an attempt has been made to support the urgent need for research in nursing. If it is recognized that a substantial part of the professional activity of nurses at all levels and in all spheres is based on convention rather than substantive knowledge, the need to extend that knowledge cannot be denied and the responsibility for research support cannot be evaded.

Research activity requires knowledge of the scientific method; the research process consists of a series of steps which is subject to scientific rules. Knowledge of the scientific method can be acquired and need not be the province of individuals who work in academic settings. All nurses must develop an awareness of research and recognize its relevance to nursing.

More direct involvement in research at different levels should be encouraged and valued. Uncertainty should be overcome by seeking help rather than by escapism and avoidance. Qualified researchers can help a great deal by teaching, explaining, and communicating intelligibly. The reservations about the investment of manpower and finance in research must be viewed sympathetically and the long-term benefits, as well as the immediate gains, of a research-oriented environment should be allowed to enter into the debate quite apart from the possibility of usable research results.

The future of nursing depends to no small extent on the development of research. There is reason not only for anxiety but also for hope. The anxiety is based on evidence of apathy and this is linked with limited resources. There is, moreover, a dearth of demonstrable benefits of research for nursing which is partly due to the lack of research findings and this can be generalized over a wider area. Most research in nursing has been undertaken single-handedly by researchers who were limited by time and finance. Their small studies require replication, which means precise and careful repetition to see if the findings can be reproduced elsewhere. Moreover, researchers have not always presented their results in a form which is appropriate for nurses in general and these results have, therefore, often been ignored. One major gap seems to be the translation of research findings into practice, an issue addressed by Hunt (1987).

Hope lies in the fact that the difficulties are being recognized and more nurses are beginning to develop a genuine interest and a measure of knowledge in research activity. More nurses ask questions and more attempt to search for an answer. Opportunities for research training are likely to increase and research involvement is beginning to be recognized as a legitimate part of professional activity.

The implementation of Project 2000 (United Kingdom Central Council for Nursing, Midwifery and Health Visiting, 1986) should provide not only incentives but also support for the development of research awareness during the process of professional preparation. Its notion of the 'knowledgeable doer' is particularly relevant.

If academic researchers can become more sensitive to professional needs and if professionals can become more sensitive to the need for scientific enquiry, the future for professional nursing – for the care of patients, for the education of nurses, and for the management of nursing services – is exciting and justifies optimism.

REFERENCES

Clark E. (1987) *Research Awareness, Module 2, Sources of Nursing Knowledge*, Distance Learning Centre, South Bank Polytechnic, London.

Committee on Nursing (1972) *Report of the Committee on Nursing*, HMSO, London.

Cormack D. (1979) Knowledge for What? Janforum, *Journal of Advanced Nursing*, **4**, 93–4.

Hunt M. (1987) The process of translating research findings into nursing Practice, *Journal of Advanced Nursing*, **12**, 101–10.

International Council of Nurses (1985) *Guidelines for Nursing Research Development*, ICN, Geneva.

Macleod Clark J. & Hockey L. (1989) *Further Research for Nursing*, Scutari Press, London.

Treece E.W. & Treece J.W. (1982) *Elements of Research in Nursing*, The C.V. Mosby Company, St. Louis, U.S.A.

United Kindgom Central Council for Nursing, Midwifery and Health Visiting (1983), *Nursing Research, The Role of the UKCC*, UKCC, London.

United Kingdom Central Council for Nursing, Midwifery and Health Visiting (1984), *Code of Professional Conduct for the Nurse, Midwife and Health Visitor*, UKCC, London.
United Kingdom Central Council for Nursing, Midwifery and Health Visiting (1986), *Project 2000: a new preparation for practice*, UKCC, London.

Chapter 2
The Development of Research in Nursing
Annie Altschul

It is hard to believe, now that so much is written about nursing research, that the subject has a relatively short history in Great Britain and a not very much longer one elsewhere. At present, the main concern of nurse researchers is that not all nurses read or use research reports; thirty years ago few nurses had even heard of nursing research.

INFORMATION GATHERING

One objective of nursing research is to provide baseline data for those who plan or manage nursing care and nursing services. Florence Nightingale (1820–1910) was well aware of the need for factual information. She could never have persuaded governments to make the sweeping changes they did in the military health services and in the British Colonies if she had not based her recommendations on extensive and thorough investigation and statistical analysis. However, little progress was made in the 50 years that followed. When Virginia Henderson (1970, 1972) attempted, retrospectively, to document the nursing literature for the first half of the twentieth century she was able to publish an annotated guide to 'reported studies, research methods, historical and biographical material' for the 50-year period in just two volumes. The author index for both volumes covers a mere 321 pages.

Subsequently, separate volumes were needed to cover periods of four, two and one year respectively, demonstrating how rapidly the subject expanded. Between 1950 and 1960 a large amount of so-called research was carried out almost simultaneously in different parts of the UK into different aspects of nursing. Reading some of the reports now makes one hesitant to apply the word 'research' to most of the investigations carried out; such reports are often devoid of any references and lack theoretical introductions. There may also be little attempt to justify the sampling procedures and what statistical treatment there is can be strongly criticized. It would be wrong, however, to dismiss this early research work on the grounds of lack of scientific rigour. There was, at that time, very little literature to refer to. The researchers of the 1950s are the people whose works have become classics, whose research is still quoted, and whose methods and findings have provided the starting point for much of the work which has been carried out since.

Work studies

One of the most surprising pieces of research, in retrospect, was a study by Skellern (1951), a ward sister who, single-handedly, studied administrative and teaching problems in general hospital wards. Her study was sponsored by the

Royal College of Nursing and the report is available from the RCN library. Although it was followed by a spate of large-scale work studies up and down the country, little acknowledgement was made of Skellern's pioneering efforts.

That all was not well in the organization of nursing work in hospital wards, was widely acknowledged. The report of the working party of the Ministry of Health and the Department of Health for Scotland (1955) on *Recruitment and Training of Nurses* showed that the whole organization of nurses' work needed to be reconsidered. Meanwhile a number of work studies, or, as they were referred to at the time, 'job analyses' had been carried out. The Nuffield Provincial Hospital Trust (1951, 1955, 1958) had, over the years, published studies on the function and design of hospitals – studies in which nurses had co-operated. The design of experimental wards in Greenock in Scotland, for example, and in Musgrave Park Hospital, Northern Ireland, were based partly on a study of nurses' movements in assembling equipment and carrying out nursing care.

The report of the Nuffield Provincial Hospital Trust (1951) relating to job analysis, was carried out under the auspices of the Nuffield Trust in General Hospital Wards and was an extremely influential document; nurses were members of the advisory and study teams. The report presented a very convincing picture of what nurses did and how. It demonstrated that very different work patterns existed in similar wards, pinpointing maldistribution of resources and it received a great deal of publicity. The Royal College of Nursing set up a working party to study the report and make recommendations for future policy.

One of the headings the working party had used in the report was 'What is the proper task of the nurse?', another was 'Conserving nursing skills'. People who nowadays deplore the fact that research findings are not always acted upon may pause a moment to contemplate the damage to the nursing profession which has resulted from acting upon the report of the Nuffield Provincial Hospital Trust (1953). Ever since then, nurses have been attempting to distinguish between basic care and technical care, a distinction which has led to a downgrading in the prestige of basic care, the very aspect of care which is most important to patients. People have talked ever since about 'non-nursing tasks', and have delegated to non-nurses some of the most satisfying and most skilled of nursing functions, such as the serving of food and the concern for a hygienic environment for the patient. The delegation of so-called 'basic care' such as bathing and washing patients has created problems not only of standards of care, but also in the area of professional and industrial relationships.

Perhaps one of the most damaging consequences of the report was to delegate documentation to clerical staff, depriving nurses of the very knowledge about patients which is essential to the planning of nursing care. One cannot help but wonder if the need to develop the 'nursing process' would ever have arisen if nurses had not opted out of record keeping, especially during the admission procedure of patients.

None of the adverse consequences of the Nuffield report should be blamed on the researchers, however; they are the result of taking action, sometimes inappropriately, without full consideration of the consequences that might result.

In both general hospitals and psychiatric hospitals, job analysis was the order of the day. Three work studies were published almost simultaneously (Manchester Regional Hospital Board 1955; Oppenheim & Eeman 1955; Maddox 1957). All of them showed how differently nurses in wards which on the surface were similar worked, and all acknowledged the difficulty inherent in describing what nurses do or do not do without knowing what they think or why they are doing it. The studies also revealed how little of their time nurses spend in direct contact with patients. They demonstrated differences between what student nurses were taught and what they actually did. They also questioned what was the proper function of the qualified mental nurse. It will be readily seen that none of the questions raised have yet been satisfactorily answered.

Work studies take as their starting point the geographical location in which nurses work and they document what nurses actually do. The findings often come as a surprise to the people who are the subjects of observation because, subjectively, time measurably spent on certain tasks seems quite different from that reported by the observer. The importance of a task distorts the length of time it seems to take, as does the degree to which one likes or dislikes a job. Psychiatric nurses, for example, underestimate the amount of time they spend listening to patients' problems, perhaps because of the importance they attach to this, and they overestimate the time spent locking and unlocking doors, perhaps because they dislike it. An estimate or a measurement of how much time nurses spend on domestic work or on record keeping cannot, by itself, determine what the nurse ought to do or even whether she is the best person to do it.

The role of the nurse

An attempt to answer questions about the proper function of various grades of nurses led to the research carried out by the Dan Mason Nursing Research Committee (1956, 1960). Meanwhile, the nursing profession had added to its problems by creating a new category of nurse, initially called the 'assistant nurse', whose work was studied by Bennett (1955) and by the Standing Advisory Committee of the Central Health Services Council (1954). The main problems for nursing, however, appeared to be concern not about what nurses did when they were at work, but the reasons why nurses were so difficult to recruit, why they frequently left after a short time, and why some of those nurses who stayed had high sickness or absenteeism rates. Studies of these problems have dominated the research scene for the last 30 years.

Recruitment and wastage

McGuire (1969) summarized the research into recruitment and wastage up to the late sixties, but much more recent research also exists. Research into absenteeism and sickness is particularly complex because accurate record keeping is necessary before the many variables involved can be studied. Record keeping is, however, complicated by the fact that criteria for deciding why a person is away from work keep changing. Whether a doctor's certificate is needed or not, for example, changes the whole picture; whether days off precede or follow a period of absenteeism and should be included or excluded is also not always clear. Those involved in nursing education in the last 20 years have found research into recruitment and wastage particularly relevant, and linked to this is research into selection of candidates.

In order to succeed in nursing, a certain level of ability appears to be necessary and reports have suggested that personality factors should be taken into account. Psychology offers a wealth of research in this field but so far nursing research has failed to show up any significant link between personality measurements and success in nursing. Perhaps this too is due to the fact that criteria for describing what is a 'good' nurse are difficult to develop. As early as 1949, Sawers attempted a survey of psychological tests to be used as an aid in selecting nursing candidates.

Nursing establishment

Nurse managers have been primarily interested in manpower problems which are related to selection and retention of nurses and to their training. How many nurses are needed in any particular institution is a question many people would like to have answered. Politicians would like to know because of their concern with budgeting; nurse managers need to know because they have the responsibility for the deployment of staff, and practising nurses need to know because they are required to monitor the quality of care they are able to give.

A variety of research approaches have been tried in order to estimate what the nursing establishment ought to be in the various types of Health Service agencies, in the various specialities, and in various circumstances. The most common approaches are the study of nursing dependency of patients (Barr & Moores 1972, Scottish Health Service Studies No 9 1967) and the study of the workload itself, with a measurement of the time it takes to perform the work satisfactorily. The workload depends not only on the patient's need for care, but also on ward design, on the development of suitable equipment, and on the amount of work which needs to be done but which may not be directly related to individual patients.

Attempts have been made to identify what special needs exist, for example, in obstetric wards or in psychiatric wards and what effect teaching responsibilities of trained staff have on the workload. Recent research has addressed the question of the skill mix appropriate for different types of hospital wards and for work in the community.

It has always been of importance to determine whether the employment of fewer, highly qualified, nurses gives better value for money than the employment of more, less highly trained, staff on a lower point of the salary scale. For a long time it was assumed that the clinical practice performed by student nurses was a relatively cheap way of getting the work done. However, the system of nurse-training in which service needs determine what clinical experience students gain, has long been criticized. It is now recognized that student labour is no longer cheap. Changes in nursing education, now taking place, make it imperative to use research findings in order to make the right decisions about the employment of support workers and their training. Research (Hardie 1980) has also revealed anomalies in the deployment of enrolled nurses and nursing auxiliaries, who at various times are used as unskilled workers, but, when shortage of other nurses arise, are required to shoulder responsibilities for which they have not been prepared. The imminent discontinuation of enrolled nurse training reinforces the need to research the problem of skill mix.

Nursing standards, quality assurance

Without some knowledge of the amount of work to be carried out in any particular ward, it is difficult to assess how well the staff perform their work. Measurement of the quality of work is sometimes referred to as nursing audit. Some recent research into the value of nursing audit has added to our knowledge of staffing patterns (Huczynski 1976).

While all nurses aim to deliver high quality of care to their patients, the responsibility for monitoring the quality of care is that of nurse managers. In the current climate of market forces and cost effectiveness, general managers are also involved in setting standards and checking whether they are being met. The growing awareness of nurses' own professionalism means that nurses increasingly wish to be accountable to patients and clients for the standard of their work. The importance of quality assurance work is recognized by the Department of Health (1989).

The Royal College of Nursing has been particularly active in researching the issue of standards of care and in publicizing existing research (Kitson 1989). Pearson (1987) has given one example of the way in which research into the establishment of quality of care can be pursued. This paper has shown that planners need information, and that researchers have so far provided it by studying the jobs and the people who perform them.

There are, however, other influences at work which determine the path which research has taken. The most important influence has been the sheer determination of some pioneers in nursing to ask questions about nursing practice as they found it, to challenge traditional methods of delivering care, and to allow their curiosity free rein.

RESEARCHING PATIENTS' OPINIONS AND NEEDS

Carter (1953), in a discussion of the very first issue of a new journal, *Nursing Research*, urged nurses to collaborate both for the discovery and for the solving of problems. 'They owe it to their patients', she said. The International Council of Nurses (1956, 1960) organized conferences on the planning of nursing studies to help nurses to learn how to investigate nursing problems. The reports of these two conferences can still offer helpful advice to novice researchers today.

British nurses were also getting together, often in each other's homes, to talk about research interests they had developed, problems they were encountering, and findings that had excited them. The first 'Nursing Research Interest Group' was created in London in this informal way. Research interest groups now exist in many parts of the country, playing an important part in creating interest and helping disseminate research findings.

Significant landmarks in research into nursing problems were the founding of a research unit in 1959 to investigate 'geriatric nursing problems in hospital'. Doreen Norton, the nurse appointed to the unit, had been tireless since even before that date in not only describing practical nursing problems in need of a solution, but also in persuading nurses to take innovative action as well as evaluating the effect of nursing intervention, especially with the elderly. The report of the investigation, published in 1962, was reissued in 1975 in response to the large demand from researchers who recognized that the topic is as relevant today as it was in 1962 (Norton *et al.* 1975).

Another important step in the development of research into clinical nursing problems was the appointment of a Research Officer to the Royal College of Nursing in 1955. Marjorie Simpson (1982), who held this position, and Winifred Raphael, were early researchers who took as their starting point the needs of patients and the evaluation of quality of care. The Royal College of Nursing's Study of Nursing Care (McFarlane 1970), a project which comprised 11 studies, each designed to develop tools for the evaluation of care, initiated many of the presently most influential researchers into their role. These studies produced sufficient research ideas and preliminary findings to form a basis for research for a long time to come.

The creation of Research Liaison Officers in some health authorities has generated interest among practising nurses in reading about research applicable to their own work situation and in carrying out their own investigations. Increasingly, nurses aim to find a sound research base for specific nursing actions and also to demonstrate willingness to abandon practices based purely on tradition.

Before leaving the field of nursing research related to patient needs and nursing practice, mention must be made of developments in psychiatric nursing. The 1950s were important years for psychiatric nurses everywhere because research made nurses aware of their influence on patient behaviour. Some of the studies in the US demonstrated that patients were more disturbed when nurses disagreed with doctors; they also showed that nurses could influence the incidence of incontinence, and that nurses could successfully communicate with very withdrawn schizophrenic patients (Stanton & Schwartz 1954; Greenblatt *et al.* 1955; Schwartz & Shockley 1956; Peplau 1957).

In the UK, research at the Cassell Hospital (Barnes 1968) and Tavistock Clinic, and the Henderson Hospital, all pointed to the need for research into nurse-patient relationships, but research into this area by nurses has only fairly recently begun.

More recent nursing research in the field of psychiatric care has dealt with the effectiveness of therapeutic communities and with the influence of ward atmosphere on patients (Sugden 1981). Preparation of patients for life in the community after living in the shelter of an institution is a fertile research field for nurses involved in behavioural therapy (Barker & Fraser 1985). Psychiatric nurses in hospital and in the community work in multidisciplinary teams. It is appropriate that they should be engaged in co-operative research with members of other disciplines. Community psychiatric nurses exercise increasing influence on the outcome of the policy to keep mentally disordered people in the community. Recently, their work has received considerable attention by researchers (Pollock 1989).

LEARNING TO RESEARCH

There is a third thread of influence in the development of nursing research, namely the influence which has arisen from changes in nursing education.

Research in universities

Carter (1954) completed a survey of British nurses, with university degrees and diplomas, and of the nurse tutors' course in Edinburgh. Her report strongly recommended the same opportunity for higher education for nurses as that available to other professions. She deplored the fact that the 'disciplined mental equipment of the graduate' was not understood in nursing circles as an asset in professional practice. Very soon after Carter reported, the University of Edinburgh did indeed open its doors to nurses; by 1956 the first nurse tutor students and by 1960 the first undergraduate nursing students had commenced their studies. In 1960 the first PhD degrees were awarded to nurses in Edinburgh.

University education for nurses is now fairly well established and the importance of this development for research in nursing is twofold. First, it is normal for all university students to be introduced to research in their own subject, to be expected to read research reports, and to refer to research in all their written work. For many university students, it is also expected that they carry out small research projects themselves and write a short dissertation. In some subjects, courses in research methods and statistics are part of the curriculum. There are now a large number of nurses who have had at least this minimal amount of exposure to research. Second, the function of universities is to advance knowledge. The reputation of a university department stands or falls not only by the performance of its students but by the research activities of its staff, and by the facilities it offers to postgraduate students and others to pursue research. The upturn in the research output in the UK in the last 20 years is very largely the result of the increased number of students who have produced PhD and MPhil theses and of university lecturers who have carried out research and encouraged others to do so.

The research studies carried out by postgraduate students are inevitably small in scale and are the outcome of individual effort. It was pointed out by Simpson (1971) that such a profusion of small studies was not really the most effective way for knowledge to advance.

Research units

The greatest impact on nursing in the last few years has undoubtedly come from nursing research units, of which several have now been established in the UK. Research units are more securely financed than are individual researchers: they are able to plan long-term research projects; they are able to engage in co-operative effort. They can ensure that consecutive research projects build on each other, and they are not constrained in their methodology by academic convention in the way research for higher degrees often is.

Continued funding of research units is, however, dependent on the financial circumstances of the government research councils or other funding bodies. The quality of their research output and of publications is under continuous scrutiny. They also have to demonstrate that their work satisfies the demands of consumers (Rothschild 1982). Some degree of specialization has become inevitable in order to make the most effective use of resources. It may be that, in future, specialization of research units will no longer be determined by professional identity (for example, nursing research) or by academic discipline (for example, sociology or psychology) and that instead they will be set up to investigate specific health topics on a multidisciplinary basis. Research topics which lend themselves to such an approach are beginning to emerge: for example, in pain management, continence, patient education, and terminal care.

We are fortunate in the UK in having found a number of publishers willing to accept PhD or MPhil theses for publication – in spite of the fact that, commercially, this is not very profitable. The Royal College of Nursing has also contributed in no small way to the development of nursing research in making all theses available in the Steinberg Collection of Nursing Research.

It is now not at all difficult for nurse researchers to check for themselves what research in their area of interest has already been published or is in the process of being carried out; registers of research and cumulative indices are readily available and librarians are now more than willing to help (see Chapter 9).

Conferences, presentation of papers

Great changes have taken place during the last three decades in the involvement of nurses in local, national and international conferences. It used to be rare for nurses to attend conferences and almost unheard of for nurses to be included in the list of speakers. The opportunity to attend conferences now exists, whatever the special interest of any individual nurse. Nursing research conferences are of particular value to those who are concerned with clarification of methodology, and for those who seek the opportunity to talk about their own research to an interested peer group.

For the same reason, publication of the proceedings of research conferences is also helpful. However, as the volume of nursing research grows, the era for conferences or journals to be called simply 'nursing research' seems to be coming to an end. The range of topics at conferences is becoming so large that it is difficult to identify which particular audience is being addressed. Individual nurses find it difficult to follow the sometimes complex timetables of conferences that cater for diverse interest groups and have to accommodate large numbers of concurrent sessions. Inevitably, the quality of presentations becomes uneven. Novices may tend to feel confused; experts may be disappointed. 'Nursing research journals' themselves cover too large a range of topics, too wide a span of methods, too great a difference in levels, to continue to be generally useful.

Conferences and journals which deal with specific topics of interest, not only to nurses but also to other health professionals, would now seem to be needed. A focus on such topics as cancer, AIDS or Alzheimer's disease are examples of the way specialized interest groups may be catered for. Avoiding the medical model, one might look at topics such as stress management, child abuse, nutrition, infection control. Such conferences and journals could have contributors from members of a variety of disciplines. The time has come when nurses should no longer be satisfied with attending *nursing* conferences, with reading *nursing* journals and contributing to these, but when they should offer their contributions to other disciplines and invite others to participate in nursing events.

International co-operation: transcultural research

Many research reports caution the reader against generalization from the findings, believing that they might be based on too small a sample, or that the specific setting in which data were collected may not apply to different geographical locations, or different social or cultural groups. In order to test the validity of any piece of research for different populations, the answer may not lie in the use of bigger samples but in replication of the research with different samples. There is a growing interest in establishing international co-operation in research and in carrying out transcultural research projects. The World Health Organization has initiated some transcultural nursing research (1987) using collaborating centres in England and Scotland.

An important contribution to international co-operation is the wider dissemination of research reports and the effort made by researchers to include in their literature search, and in their list of citations, references from countries other than their own.

CONCLUSION

From very small beginnings we have now moved to a stage in the development of research when we have, in this country, a fair number of well-prepared researchers, and a large number of keen, enthusiastic nurses, many of them graduates, who are trained to think and to ask questions, who read and are able to write, who have a thirst for knowledge, and insatiable curiosity. We have people of varied academic backgrounds who bring into nursing the research approaches and skills learnt in the study of their disciplines. We have a growing body of knowledge about nurses and about nursing, and an increasing number of nurses in clinical practice, teaching and administration who are willing to evaluate research findings and make use of them in their daily work.

With a number of thriving research units now well established, we have the opportunity, in the future, to co-ordinate research efforts, and to build upon previous work. The future looks promising for nursing research.

REFERENCES

Barker P. & Fraser D. (1985) *The Nurse as a Therapist*, Croom Helm, Beckenham.

Barnes E. (1968) *Psychosocial Nursing*, Tavistock Publications, London.

Barr A. & Moores B. (1972) *Nursing Dependency As A Basic For Staff Deployment.* Oxford Regional Hospital Board.

Bennett B.A. (1955) State enrolled assistant nurses in England, Wales and Scotland. *Practice Nurses Digest* **2**, 3-6.

Carter G. (1953) On being confronted with the first issue of Nursing Research. *Nursing Times* **49**, 4-5.

Carter G. (1954) University training for leadership and its relation to the nursing profession. *Nursing Mirror* **98**, (21) 1391.

Central Health Services Council (1954) *Report on the Position of the Enrolled Assistant Nurse Within the National Health Service.* HMSO, London.

Dan Mason Nursing Research Committee of Great Britain (1956) *The Work of Recently Qualified Nurses*, Dan Mason, London.

Dan Mason Nursing Research Committee of Great Britain (1960) *The Work, Responsibility and Status of the Staff Nurse*, Dan Mason, London.

Department of Health (1989) *A Strategy for Nursing*, London, Department of Health.

Greenblatt M., York R. & Brown E. (1955) *From Custodial to Therapeutic Care in Mental Hospitals*, Russell Sage, New York.

Hardie K.M. (1980) *Auxiliaries in Nursing: Implication for the Division of Nurses' Labour*, Unpublished PhD. Thesis, Edinburgh.

Henderson V. *Nursing Studies Index*. Vol. 1, 1900-1929 (published 1972) Vol. 2, 1930-1949 (published 1970). Lippincott, Philadelphia.

Huczynski A. (1976) *Doncaster Nursing Management Audit, Evaluation Study*. Nursing Research Unit, University of Edinburgh.

International Council of Nurses (1956) *International Conference on the Planning of Nursing Studies*, Sevres, France. International Council of Nurses.

International Council Of Nurses (1960) *Learning to Investigate Nursing Problems*, Delhi, India. International Council of Nurses.

Kitson A.L. (1989) *Standards of Care. A Framework for Quality*, Scutari Press, Harrow.
McFarlane J.K. (1970) *The Proper Study of the Nurse*, Royal College of Nursing, London.
McGuire J.M. (1969) *Threshold to Nursing*, Bell, London.
Maddox H. (1957) *The Work of Mental Nurses*. Birmingham University.
Manchester Regional Hospital Board (1955) *The Work of the Mental Nurse*. Manchester University Press, Manchester.
Ministry of Health and Department of Health for Scotland (1955) *Report of the Working Party on the Recruitment and Training of Nurses*. HMSO, London.
Norton D., McLaren R. & Exton-Smith A. (1975) *An Investigation of Geriatric Nursing Problems in Hospital*. Churchill Livingstone, Edinburgh.
Nuffield Provincial Hospital Trust (1951, 1955, 1958) *Studies in the Function and Design of Hospitals*, The Trust, London.
Nuffield Provincial Hospital Trust (1953) *The Work of Nurses in Hospital Wards. Report of a job analysis*. The Trust, London.
Oppenheim A.N. & Eeman B. (1955) *The Function and Training of Mental Nurses*. Chapman, London.
Pearson A. (1987) Nursing and Quality. In *Nursing Quality Measurement: Quality Assurance Methods For Peer Review*. Ed. by A. Pearson, pp. 1–14. John Wiley, Chichester.
Peplau H. (1957) *Therapeutic Concepts (in National League for Nursing, Aspects of Psychiatric Nursing)*. The League, New York.
Pollock L. (1989) *Community Psychiatric Nursing, Myth or Reality*. Scutari Press, Harrow.
Rothschild N.M. (1982) *Enquiry into the Social Science Research Council*, DES Cmmd. paper 8554.
Sawers J. (1949) *Psychological Tests as an aid to the Selection of Nursing Candidates. A survey of their development in the United States*. Report submitted to the Education Committee of the Florence Nightingale International Foundation, London.
Schwartz M.S. & Shockley E.L. (1956) *The Nurse and the Mental Patient*. Russell Sage Foundation, New York.
Scottish Health Service Studies No. 9 (1967) *Nursing Workload per Patient as a Basis for Staffing*. Work Study Department, North Eastern Regional Hospital Board. Scottish Home and Health Department, Edinburgh.
Simpson M.M. (1971) Research in nursing: the first steps. *Nursing Mirror* **132**, 11, 22–7.
Simpson M. (1982) *If I Could Alter One Thing*. The First Winifred Raphael Memorial Lecture. Royal College of Nursing, London.
Skellern E. (1951) A nursing investigation. *Nursing Times* **47**, 792.
Stanton A. & Schwartz M. (1954) *The Mental Hospital*. Tavistock Publications, London.
Sugden J. (1981) *Nursing Activity and Some Variables in the Psychiatric Treatment Process*, Unpublished M. Phil, thesis, Edinburgh.
World Health Organization (1987) *People's Needs for Nursing Care. A European Study*. World Health Organization, Regional Office for Europe, Copenhagen.

Chapter 3
Agencies Supportive to Nursing Research
Senga Bond

This chapter is devoted to sources of support for nurses who wish to carry out research. Of course, research efforts extend from large-scale multidisciplinary, multicentre projects involving major financial and manpower resources, to those which can be done by a single individual, requiring little more resources than a notebook and pencil and sufficient time. Some forms of assistance are appropriate for both types, and all research workers, whatever the stage of their research career, require support of some kind.

Let us assume that you have the motivation, interest, and a bright idea and want to embark on research but lack the knowledge of where to begin. The fact that you are reading this book would suggest that you are on the right track! Books such as this one are a useful source of ideas but because they are not interactive in the same way as people are, they are at best only a partial answer. If we posed the question, 'Why do I want help?' it might be answered in a number of ways, including:

Education for research;
Supervision and advice;
Kindred spirits to provide emotional sustenance;
Financial assistance;
Information resources.

EDUCATION FOR RESEARCH

Some aspects of research are now included as a (small) component of most nursing courses and there are many short 'research appreciation' courses. While you may have had some introduction to research ideas and to research studies, it may be worth considering more extended research training through a full- or part-time course. Courses in research methods are available at diploma level in many institutions of higher education and it is generally easier than it was to obtain time off work for a part-time day/evening course. The calendars of universities, polytechnics and colleges should provide details of whether such courses are available, and of entry requirements. Some courses provide an option which permits progress from diploma to higher degree level. Should an appropriate course not be available locally it may be worth considering the Open University 3rd Level Research Methods Course, Research Methods in Education and the Social Sciences (DE304). As its title suggests, this course is generally oriented towards the social rather than the biological sciences. It also forms part of an MSc which also may be taken through the Open University.

Another way of obtaining research education is to apply for one of the research studentships awarded annually by government health departments in Scotland, England and Wales, and Northern Ireland. In Scotland, these have recently been extended to include Health Services Research Fellowships so that nurses may apply within both categories. These studentships are generally advertised in the press each year for commencment at the beginning of the next academic year. The appropriate liaison person (from whom information can be obtained) for the government departments in each country is given at the end of this chapter. These studentships generally exist to enable nurses to obtain a higher degree through research, although this is not exclusively the case.

A glance through the appointments sections of the nursing press indicates that there are nurses who fill research appointments in many health authorities. One of their responsibilities is likely to be the maintenance of a list of research courses available locally. Research appreciation courses are not intended for those about to do research: they are oriented more towards 'consumers' and 'participants' in research rather than 'doers'. One advantage of doing a formal research methods course is to assist beginners in deciding whether they really have the motivation and ability to carry out research. While taking a course does delay the starting up of any project, it also lays down a good foundation from which to proceed. It is for this reason that students embarking on a higher degree by research are advised to participate in a general methods course, so that, as well as learning through using a particular method, they extend their knowledge to other methods and techniques used in research.

SUPERVISION AND ADVICE

The need for assistance could be in working up a project that inspires you but where you are not sure what to do next. To provide a formal supportive agency, this is the kind of work for which nursing personnel in the health service would be the first port of call. The person chosen should have a sufficiently broad overview of research to assist you to refine your ideas and begin to formulate possible directions for the project. It is important to bear in mind that it is not possible for any one individual to have detailed knowledge of every research problem with which they may be faced, but nurses in research appointments should be able to assist you sufficiently to enable you to consult with someone possessing a more specialist knowledge if this is warranted.

The Nursing and Health Services Research Units in universities and polytechnics, as well as the Daphne Heald Unit at the Royal College of Nursing, will be able to provide assistance in a few cases, although they could be inundated with requests for help, and their purpose is first and foremost to carry out their own research. It is important, therefore, to obtain help locally whenever this is possible and to be well prepared before consulting more widely.

It may be that there are other local resources besides nurses: these might include research workers in related fields, medical colleagues, or social or biomedical scientists. Ask your colleagues whether they know of anyone and watch out for 'local' names in publications. Personal recommendation of someone who is helpful is by far the best way of securing helpful contacts. Research interests are certainly one way of bridging professional boundaries as well as of drawing service matters into closer communication with nursing departments in universities and polytechnics. This is especially so when there is an interest in pursuing research for a higher degree, requiring academic supervision. However, academic staff are often pleased to assist in work directly associated with their own interests so long as the individual researcher involved is sufficiently able to work with only a small amount of intermittent supervision. The message is to begin where you are and to use whatever talent is available locally before proceeding further.

KINDRED SPIRITS

Another type of support, which is rather different from specific advice or supervision for your project, is to find like-minded individuals who are carrying out research and who face similar problems. It is probably a universal phenomenon that research workers at some point in developing or carrying out a project feel isolated, dejected, and ready to give up. At such times it is useful to share your experience with someone who may have gone through, or be in the process of facing, the same distress. This is when membership of an informal or formal research group may be useful. All local research interest groups serve several functions; one of their strengths is the bringing together of people who have a general interest in learning about and supporting research. On the whole, you are likely to find others with research interests very willing to help and listen, and to offer support of varying kinds.

Other benefits to be gained from membership of a local research group are hearing about current developments in research internationally, nationally, and locally and learning how others have gone about research and how they have attempted to overcome their particular difficulties. By providing an informal setting to discuss research issues generally, research meetings can be very positive occasions for those planning to begin, or who are already engaged in research. Less formal get-togethers of nurses involved in research are also useful. Sometimes an informal lunchtime gathering will be enough to air a difficulty and to regain vital energies which may be dwindling.

At a national level, the RCN research advisory groups provide occasions for hearing research workers talk about their work. This is most effectively done at the annual conference where the weekend is taken up by the presentation of research findings as well as the discussion of methodological issues in research. Special interest groups can also meet to discuss particular issues. While at the time of writing anyone is eligible to attend the RCN advisory group conference, full membership of the group itself is restricted to RCN members who have proven research ability, as evidenced by a higher degree or equivalent.

The other kind of non-nursing groups and associations you could consider joining are those with a more specific focus of interest; examples would be the Society for Tissue Viability, the British Society of Gerontology, and the Society for Research in Rehabilitation. While some of these are not specifically research groups, a major interest is the discussion of current research methods and findings in their respective fields. These groups are of major importance in keeping abreast of developments which are broader than nursing and maintaining current awareness. Membership of such a group would also bring you into contact with others who focus their interest in a narrower substantive field. In time, it is to be hoped that professional nursing groups like the RCN societies and forums may develop a more research-oriented approach in their conferences and professional meetings.

FINANCIAL ASSISTANCE

Financial assistance may be sought either for research education or for funding a specific project. Some health authorities have short-term training schemes which are open to nurses in their employment. An example of these would be the Greater Glasgow Health Board, which for many years has awarded research training opportunities to nurses. For several years, South West Thames Regional Health Authority have funded a scheme for nurses with an interest in the care of the elderly. This scheme involves liaison with appropriate staff at the University of Kent who provide assistance in the development of a specific project over a four-month period of secondment. Other local schemes are available in Health Authorities who wish to support research in nursing whereby a small number of posts are set aside to enable nurses working at the staff nurse/ward sister grades to spend part of each week carrying out a research project while for the remainder of the week they are employed in a service capacity. It is important in this kind of scheme to ascertain that, as well as being given paid time and the resources to mount the project, there is an element of education, supervision and assistance to sharpen research skills.

While these types of appointments are likely to be advertised in the local or national press, it is often less easy to ascertain what financial assistance may be available locally to attend a research course. Some Health Authorities consider it appropriate to fund research training, others do not. You may need to approach the most senior nurses to ask about current policy for funding research training. Health Authorities have the *discretion* of paying Open University fees if appropriate but on this, as in all educational matters, views and policies differ widely.

The government-sponsored research training schemes do provide full salary and fees and an allocation is made for research costs. Competition for these is likely to be considerable and the possession of a first degree or evidence of previous involvement in research is advantageous. However, there is nothing to be lost by carefully studying the requirements for admission to any courses or for any award and making an application. The Department of Health annually awards a post-doctoral research fellowship while the Medical Research Council includes nurses with a higher degree as eligible to apply for one of its Special Training Fellowships for Health Services Research.

In financial terms, far more money is available for funding individual projects than for research training. However, funding bodies are unlikely to finance research proposed by an inexperienced researcher and so a vicious circle can begin. A range of funding resources is available; the question is which to apply to.

Government research budgets are available to nurses through the Office of the Chief Scientist at the Department of Health in England and Wales; from the Scottish Home and Health Department in Scotland; and from the Department of Health and Social Services in Northern Ireland. The organization of each of these, however, is somewhat different.

Research funds are not set aside specifically for nurses but are held within an overall budget for Health Services Research. The Department of Health Yearbook of Research and Development provides an annual record of the research work sponsored and directly commissioned by the Department of Health. The Department's research committees agree on a number of themes each year as a framework for establishing and pursuing research priorities. Applicants for research grants are strongly advised to tailor their research to one of these current themes.

In Scotland, there are Project Grants and Mini-project Schemes. The former aim to provide support up to £75 000 over a three-year period; there are about 50 such projects at any one time. Again, applicants for this funding should tailor their research to meet the customer needs of a specific commission. The Mini-project Scheme aims to provide support up to £5 000 for small health services research projects, and pilot studies, which might lead to the development of applications for larger project grants. The purpose of this scheme is to encourage newcomers to enter health services research from any health profession or academic discipline.

Direct government money funds the independent Medical Research Council (MRC) and the Economic and Social Research Council (ESRC), to which appropriate submissions may be made. Nurses are likely to apply to the Health Services Research Committee of the MRC and a Small Grants Scheme for projects costing less than £20 000 exists. The addresses for these Councils are given at the end of the chapter.

Another indirect government funding source to the health services is the locally organized research scheme, detailed in Health Circular 88(6). This scheme is specifically for staff working in the NHS, in any discipline, and is a very appropriate source for nurses although disappointingly few apply for funds. Responsibility for managing the scheme is devolved to Regional Health Authorities and Boards of Governors of the postgraduate teaching hospitals, a not insubstantial budget being allocated from revenue to the scheme each year (£15.4 million in 1988–89). There is no standard pattern for the scheme and details of how to make an application should be available from the secretary to the Research Committee at the Regional Health Authority. Some limitation may be imposed on the duration of projects or the total amount of funding awarded, but it is generally possible to work within these. Expensive projects would require to be referred elsewhere, but important small grants of as little as £300 – for equipment, for example – have been given on occasion to permit a study to proceed. In Wales, the equivalent is the Welsh Scheme for the Development of Health and Social Research, administered through the University of Wales College of Medicine.

The second major source of research funding is that from the voluntary trusts and charities. The best source of information about large and small charities is the Directory of Grant Making Trusts (Charities Aid Foundation 1989). This is an invaluable, comprehensive guide to all types of charitable trust and details of the concerns and conditions of each charity are given. While few specify nursing as such, interests span much of the subject matters relevant to nurses with a large section dealing with health and medicine.

The major concerns of these charities may be linked to specific illnesses, for example, cystic fibrosis, leukaemia, heart disease, and to patients who suffer from these diseases. However, there are also those with much broader philanthropic interests, for example, the Joseph Rowntree Memorial Trust. Some limit their concerns to specific geographical areas – one was identified, for example, for Cockermouth. It would be sensible to orientate research to the specific concerns of the trust involved, rather than to the concerns of nursing per se.

A few charities have been extremely positive towards nursing; the Sainsbury Family Trust and the King's Fund are but two which have generously endowed nursing developments involving research activities. Similar charities like the Elizabeth Clark awards, and the Iolanthe Trust administered through the Royal College of Midwives, are able to provide small amounts of funding for research.

A directory of grant-giving bodies specifically for nursing is provided in the Directory of Nursing Scholarships, Bursaries and Grants (Royal College of Nursing 1974) which is in the process of much needed updating. Many of these provide small amounts of money for educational purposes but some may be prepared to finance research projects. An updated text on the same subject, Directory of Funding for Nurses, will be published in 1991 (see Institute of Nursing 1991).

Finance for research may also be attracted from industry and commerce, particularly from the pharmaceutical industry and those companies devoted to other health products. Some companies such as 3M, Smith & Nephew, and Maws, award annual scholarships, but *ad hoc* projects may also be funded. Commercial concerns could probably be more widely used than they are but sometimes ethical considerations intervene as, for example, with taking research monies from companies like Nestlé which sells milk powders to third world countries, or the tobacco industry's research fund 'The Health Promotion Research Trust'. Parahoo (1988) provides a further view of funding nursing research.

Chapter 11 in this book deals with writing a research proposal, only one facet of attracting research money. The proposal, irrespective of its scientific merits, must prove sufficiently appealing to attract sponsorship and there is an art in preparing such a submission.

INFORMATION RESOURCES

While information resources have been placed last, they are by no means least in importance. Anyone wishing to carry out research will need to know what has already been published on the topic. For this reason, libraries and information services are integral to research development. In Chapter 9, major libraries, indexing and abstracting resources are detailed.

While using abstracting and indexing journals, it is important for individual researchers to keep abreast of current literature; group efforts to share knowledge and reading can be most useful here. In some clinical and academic departments, journal clubs meet on a monthly basis to discuss recent important publications and to inform participants of useful papers and books which have been identified. By allocating particular journals to members and sharing the reading, an enormous amount of scanning can be shared and useful items located which might otherwise have been missed. Journal clubs have the added advantage of encouraging discussion, learning how others react to methods and findings, and generally sharpening research awareness. An active journal club also demonstrates to others the importance placed on knowing what is happening nationally and internationally. They are, therefore, as important for 'users' as 'doers' of research.

CONCLUSION

No matter who the participant is, or what the degree of development in their research career, some forms of support are necessary in order to carry out research. This chapter has done little more than indicate some of the sources of such support. It would be easy to consider support purely in financial terms: for reseach education or to fund a project to buy staff or materials. This is only part of the story. Just as important, however, are sources of support which are sustaining in intellectual and emotional terms. One has only to read the acknowledgements section of any thesis to find reference to the assistance given by supervisors and colleagues, not to mention long-suffering spouses. Perhaps even most important are those who provide data – patients, students, or colleagues. Often it is the generosity of others in terms of their time, intellectual application, and listening ability, as well as their skills in motivating and encouraging the writing of proposals and reports, which enable research to succeed.

The research community itself is perhaps the most important supportive agency. Researchers, by their willingness to give the same encouragement and assistance to others which they themselves have received, are an important source of mutual support.

USEFUL ADDRESSES

Deputy Chief Nursing Officer, Department of Health, Dundonald House, Upper Newtownards Road, Belfast BT4 3SF.

Nursing Officer (Research), Chief Scientist Office, Scottish Home and Health Department, St. Andrew's House, Edinburgh EH1 3DE.

Principal Nursing Officer (Research), Department of Health, Alexander Fleming House, Elephant and Castle, London SE1 6BY.

Chief Nursing Officer, Welsh Office, Cathays Park, Cardiff CF1 3NQ.

The Secretary, Medical Research Council, 20 Park Crescent, London W1N 4AL.

The Secretary, Research Grants Board, Economic and Social Research Council, Cherry Orchard East, Membrey Park, Swindon SN2 6UQ.

REFERENCES

Charities Aid Foundation (1989) *Directory of Grant Making Trusts*. Charities Aid Foundation, London.

Department of Health (1989) *Handbook of Research and Development*. HMSO, London.

Department of Health and Social Security Health Circular 88(6). Management services arrangements for locally organised and clinical research in the NHS. DHSS, London.

Institute of Nursing (1991) *Directory of Funding for Nurses*. Institute of Nursing (Radcliffe Infirmary), Oxford.

Parahoo K. (1988) Funding nursing research. *Senior Nurse*, **8** (9/10), 12–14.

Royal College of Nursing (1974) *Directory of Nursing Scholarships, Bursaries and Grants*, Royal College of Nursing, London.

Chapter 4
Moral Issues in Nursing Research
Ruth Schröck

Nursing research is a time-consuming and costly activity, and its success depends on prying successfully into other people's activities and experiences. This raises a great many moral issues. That is, the researcher needs to ask and answer questions about the proposed research or any work in hand which are directed at discovering whether what is being done is right or wrong.

What is right or wrong in any situation depends to a large extent on what different people consider to be important. In the endeavour to scrutinize dispassionately a situation in which people interact and respond to each other individually and invest effort and commitment in providing personalized nursing care, the nurse researcher faces inevitable conflicts. As a nurse, she would consider it wrong to watch a patient struggle painfully and ineffectively in reaching for a drink; for a researcher, any verbal or physical intervention might be unacceptable. The skilled nurse would protect a patient from unnecessary and potentially embarrassing or upsetting questions; the researcher must often question extensively, and deliberately range over wide areas of concern.

Whatever a nurse was able to do in alleviating the discomfort and anxiety of a patient here and now, she would undoubtedly and properly consider to be of immediate importance and value. The researcher's potential contribution to more effective nursing care can only ever be a long-term result. It is never far from most nurses' minds that time is a valuable and often severely limited commodity. Yet the researcher has to take up a considerable amount of people's time, has to remain unhurried and even comtemplative in situations where others are literally rushed off their feet.

These and other inevitable conflicts between the nursing and research perspectives are the source of many moral dilemmas. They are exacerbated when the suspicion arises that the researcher is not pursuing such potentially disturbing activities primarily for the ultimate benefit of patients, but for quite different purposes.

THE RESEARCHER'S RESPONSIBILITIES

The researcher is obliged to consider the implications of the proposed research for the participating subjects, the community, and for the status of knowledge.

The participating subjects

Norton (1975) aptly paraphrased the Nightingale dictum that the first duty of the researcher is to ensure that the research shall do the participant no harm.

It may appear obvious that the participant must be protected from suffering physical harm. The possible physical dangers may not be as apparent in nursing research as, for example, in medical drug trials or in the experimental introduction of as yet untested medical therapies. The following examples, however, might illustrate some possible dangers.

(1) A nurse researcher observes the nursing interventions following accidental or deliberate self-poisoning. It is her duty as a qualified nurse to intervene if the gastric tube has been passed incorrectly, exposing the patient to the danger of inhaling water which is about to be poured through the tube.
(2) In an experimental study designed to test ways of minimizing unnecessary invasion of privacy by accompanying apparently able patients to the toilet or bathroom, the researcher must very carefully consider the potential dangers to the members of the experimental group who may be randomly divided into those who are accompanied and those who are not.
(3) As part of a study to find criteria by which one might distinguish between effective and ineffective responses of nurses to patients' aggressive behaviour, one group of nurses is instructed to ignore minor verbal and physical outbursts of aggression. Unless the situation is carefully controlled, nurses could be exposed to physical danger.

Even more difficult than anticipating possible physical dangers is the identification of emotional harm that could be caused by the researcher's activities. Being observed, questioned, or singled out for implementing or experiencing new nursing approaches, can provoke a great deal of anxiety in both nurses and patients. It is a serious problem for the researcher to decide whether she is willing, able and in a position to deal therapeutically with the anxiety-provoking effects of, for example, an interview concerning people's feelings and thoughts about death, separation, mutilation, or permanent disability. Even just one insensitive question can cause considerable distress to respondents.

In studies which aim to discover potential areas of ignorance in either a nurse or a patient population, it would be harmful indeed to leave the respondents with the perhaps newly acquired feeling that they ought to know more than they do. The researcher must decide beforehand whether she could legitimately supply the information which her subjects have become aware of lacking through the researcher's activities.

In any kind of experimental study where a control group does not receive the special attention or intervention designed for the 'experimental group', the researcher must consider carefully how she will deal with the anxieties that this may cause. Wilson (1984) rightly points to the risk of having a treatment plan decided by randomization which places an experimental subject at a 50% chance of receiving care or treatment that might not be as effective as standard care.

There is the inevitable social effect to be considered that a researcher's presence will have on the interactions and cohesion of a group of people who participate in a study. This may be less disturbing when, for example, the chosen method of investigation entails the use of a postal questionnaire. It could have a devastating effect on the relationships of a group of people, if, say, the researcher employs a method of participant observation or utilizes the increasingly common ethnographic methodologies, unless the researcher remains sensitive to and aware of the effects her presence produces.

It must be part of the research plan to provide for some means of monitoring social effects of the research activity, and for opportunities for the participant group to regain its social cohesion at or after the departure of the researcher, if this has been affected in any way.

The community

There are aspects of research which have implications for the wider community.

The participants, be they nurses or patients, are part of a wider community, e.g. a hospital, a health centre, a college, a residence, or a profession. The community will not only be aware of the fact that some often inadequately explained and ill-understood research activities are being conducted in one of its parts, it will frequently have to contribute to realizing these activities by rescheduling events, moving staff, selecting patients, or even being temporarily deprived of the time and attention of some of its senior members.

Resentment against what may be considered to be an unjustified disturbance of the usual order of things can be very destructive. If one part of the community becomes the repeated location for research activities, often because significant members of staff in these areas encourage researchers who in turn prefer to go where they feel welcome, it can become isolated from the rest of the community. This may result in a feeling of envy in the rest of the hospital or college, and in a resistance which may become apparent later when the findings are to be implemented throughout the community.

The phenomenon of being over-researched may have negative effects on the part of the community which is being singled out for research activities. An unjustified and resented sense of elitism may develop which will contribute to its isolation. An increasing tendency to self-criticism, introspection and doubt can eventually undermine the practical effectiveness of an over-researched area or group of people. A constant stream of researchers, probably engaged in quite disparate studies, will also prevent an over-researched area from implementing any findings which could contribute to more effective nursing care. Not infrequently, such an area or group of people becomes research-wise. While not deliberately forming responses which suit the researcher's expectations, the increasing familiarity with what it is 'they are after' can distort responses in a most unwelcome way.

Researchers are usually members of a professional or academic community which supports, directs, and often finances their activities. They are accountable to their respective communities, e.g. a university department or research unit, for the use of financial and personnel resources. There can be conflicts between the demands of legitimate research activities, and other obligations, such as teaching or administration. In a totally research-orientated community, conflicts might arise between the interests of the individual researcher and the major research aims of the institution. Although research is often an individual enterprise and not infrequently a lonely pursuit, the researcher has important responsibilities to the community of which she is a part.

However, the interests and priorities of the researcher's community may seriously conflict with those of the participant's community.

A hospital or college may welcome research in order to improve its performance as a caring or teaching institution. The academic community of the researcher may be primarily more interested in the number of higher degrees which its members may obtain or in the quantity of publications which issue from the researchers.

These latter concerns influence not only the amount of time which the researcher may devote to offering adequate feedback to the participants' community and to giving appropriate help in implementing the findings, but may at the very outset determine the identification of the research questions in such a way that the answers afford high academic acclaim but little practical application.

Whether research is supported by public or private funding, the interests of the group which provides the necessary resources may raise the question of bias. Price (1989) among others points out that health service industries, as well as public departments or agencies, have a vested interest in many areas of medical and nursing research.

Any 'commissioned' research may be affected by the expectations of those who cause it to be carried out. A particularly difficult problem for the researcher arises when the commissioning agency embargoes the report or insists on a form of presentation which makes the research findings appear more favourable to its purposes than they really are.

The status of knowledge

Not all research is necessary and not all research activities lead to an increase in knowledge.

Some important questions cannot be answered by empirical research. No matter how much of it is done, if an answer to a question like 'what is nursing' is required, empirical research can make only a very limited contribution. There is a vast amount of descriptive research which shows what sort of things nurses do. Most of this information comes from work studies. But even another hundred such studies could not answer questions such as, 'Is everything that nurses do "nursing"? Could and do other people do these things? If they do, are these activities still "nursing"?' These are conceptual questions which need to be analysed in a different way, if an answer is to be found.

The moral dilemmas discussed in this chapter cannot be solved by empirical research either. What is right and what is wrong cannot be decided by descriptive or experimental research. Only analysis and discussion can lead to the formulation of principles or criteria by which a logical, rational and convincing answer may be found.

Researchers need to distinguish between various kinds of knowledge. Empirical knowledge is only one way in which a human event, situation or experience can be examined. What the experience of being terminally ill or of suffering frightening hallucinations really means to the individual may perhaps be ascertained more clearly by reading such a person's poetry, looking at pictures painted by a dying or frightened man or woman, or listening to music composed by a person who had experienced extreme fear or terror. The researcher must also make an important judgement in trying to anticipate what new knowledge the proposed study may produce. As areas or groups of people can be over-researched, so topics or questions can be repeated endlessly with no appreciable increase in knowledge. It is known from a vast research literature that people who are adequately informed suffer less anxiety; patients feel they do not know enough about their illness and treatment; nurses do not inform patients due either to ignorance or lack of competence in how to do so effectively; some clearly identifiable institutional settings are more conducive to open communications than others. Any study investigating these aspects of the experience of being ill does not contribute anything to new knowledge about these matters.

It is the responsibility of the researcher not to repeat unnecessarily what has already been substantiated by others.

MORAL CODES AND GUIDELINES

The responsibilities of the researcher are recognized in moral codes and guidelines which set out the researcher's obligations to the subjects of the study, to sponsors and employers, to colleagues, and to the development and promotion of knowledge.

The earliest guidelines on ethical values in nursing research were developed and published by the American Nurses' Association (ANA) (1968). In examining the investigative role of the researcher and the role of the nurse practitioner, the guidelines touch briefly on some of the inherent conflicts that may arise. The most prominent concern is with the protection of human rights by ensuring the participant's right to privacy, to self-determination, to conservation of personal resources, to freedom from arbitrary hurt, and to freedom from intrinsic risk of injury. The rights of minors and incompetent persons are considered and the matter of consent is discussed. A section deals with drugs used in research and, perhaps a little unexpectedly, another refers to animals in research.

The Canadian Nurses' Association (CNA) 1972) subsequently brought out similar guidelines aimed primarily at nurses doing research.

More comprehensive in that not only nurses undertaking research but also those in positions of authority and those practising in places where research is carried out are addressed, are the guidelines produced by the Royal College of Nursing (RCN) of the United Kingdom (1977). Following a brief preamble, the first part of the RCN guidelines relates to points which nurses undertaking research need to consider. The aspects which are mentioned can be summarized as follows:

(1) The research must be necessary and must contribute to further knowledge;
(2) The subjects must receive full explanations of what their participation might entail and must be told explicitly that they have the right to refuse;
(3) Consent must be obtained, if necessary, from a relative or legal guardian;
(4) Subjects must be protected against physical, emotional, mental, or social injury;
(5) Confidentiality must be assured and maintained;
(6) The researcher must be qualified to carry out the investigation, must make public the results of the inquiry, and must attempt to prevent their misuse;
(7) The contract between the sponsor of the research and the researcher must make explicit their mutual obligations and must state clearly the remit for the work to be undertaken;
(8) Clear arrangements must be made as to the researcher's duties and responsibilities in the place where the research is carried out.

The second part of the RCN guidelines is directed at nurses in positions of

authority where research is to be carried out. It provides comments on sa.
or commissioning research within the organization, and emphasizes that c
to participate cannot be given on behalf of other people. The researcher's re.
for anonymity or confidentiality of data must be respected, and any information
obtained as part of the research programme must not be used for other purposes
within the organization. However, every effort should be made to utilize relevant
findings.

In part three of the guidelines, nurses who are practising in places where
research is being carried out are reminded of their responsibilities as practitioners,
especially in safeguarding patients'/clients' rights and well-being.

Nurses who agree to assist with the collection of data are bound by the same
obligations as the researcher, especially in being accurate and honest. The
possible conflict, at times, between the demands of being a practitioner and a
researcher is mentioned. Information which nurses obtain in their role as
practitioners must be treated with the same confidentiality as is the practice when
no research is being carried out. It must not be made available to the researcher
unless this has been previously agreed.

The common elements in these codes of conduct mentioned above are the
rights of the subject, the obligations of the researcher, and the considerations of
the setting in which research is carried out.

Points of omission in the moral codes and guidelines

Although the right of the patient to withdraw from participating in a research
project is usually emphasized, the nurse's right to withdraw is not made quite so
explicit. However, the RCN code (1977) lays the responsibility on the researcher
that 'he/she must make explicit the subject's right to refuse to participate or to
withdraw at any stage of the project, and (that) this right must be respected.' Less
clear is to what extent nurses have the right to assist patients to withdraw from the
project. It is accepted that nurses should satisfy themselves that patients
understand what is going on and that they are entitled to withdraw at any time.
Nurses are obliged to report any adverse effects on patients to either the
researcher or an appropriate authority. But whether nurses are also morally
obliged to assist the patient in making his or her wish to withdraw clear to the right
person, and in an appropriate form, is left open. It could well be the case that a
patient, though adversely affected, feels inhibited to make his wish known, either
because he does not wish to appear unco-operative or ungrateful, or he
anticipates, rightly or wrongly, that important people may be displeased. Someone
is needed to act on the patient's behalf. Relatives and friends may share the
patient's reluctance to step out of line. Is it the nurse's obligation to act as the
patient's advocate in this situation?

The RCN guidelines (1977) point out that nurses who participate as data
collectors in addition to their usual duties must make it known, if these extra
activities become detrimental to their normal work.

More discussion is needed to identify situations in which nurses function as
unknowing and unpaid data collectors, especially in areas designated for medical
research. Apart from the justified point made by the RCN guidelines that the
additional work may detract from the primary caring functions of the nurse, a
nurse who is unaware of the purpose of collecting particular kinds of information,

or preserving certain kinds of specimen, or conducting procedures in a prescribed way, may produce unreliable data for the researcher and may contribute unwittingly to distorted results.

The obligation of the researcher who utilizes such assistance in data collection to ensure herself of the reliability of the information by methodical monitoring of the accuracy and conscientiousness of the (perhaps unwilling) data collectors is not mentioned in any of the guidelines.

What might be termed the intellectual honesty of the researcher is mentioned in various ways in the moral codes governing the conduct of nursing research. All three codes discussed in this chapter refer to the competence of the researcher. The ANA guidelines on ethical values (1968) state that 'The investigator is a registered nurse who has achieved the educational and technical competence to perform the conceptualizing supervisory, collaborative, and evaluative functions inherent in the investigative role.' The Canadian Nurses' Association (1972) emphasizes in addition that 'the researcher has responsibility to acknowledge personal limitations . . .'.

However, only the RCN guidelines (1977) make any reference to those learning to do research. This is confined to the observation that they should only work under the guidance of an experienced researcher.

With the undoubtedly welcome increase of nursing courses at both basic and post-basic level which incorporate some concern with nursing research in the students' programme, it may be necessary to examine more specifically the various approaches to students' projects and dissertations which are designed to give the student the opportunity of learning some research skills.

There is undoubtedly some misuse of time-consuming and inappropriate fieldwork. Many fundamental research skills can be acquired to some extent in college-based activities without the need to set up elaborate and often impractical fieldwork projects. One of the major constraints in successfully completing the necessary fieldwork for even the most modest project, lies in the limited time available to most students to pursue these 'research' activities in addition to their other course commitments. Not only will such a student be dissatisfied with the results, feeling frustrated by what appear to be insurmountable difficulties, but it may also prevent him or her from engaging in any further research.

Since students' time and financial resources are limited, areas that are geographically close have to be utilized for the planned project. The dangers of an area or a group of people becoming over-researched have already been mentioned. The possibility that a constant succession of still inept student researchers may produce difficulties for experienced researchers to gain entry to the field must also be borne in mind.

That a researcher must not manipulate data to suit his or her anticipated outcome of the research may be presumed in the statement, 'The researcher is also obliged to maintain objectivity and fidelity to . . . scientific and ethical premises in reporting findings' (ANA 1968). But apart from actually falsifying data or manipulating them by leaving aside those which do not seem to fit, it is not an uncommon practice to report only on the successful aspects of the research. Not only does such reporting give the impression that most researchers have a perfectly clear plan which is executed smoothly without any setbacks; by not reporting on the delays, ineffective approaches, or inappropriate tools, the researcher compels others to repeat mistakes quite unnecessarily.

The RCN guidelines (1977) point out the researcher's obligation to report negative evidence; although it may be implied in the other codes, it does seem to be a point which might need more explicit discussion rather than less. Reporting and publishing may first come to mind when one endeavours to examine the idea of scientific accountability – something which is raised in rather general terms in the three codes. It has already been pointed out that researchers are accountable to their academic or research community for the use of resources and generally for the ways in which they pursue the aims of their respective institutions. Both the American and the Canadian codes introduce the notion that the researcher is accountable for the scientific standards of his or her work to academic or research colleagues, that is, to his or her peers: 'The investigator is accountable to his peer group, both within and without the profession of nursing . . . a review committee of peers, not part of the investigational team, is a marked asset in any investigation' (ANA 1968); 'In order to ensure the integrity of the investigation, the researcher must present the project for review to a group of professional peers' (CNA 1972).

The RCN guidelines (1977) refer in a similar manner to the researcher's responsibility towards colleagues by pointing out that she 'has an obligation to make sure that professional colleagues with a responsibility for the subject are informed of the proposed research.' At the very least, one might interpret the subject to mean the academic or research discipline in which the researcher works. The RCN statement is not only narrower in referring to information rather than review, it could also be interpreted as relating to the subject, the participant in the study.

How important properly conducted peer reviews might be in helping the researcher to fulfil her responsibility 'for the advancement of the theory and methods of the science in which he/she is working' (RCN 1977) is made much clearer in an article by Mackay and Soule (1975). These authors examine more closely the purposes of peer reviews which are:

(1) To identify the weaknesses in design and methodology;
(2) To contribute thinking directed toward the central theory or clinical question being examined;
(3) To reveal potential moral dilemmas;
(4) To ascertain possible legal implications;
(5) To give expert judgement on whether the study is scientifically sound and able to answer the questions it asks;
(6) To judge the effect of the study on the planned project environment;
(7) To evaluate the investigator's ability and expertise to carry out the project, and his or her willingness to be accountable.

Scientific accountability appears to be a much wider concept, going far beyond the obligation to report and to publish the research findings. The work of the researcher, from the planning to the publication stage, must be open to competent scrutiny and constructive criticism.

ETHICAL COMMITTEES AND OTHER PROTECTIVE BODIES

Ethical committees are usually set up by the medical profession to vet medical research projects. Their primary purpose is the protection of the potential subjects of medical research. They may operate at Area Health Authority level, at hospital level – especially in teaching hospitals and university clinics – as a subcommittee of the British Medical Association, or as parts of governmental bodies. With the increase in social science and nursing research in health care settings, almost all research proposals of non-medical staff or researchers, which involve the use of patients as subjects in the study, must be approved by the appropriate ethical committee.

Some ethical committees include a lay member who represents the views of the public; not very many as yet are representative of the multi-professional research which it has become their task to adjudge. There is also some concern that an ethical committee may withhold approval of a project less in order to protect potential subjects, but rather more to either demonstrate its power or simply to support the kind of research with which its members are most familiar (Pollock & Tilley 1988).

Since specific proposals involve the identification of individuals and particular areas, ethical committees are rightly sensitive to the need for confidentiality. On the other hand, if the impression of secrecy is created, the very people an ethical committee aims to protect may begin to doubt its intentions and effectiveness (Stimson & Stimson 1978).

Community Health Councils can ask questions of any ethical committee in their area, and can investigate, to some extent, disturbing aspects of research which come to their notice. Statutory bodies like the Scottish Mental Welfare Commission protect the rights of particular patient groups and would examine carefully allegations of neglect, ill treatment, or unwilling participation resulting from ill-conceived or poorly conducted research.

Voluntary organizations devoted to providing help and advice to patients generally, such as the Patients' Association, or to particular groups of patients, such as the Schizophrenia Fellowship, and Mind, have become increasingly alert to potential infringements of patients' rights and are competent in pursuing searching inquiries on behalf of individuals or groups of people.

The Society for the Study of Medical Ethics, based in London, is an independent body and a non-partisan organization, set up for the study of moral issues raised by the practice of medicine and that of other health care professions. It provides an information service on research on moral issues in health care including those raised by research activities.

In the last resort, a citizen can instigate legal proceedings in the endeavour to protect himself or herself against unwarranted invasion of privacy, illegal compulsion, breaches of confidentiality, or potential damage. Alleged results of negligence, ill treatment, deprivation or any other harm resulting from research activities could undoubtedly lead to criminal proceedings regardless of the fact that the complainant may have consented to participate in a particular study, or that others may have done so on his or her behalf. That legal proceedings of this kind are still comparatively rare in the United Kingdom may be testimony to the integrity of both researchers and practitioners in the health care professions.

There is little doubt, however, that the individual researcher's sensitivity to the moral implications of research and a firm adherence to a professional code of practice are the only sound foundations on which the security and well-being of all who participate in research, or contribute to it in any form, can rest.

References

American Nurses' Association (1968) The nurse in research, ANA guidelines on ethical values. *American Journal of Nursing*, **68**, No. 7, 1504-7.

Canadian Nurses' Association (1972) Ethics of nursing research. *The Canadian Nurse*, **68**, No. 9, 23-5.

MacKay R.C. & Soule J.A. (1975) Nurses as investigators: some ethical and legal issues. *The Canadian Nurse*, **71**, No. 9, 26-9.

Norton D. (1975) The research ethic. *Nursing Times*, **71** No. 52, 2048-9.

Price B. (1989) The thorny path of nursing research. *Nursing Times*, **85**, No. 23, 62-3.

Pollock L. & Tilley S. (1988) Submitting for approval. *Senior Nurse*, **8** No. 5, 24-5.

Royal College of Nursing of the United Kingdom (1977) *Ethics related to research in nursing*. Royal College of Nursing, London.

Stimson G. & Stimson C. (1978) *Health rights handbook: a guide to medical care*. Prism Press, Dorchester.

Wilson H.S. (1984) Research reflections: making the scientific ethical. *The Journal of Nursing Administration*, **14**, No. 11, 6-7.

Chapter 5
Common Terms and Concepts in Nursing Research
Allan S. Presly

This chapter introduces and defines a number of commonly used terms and
concepts likely to be encountered in a representative selection of research which
is of interest to nurses. They will be introduced in the sequence in which they are
likely to be met in a research report, but, obviously, by no means all of these terms
will occur in any single research report.

RESEARCH

Research is a form of systematic inquiry. It sets out to answer questions through
assessing, summarizing and drawing conclusions from what are often very large
amounts of information. The intention is to reach as unambiguous conclusions as
possible and to minimize the extent to which the reader has to interpret the results.
Ideally, therefore, any two people studying the results of a piece of research should
agree with the researcher's conclusions. It has to be said, however, that this is very
difficult to achieve in practice! The research report must make clear the
procedures used, the results obtained, and the conclusions drawn. The golden
rule should be that the report contains enough information to enable the research
to be repeated exactly by someone else wishing to answer the same question in the
same way. This repetition is called a *replication*.

Replication

In all sciences, replication serves at least two purposes. Each replication under the
same conditions further establishes the reliability of previous results. Secondly,
the same results might be replicated under *different* conditions. This would again
increase confidence in the reliability of the original results, but it would also serve
to establish their generality.

Retrospective and prospective research

Research may be *retrospective* or *prospective*. Retrospective research refers to
the investigation of events which have already happened; for example, you might
set out to discover how many patients with urinary tract infections were admitted
last year to hospital X. Prospective research sets out to investigate events which
are yet to happen; in this case, you might set out to discover how many patients
with urinary tract infections will be admitted to hospital in the coming year. The
advantage of prospective research is that it can be planned in advance, for
example, who and what is to be assessed and how the information is to be
recorded. In retrospective research, the researcher has to depend on information
which may have been recorded by a large variety of people who did not know it

was likely to be needed for research purposes. The accuracy of such information can leave a lot to be desired! In either case, the results of the research will refer to some defined *population*.

POPULATION

Population literally means 'all the people' and in research the term is most commonly used to refer to a specific group of people. However, in a research context, population refers to all the members or objects of any defined group from which measurements might be taken or about which information might be collected.

A research population refers to the entire group to which the results of the research are to apply. A population could thus consist of all people of a specified age group whose blood pressure was to be measured, a whole series of laboratory animals on which a new drug was to be tested, or all the items of equipment – for example, syringes, incontinence pads, or lifting aids – whose efficiency was to be assessed. Membership of any given population should be specified clearly so that there is no doubt as to how widely the research findings can be generalized.

It is, of course, rarely possible to assess all the members of a given population. It might be possible to assess all known patients suffering from a rare condition, as was done in Scotland, for example, for babies who suffered damage due to their mothers being given the drug thalidomide. It would not, however, be possible to investigate all those patients with a diagnosis of, say, 'senile dementia'. Thus a *sample* of the population usually has to be taken.

SAMPLING

The sample must reflect, as far as possible, every aspect of the population from which it is selected. Suppose one wanted to study some aspect of patients with a common disease who were admitted to one hospital over a year. The population would be all the patients so defined, but if their number was very large, the researcher would probably decide to assess only a sample of them. The sample selected would, for example, have to show the same age range, the same proportion of males to females, the same proportion of urban to rural residents, and the same proportions from each admission ward concerned.

Random sample

One way of ensuring that a sample is representative of a population is to select a *random sample* in which all the patients in the specified population have an equal chance of being included and every possible sample has an equal chance of being drawn. Suppose a random sample of 10 patients out of a total of 100 is required. One might write down a series of 10 numbers, between 1 and 100 'out of one's head', but this is very unlikely to be truly random due to a variety of subtle biases and prejudices which influence us. It is very likely, for example, that between 1 and 10, the numbers 3 and 7 which have special significance for many of us, would appear in many people's selections, and would thus have a greater chance of being included than other numbers. The final list would not then be random. Fortunately, this task is simplified by the availability of published lists or computer programmes for random numbers which allow the selection of 10 patients from the 100 without introducing bias to the selection. Given that the sample is truly random and as large as possible, it can then be said also to apply to the population from which the sample was taken. It is generally accepted that the larger the sample the better.

Stratified sample

Sometimes it may be appropriate to arrange things so that some characteristics of the sample are left to chance, while others are specifically selected. This is sometimes referred to as a *stratified sample*. One might want to ensure in advance that the sample contains the correct proportion of the over- and under-50s, or of males and females, if these factors – age and sex – were considered to have a particularly important bearing on the outcome of the research. Within each subgroup so selected, however – for example, the over- and under-50s – the subjects would still be chosen at random. Whatever type of sampling is used, the members of the sample are generally referred to as the *subjects* of the research.

CORRELATIONAL RESEARCH

Some research is of the *descriptive* or 'look and see' type. The research might, for example, investigate whether the amount of time spent in hospital following a particular operation is related to the age of the patients, that is: 'Do older people take longer to recover from this operation?'. A random sample of patients who had undergone the operation could be selected, their ages noted, and the length of time they stayed in hospital post-operatively calculated. A measure of the relationship between the two sets of figures is called a *correlation*. If there is a clear relationship, it can be concluded that age does have an apparent bearing on recovery time, older patients being more likely to stay longer in hospital.

Can it also be concluded that older people take longer to recover from the operation? It can not. All that can be said is that there is an association between the two things measured, referred to as *variables*, which needs to be explained. It cannot be concluded that one causes the other, that is, that increasing age is a cause of longer stays in hospital. The difficulty with this type of research is that both the variables being measured may be connected to a third factor which may account for the relationship between them. In this example, older people are more likely to be widowed or to live alone. As a result, staff may be more reluctant to discharge older patients as quickly where there is no support at home, even though their physical condition may be as good as that of younger people. Here, living alone is a possible explanation of the connection between age and longer stays in hospital. It cannot simply be said that older people take longer to recover from the operation, although, as seen above, there is a correlation between age and length of stay in hospital.

EXPERIMENTAL RESEARCH AND TESTING HYPOTHESES

Another type of research is often referred to as *experimental research* where the researcher sets out to test a *hypothesis*. A hypothesis is a type of prediction which is usually derived from a survey and analysis of previously published research. It is a statement of the kind: 'If X is done to this sample, then Y will follow' (or, more correctly, if X was not done Y would not have happened). It can then be concluded that X caused Y to happen. This is the main advantage of experimental research over the descriptive type in that it makes *causal relationships* much clearer. The researcher in this case does not simply observe what happens or has happened, she introduces some form of *control* into the situation.

Dependent and independent variables

The experimenter, for example, might set out to test the hypothesis: 'If a new method of teaching physiology is introduced into the School of Nursing, then nurses' exam marks will improve'. Here, an experiment is set up where the researcher deliberately manipulates or controls one major factor or variable, the type of teaching, referred to as an *independent variable*, in order to assess its effects on another factor, exam marks, referred to as the *dependent variable*. This type of research is frequently used in the evaluation of new drugs or methods of treatment as it is more likely to allow the researcher to say that one thing causes another than does the correlation type. It makes it less likely that alternative explanations of the kind noted in the previous example regarding recovery from operations can be put forward to explain the results. Research of this type generally follows one of a number of plans which are decided in advance. Such a plan is called the *design* of the experiment (see Chapter 16).

PILOT STUDY

Before the research proper, a *pilot study* may be carried out. This takes the form of a small-scale trial of the research method, to ensure that the design is feasible. A pilot study may be on a small number of subjects only, but might help to determine a variety of practical questions: Can the subjects understand what is being asked of them? Does the nurse understand the new procedure which is to be tested? Are a large enough number of the type of subjects required likely to appear within the time available? Is the information needed always available from case records? How long is the new procedure likely to take? Does a new drug have undesirable side-effects?

MEASUREMENT

Scales of measurement

Following selection of subjects, some kind of assessment or *measurement* will usually be carried out on each one. Such measurement may be only *qualitative*. Subjects of the research are differentiated only by possessing or not possessing a given characteristic, for example, pass/fail, recovered/died, single/married/ widowed/divorced. The subjects are divided into a number of categories, but the differences between these categories are not measurable in any real sense. This is referred to as a *nominal scale*. A more informative measurement is an *ordinal scale*. Here, subjects can be categorized more precisely, at least in terms of rank order from greatest to least, or best to worst. Examples might be the grading of essays on a scale of A–E, or grading according to social class. Again, however, there is no precisely measurable difference between any two grades.

If the temperatures of a group of subjects are taken, however, measurement becomes genuinely *quantatative* in the sense that any level between the known upper and lower extremes is possible. Precise statements of difference can now be made: the difference or interval between 10 and 11 degrees Centigrade is the same as the difference between 11 and 12 degrees. Where this is so, the scale is an *interval scale*. Where, additionally, a scale has a true zero point, the scale becomes a *ratio scale*. This would be the case for measures of height and weight, but not for temperature, where the zero point is arbitrary.

Reliability

Measurement must give a *reliable* result whether done by observation and recorded on a simple rating scale – for example, the patient looks 'more cheerful', by checking or counting, for example, the number of times a patient is incontinent – or by technical means, for example, blood pressure or temperature. The same results must be achieved, as far as possible, regardless of who is doing the measuring, so that several nurses weighing the same patient on the same set of scales in quick succession, should get the same result each time, or very nearly so. *Inter-rater* or *inter-observer reliability* should thus exist.

With an accurate or reliable method of measurement, any influence or bias on the part of the person(s) doing the measuring is reduced to a minimum. This is relatively easy with measures such as height, weight, temperature, and so on, because of the technical means available for such measurement. However, research frequently involves assessing or measuring variables which are much harder to quantify. It may be necessary for a nurse to assess how depressed a patient is, whether his colour is better, whether he can move more easily, or the degree of pain he has experienced. There are no absolute standards or technical aids for measuring these parameters, and eliminating inter-observer influences or inaccuracy due to different raters can be very difficult.

Operational definitions

Reasonably reliable judgments, however, can still be made if precise definitions of what is meant by such things as degrees of depression or mobility are provided. These precise definitions are sometimes referred to as *operational definitions*. These are necessary because the same term can often have different meanings for different researchers. 'Intelligence' is a good example. Although it is a concept of great value, there are many varied and even contradictory definitions of it. For a particular research project, therefore, an operational definition usually has to be arrived at. This might be 'intelligence as measured on Test A'. This does not mean this is the exact or the only definition. It does mean that for the purposes of this research, this definition can be conveniently agreed upon.

A second sense in which measurements must be accurate (reliable) is that given an unchanging condition, the measurement should give constant results over time. It might be known that a given dose of a drug should show up as a given concentration in a urine specimen. If the treatment is not changed, the estimates of this concentration should remain the same. If not, then explanations for this would have to be sought, and one obvious one might be that the method chosen to measure the concentration is unreliable. Whatever the type of measurement used, the research report ought to include an assessment of how reliable the measurements quoted are, and this is one area where statistical methods might well be used (see Chapter 28).

Validity

Another essential feature of all measurement used in research is that it must be *valid* – researchers should be able to predict accurately on the basis of the measures taken. Given that a reliable method of measuring blood pressure exists, such information will only be of value if it allows predictions to be made. Measurement of blood pressure is only valid to the extent that it allows identification of what treatment is necessary if blood pressure is too high or too low, and what will happen if the treatment is applied. Measurement of intelligence is only valid to the extent that it will allow predictions to be made about the research subjects, for example, what type of school class they are best suited to, what type of job to try for, and so on. A good example of the question of *predictive validity* can be found in the article by Lothian (1989) where he considers the value of a number of scales which claim to assess the risk of developing pressure sores.

PROCEDURE

Having selected subjects and decided upon measures, a research report should describe accurately the *procedure* followed. The reported procedures should include when the measures were taken and by whom, under what conditions, and how the results were recorded. This is of considerable importance, because it will enable the research to be repeated in precisely the same way by others, if necessary. If more than one sample is involved in the research, it is also essential to know that exactly the same procedure was followed in each case. Research frequently involves a comparison of one group with another, where, for example, a new drug is applied to one group and compared with the effects of an established one applied to another similar group. Clearly, if it is to be claimed that the new treatment is superior to the old, the treatment procedure must be identical for each group except for the single difference of the drug given.

RESULTS

A research report will then present *results* based on analysis of the *data* collected (see Part II, Section D). Data are the raw materials from which conclusions will be drawn and will often consist of lists of tables or information, in quantified form, containing such things as heights, weights, ratings, scores, test results or percentages. To make sense of these data, especially if the research project is on a large scale, it will often be necessary to make some use of *statistical methods* (see Chapter 28). First of all, these will enable the researcher to summarize and present a large quantity of results by means such as easily understood averages, graphs, and histograms. Second, they will help the researcher arrive at legitimate conclusions and reduce the element of subjective bias which anyone analysing the research findings will inevitably bring to them.

In most cases, the results of research projects do not work out in such a way as to allow clear-cut or definite conclusions to be drawn. Although not often phrased as if this were so, most research findings are simply statements of *probability* and should, strictly speaking, be stated as such; for example, 'the probability is less than one in 20 that this result could have occurred by chance'. That is, the researcher should state what degree of *confidence* can be placed in the results. It would mean, in effect, that if the same research were repeated 20 times under exactly the same conditions, the same result would be expected in at least 19 of them (or if repeated 100 times in at least 95). Thus it is evident that the higher the level of confidence which the statistical analysis will allow to be stated, the more certain one can be that the results could not have occurred by chance.

GENERALIZATION

The purpose of nearly all research is to allow general statements about whole populations to be made. The extent to which the researcher can *generalize* on the basis of one piece of research will depend on the large number of factors outlined above and the extent to which they have been taken into account. Thus if a research project claims to have proved that treatment A is superior to treatment B for condition X, then before this is accepted, there are a number of questions which must be asked.

(1) Were the samples of patients given treatment A and B representative of all patients for whom treatments A and B might be appropriate? Were they selected at random? If the treatment could potentially be applied to all adults, then a research sample not quite representative of all the adult population – for example, on average older, or with more males than females – would not invalidate the research altogether. It would be necessary, however, to be more cautious about the claims of the researchers that the results apply to all adults.
(2) Were all the factors which might affect the results controlled for? That is, were all the research patients treated under the same conditions by the same people, applying the same procedure?
(3) Were the measures of the treatment's effects reliable and valid? Does the research report give enough information on this to be able to judge?
(4) Were the results of the research presented in full? Were appropriate statistical methods used? Researchers unfamiliar with statistical methods should seek expert advice on this subject.
(5) Were the results stated with a high level of confidence?
(6) Possibly most important of all, does the research report give enough information for others to be able to repeat the research if they wish to?

The same questions, suitably modified, can be applied to any research report, and only if these conditions are met can the conclusions be accepted. It will also be evident that, given the above, research is a difficult exercise. No one ever performed the perfect piece of research, nor is anyone ever likely to!

REFERENCE

Lothian P. (1989) Identifying and protecting patients who may get pressure sores. *Nursing Standard*, **4**, (4), 26–9.

Chapter 6
Teaching and Learning the Research Process
Phyllis J. Runciman

Teaching and learning about the research process can be an interesting challenge. In some respects, the challenge for teachers in this area of nursing education is no different from the challenge in others. It is to create a good climate for learning and to provide overall a high quality educational experience for students.

A look at the history of the development of nursing research suggests that a great deal has been achieved through education. In reality, however, it has to be acknowledged that attitudes towards research and its relevance within nursing still vary a great deal. The study of research at basic and post-basic levels may well be eagerly anticipated by some students and teachers, but it will also be regarded with considerable apprehension by others.

This chapter is therefore intended principally for nurses involved in planning research-related input in a variety of educational experiences which aim to develop research awareness and research skills. It raises a number of questions worth considering and makes some suggestions about approaches to teaching and learning based upon principles of adult education.

COURSES – WHAT'S IN A NAME!

It is not unusual for research courses to be described as basic or introductory, research awareness or appreciation courses, or research methods courses. This labelling is sometimes regarded as implying a hierarchy of knowledge and skill with research methods courses demanding skills of a higher order than basic or research awareness courses, and emphasizing the nurse as someone who undertakes research as a 'doer' rather than as a 'consumer'; that is, as someone who uses research appropriately to inform practice.

The distinction between courses, however, and between the nurse as 'doer' and 'consumer' is not altogether clear cut. Introductory and research awareness courses can make considerable demands upon a student's powers of analysis and they will deal to a certain extent with issues surrounding research design and methods. They will provide a framework within which to develop skills both as an active participant in research projects and as a knowledgeable consumer of research.

Clark (1987 p.371) lists a number of roles for a research aware nurse, roles which she suggests can be integrated easily within existing practice:

'– raising problems and questions for research
 – co-operating with researchers in an informed way
 – seeking out and critically evaluating published research studies
 – using research findings

– communicating with others and sharing the task of keeping abreast of new developments.'

Here, the emphasis is arguably more on being a consumer of research and on making nursing practice research-based and up-to-date. A research awareness course geared towards developing these abilities would need to encompass knowledge of the research process and research terminology; how to use libraries and access information efficiently and how to read research literature critically; knowledge of constraints upon and opportunities for using research findings, and exploration of the practical difficulties of changing accepted, traditional and ritual practice. These abilities, plus a growing understanding of one's own attitudes and the attitudes of others to research, are of equal value and importance to the nurse who will carry out research.

In terms of course planning, therefore, decisions about the exact title and content of a course, about the skills to be developed, and the level of academic challenge within it, will emerge as certain questions are explored, including: Who are the learners? What are their learning needs? Which competencies and course aims are relevant? What time is available? Which modes of study are preferred and possible? What approaches to teaching, learning, assessment, and evaluation will be adopted? What resources are available?

As the range and number of research courses grows, and as the concept of credit rating for educational programmes develops, it becomes increasingly important to indicate clearly the aims, content, expected outcome, and academic level of courses. This will allow potential students to select appropriately, avoiding unnecessary duplication, to build up steadily knowledge and skills, and to move flexibly within credit accumulation and transfer schemes.

WHO ARE THE LEARNERS?

The assumption may be made at the start of a course on nursing research that course participants will have had little or no research training or experience. Given the comparatively recent nature of developments in research training for nurses, this might still be expected, particularly within post-basic education. This assumption, however, that learners will have had *no* research experience should be examined.

The question to ask is this: what might represent research experience? If one starts from the perspective of experience rather than training, it is likely that all learners will be able to identify having had research experience of some kind. For example, research still tends to be perceived as something other people do and in which other people get involved; it is also perceived as difficult, esoteric, and academic. However, if one asks the question, 'have you ever been interviewed on the doorstep or in the street?' it quickly becomes apparent that we all live, day-to-day, within a research environment.

Debate about these different forms of participation in research can be both lively and instructive. It helps learners to think of research in more personal terms and it can lower barriers to learning. Such debate can also pinpoint important areas of concern: for example, how, as a researcher, do you obtain informed consent, and how free are members of the public, as subjects, to say no to participation in doorstep data collection? Moving freely across work and non-work boundaries seems to be useful for breaking down barriers towards learning about research within nursing, particularly for more experienced nurses on post-basic courses, some of whom regard research as a worrying and not particularly enticing subject for study.

Similarly, the assumption that students entering basic programmes will have had little or no research experience or training should also be questioned. Increasingly, in schools, individual and group project work may provide excellent foundation experience of the research process and it is interesting to explore with students at an early stage the exact nature of project work undertaken in school or other pre-nursing education.

Two of the first principles, therefore, from which to work are: getting to know the learners and the context for their learning, and establishing existing levels of knowledge and skills.

If groups are small, it may be possible for student and teacher together, on a one-to-one basis, to explore and identify baseline knowledge and experience and to establish individual learning goals. With larger groups, this may not be feasible. One way round the problem is to devise a simple questionnaire which would allow the learner to reflect upon past experience, on personal and professional involvement in 'using' or 'doing' research, and to state what they hope to gain from the learning opportunity now available.

In the writer's experience, using such a questionnaire at the start of a course can be helpful in a number of ways. Responses can be compared in either pairs or small groups. With the agreement of the students, responses from the whole group can be analysed and feedback given. The forms of analysis and presentation of results can become a learning opportunity. At the end of the course, the questionnaire might be reviewed as a tool for reflection to generate comment for course evaluation by students.

It is possible, for example, to find that in a group of post-basic diploma students there will be a wide range of existing knowledge and skills. Some may have little experience; others may have received research training through undergraduate studies, summer schools, or evening classes; a few may already possess masters level qualifications and have had extensive research training including the completion of research projects, dissertations, and theses.

Several issues may have to be considered as a result of information offered in a pre-course or start-of-course questionnaire, such as exemption from certain course work, teaching and learning in mixed ability groups, and the extent to which a flexible approach can be adopted towards course content. To ignore, for example, the fact that many experienced nurses wish to investigate questions which concern them at work, or that many will be expected by their nurse managers to undertake research at the end of the course, could mean that students become demotivated and frustrated. Or they may be exposed to the risks of entering ill-prepared into major areas of inquiry, especially if under pressure from nurse managers to produce much needed evidence to support developments in nursing care and services.

Some experienced nurses may already be sensitive to the need within all research for careful planning and adequate resources and supervision. Many are not, and within what is labelled as a research awareness course, it may be important to deal with the basic essentials and points for caution about undertaking research in day-to-day practice. Ignoring the possibility of the active involvement of students in research can be counterproductive.

STUDENT-CENTRED APPROACHES

Student-centred approaches are increasingly favoured in nursing education. Individual and group activities for students, and facilitative rather than didactic teaching methods, are recommended (Jarvis 1988). These approaches are in line with the principles of adult education already referred to: that adults should be given opportunities to use their previous knowledge and experiences as a resource within the new learning situation. They also relate to the further principle that adults should be allowed and encouraged to participate actively in the learning process. How can this be achieved? There are, in fact, many readily available opportunities for developing research-based student-centred learning activities. A few examples are given here.

Using libraries

The preparation of a short annotated bibliography of research-related literature on a topic of personal interest, and relevance to practice, can be a valuable exercise for several reasons. Students will be required to work with library staff; to find their way around a library and become aware of its resources; to use indexing and abstracting systems; to find, select, and read relevant literature; to present concise annotations; and to write references correctly. The complete bibliographies can be made available and can then become a resource for the whole group.

Developing the ability to read, summarize and critically appraise research-based publications is a challenging area for teaching and learning. Publications vary greatly in length, complexity, and readability, and not all are well written. Both short and long articles may be equally difficult to summarize and to critique. Students may not be accustomed to reading research material and reactions to the task might vary from 'novel challenge' to 'nightmare chore of doubtful relevance'.

Through the critiquing process, a study is carefully evaluated for both its strengths and weaknesses in terms of scientific merit and professional relevance. Some would question the extent to which one can become an adequate critiquer without significant experience of the research process itself. The task is certainly not an easy one and it takes time to acquire broad knowledge of the principles of investigation. It might be that the ability to read a research article with sufficient understanding to be able to summarize it adequately, identifying the elements of the research process within it, is the first skill to be acquired before moving into the complexities of critical appraisal.

Gradually building up a carefully selected portfolio of journal articles and reports for teaching and learning can be useful. Articles can be selected to illustrate relative strengths and limitations in terms of readability, relevance, presentation, adequacy of literature review, methodological issues, and the use and application of findings. Many research textbooks also now include helpful sections, with examples, of critical appraisal of research publications (Nieswiadomy 1987; Polit & Hungler 1989).

Another possible student-centred activity based upon publications is the preparation of posters. Poster sessions are now common at research conferences as a way of communicating research information. The preparation of posters within courses is suggested by Sweeney (1984) as an effective and enjoyable way of analysing, summarizing and visually presenting essential concepts and results from selected studies.

Given sufficient time, a group-based exercise to plan, prepare, and present a literature review on a practice-related topic can also be challenging and stimulating.

Collecting data

Much can be learnt about research design and methods through lectures, from research textbooks, and from critical appraisal of research publications/reports and articles. It should also be possible, however, to devise exercises and assignments which provide hands-on or direct experience of using existing research tools, or of designing new tools, and of collecting and analysing data. What is being referred to here is a small scale learning task contained within a relatively 'safe' learning environment. This should be distinguished from more extensive projects, about which there are words of caution later in the chapter.

In our personal and professional lives, it is likely that hardly a month goes by without participation in some form of survey or another. By telephone, on the doorstep, while shopping, and through the mail, information is sought by interview and questionnaire. From comprehensive census forms to small scale consumer surveys, useful knowledge of research methods can be gained. Such experiences of participating in research and providing data can be examined and debated. Exploring the following questions, for example, can be revealing: Were you aware of the purpose of the interview or questionnaire? Who would use the information? Did you feel under pressure to provide the information? How, if at all, was your consent to participation obtained? Were the questions easy or difficult to answer? Did you answer them all and, if not, why not? How long was the interview or questionnaire? Were any incentives offered? Did you get any offer of feedback or study results? Do you think that the data you gave was valid and reliable?

Answers to these questions help to build up knowledge, grounded in experience, of the overall planning of research, of sampling, and of many key moral issues which must be considered whatever the nature and scale of the data collection.

Because the questionnaire is such a familiar research tool, it can be useful to spend time on the critical examination of several questionnaires, comparing them in terms of presentation and content. It is possible to gather a file of questionnaires in a comparatively short time. Students themselves may be invited to do this. Once collected, the questionnaires can be scrutinized in terms of length, form of questions, ease of completion, attractiveness of presentation, etc. From such an exercise, features not previously consciously noticed become evident, such as colour of paper, clarity of typeface, the amount of writing per page, the adequacy of the opening preamble and instructions, and the final thanks.

An exercise geared towards noticing the design of questionnaires can also be a helpful first stage for an attempt at devising a questionnaire which might be piloted within the group itself. This kind of exercise quickly challenges the notion that questionnaires are easy to put together. It also demonstrates the principles of careful planning and piloting, the need for adequate time and resources, and the importance of the relationship between research question, study design, and methods.

Similar exercises can be devised to illustrate other methods such as interviewing, observation, or the critical incident technique (see Chapters 22–25). Where data are collected from peers, careful attention still needs to be paid to ethical issues and the various ways of obtaining informed consent can be explored. Attempts can also be made to demystify statistics by using and analysing data generated from within, or available to the group itself in their day-to-day work (see Chapters 27–28).

Provided that sufficient attention is given to the aims of the exercises and to whether the aims can be readily achieved in the amount of time available, this kind of learning, by doing and from reflection upon experience, can be lively. It can also clearly illustrate another first principle: namely, that expert help should always be sought both at an early stage in the planning of research, and at appropriate points throughout the development of a research project.

Research discussion groups

Another useful way to learn about research methods and data analysis is to invite researchers themselves to bring to the group completed research tools representing data in various shapes, forms, and stages of analysis. Completed and used tools are generally more revealing than blank and unused tools. Dealing with the maverick response to a question, the dilemma of incomplete data, how to analyse the content of a lengthy interview, and the relative merits and limitations of computer versus hand analysis of data, can in this way become live issues for learners.

Opportunities to hear about personal experiences of carrying out research can be stimulating and helpful for many reasons. Researchers themselves often present, with enthusiasm, a credible and realistic picture of the pleasures and the pitfalls of undertaking research. Researchers who have been through the slow and sometimes frustrating process of sharing their research with colleagues in practice, management, and education, can helpfully debate issues such as why research is or is not used, how it might most appropriately be used, and the respective responsibilities of researcher and practising nurse in doing so.

Project work

It is now many years since Hunt and Hicks (1983) described the project work undertaken by students in many post-basic courses as 'over-ambitious and poorly structured'. Problems with projects still exist, however, as the following dialogue between the writer and an applicant for a post-basic diploma suggests:

PR: 'Have you had any research training so far?'
WARD SISTER: 'Yes. I've done the course for experienced ward sisters. We had a lecture on research and then we did a research project.'
PR: 'And how did it go?'
WARD SISTER: 'Terrible. I really wasn't sure what I was doing half the time.'

Project work, undertaken individually or in groups, can be valuable for learning in basic and post-basic courses, but like any other educational experience, it requires careful planning. Key questions to consider are: 'What is the purpose of the project and how does this relate to the overall aims of the course? What are its expected learning outcomes? What activities will the student have to undertake? Does the student have the essential baseline knowledge and skill to carry out the work? What are the possible resource and cost implications of project work? How long might project activities take to complete and what time is available? Is there adequate support available for each student? Do the project supervisors have the research expertise needed for the nature and scope of projects? Have guidelines for supervisors been drawn up and have they been debated? How clear are the project guidelines which are made available to students in writing? How will the project work be assessed and by whom? How will the learning experience be evaluated by students and how will the teaching, supervision and assessment be monitored within the course?'.

By working through these questions during curriculum development, it should become apparent to course planning teams whether project work is desirable and feasible.

Project work can take many forms and some activities already referred to in this chapter could be developed as individual or group projects. The form of 'learning-by-doing' project which causes greatest concern is the one in which students are expected to plan and undertake a complete research study, including collection, analysis and presentation of new data. It is in this type of project that students are most vulnerable. Adequate supervision is essential. Without it, students may quickly find themselves out of their depth, undertaking poorly planned work of too large a scale which cannot be completed in the time available, and which fails to address adequately moral issues. Supervisors have an important responsibility for ensuring, in a learning situation, that the rights of research subjects, whether patients, fellow health professionals, general public or student peers, and the duties and obligations of researchers, are carefully and thoroughly examined (see Chapter 4). In developing guidelines for supervisors, it can be helpful to refer to research publications which include sections on the supervision process and the relationship between student and supervisor; existing guidelines from bodies such as research councils or universities can also be used or adapted.

Project work can also be developed around replication of existing research and from the research interests of teaching staff. In the latter case, students may benefit directly and relatively quickly from the existing knowledge and expertise of the researcher in a particular area of enquiry. The teacher, as supervisor, however, would need to be aware of issues of control and ownership: of the possibility of giving direction which stifles creativity, for example and of the fact that the final work should belong to the student, not the teacher.

If project work is thought to be useful, a range of options should therefore be considered. Collection and analysis of data is only one part of one possible 'learning-by-doing' approach. Hunt and Hicks (1983) remind us that locating and making use of available information will provide opportunities to learn equally fundamental and worthwhile skills.

Armitage and Rees (1988a, 1988b) provide a checklist of points to consider and questions to answer in relation to projects and their supervision. They point out that such work can be exciting and illuminating for students and supervisors. If the project is based on personal interests and aspects of nursing practice about which the student is curious or concerned, then motivation will be high, understanding of the topic will develop, and confidence in research skill will grow. If a project is poorly planned and inadequately supervised, the work may be frustrating and a far-from-satisfactory educational experience for student and teacher.

There are, therefore, many possible approaches to 'learning-by-doing'. The pitfalls and merits of each are helpfully explored by Mander (1988) in her article on encouraging students to be research-minded. She suggests, for example, that inexperienced and novice investigators can produce poor quality research and muddy the waters for those who follow. The value of learning tasks which are based on the construction and use of a particular data collection tool could be questioned in terms of what students will learn from them about 'research as a process'. Learning-by-critiquing might be valuable for some students but others may treat such an exercise superficially; some tend to find critical appraisal so daunting and anxiety-provoking that they fail to learn much from the exercise at all. Similarly, 'learning-by-proposing-to-do' has the advantage of giving students first-hand experience of literature reviews, formulating a research question, outlining design and methods, and of planning and budgeting. This approach could be criticized, however, for its artificiality in stopping short of data collection and analysis and for reinforcing the perception of the 'doers' as a group separate from other nurses interested in research.

CONCLUSION

Research is now firmly part of the teaching and learning agenda within nurse education and developments have been remarkable in a comparatively short period of time. In this concluding section, several general issues and a number of key questions are presented for debate.

Competence

Competence in research, as in other areas of nursing, develops over time. Teachers and students need to be reminded every so often that knowledge grows, skills develop, and attitudes are challenged and changed throughout a professional lifetime. As the commitment to fostering research awareness and an understanding of the principles of inquiry grows within nurse education, there will be a need to temper haste with caution and to review regularly the aims, processes, and outcomes of teaching and learning in research.

Research base to the curriculum

What exactly does this phrase mean? To what extent is research a core theme which runs through the whole course? Are research findings integrated well into teaching and into practice? Is research teaching still imported or farmed out? (Mander 1988). Specific research input is helpful, but ideally this should be supported by the whole teaching team. To what extent is educational research (see Chapter 33) used to inform course planning and monitoring, and curriculum development? Have key people been identified to act as facilitators and co-ordinators for developing research-related teaching? What opportunities are available for staff development in research and to what extent is this regarded as a priority?

Currently favoured approaches to teaching, learning and assessment should be put under the microscope regularly. For example, self-directed and experiential learning are currently in vogue but what exactly do these terms mean and how valuable are such approaches? (Weil & McGill 1989). Formal lectures and cook-book approaches to teaching the research process tend to be criticized as too mechanistic, but how justified is this criticism? A carefully planned, clearly presented lecture can be highly instructive, thoroughly satisfying, and fun to hear. Learning-by-doing, on the other hand, can be a perplexing muddle. Assessment procedures also contribute significantly to learning. Is self-assessment encouraged? What forms does it take? Are students helped to reflect actively on the processes of their own learning?

Another important area for debate surrounds questions about where, when, and how students should learn about complex issues such as the relationship between research, theory development, and the quality of care received by consumers of health care.

Networking

One welcome area of development is the growth in the amount and range of research support available through nursing and multidisciplinary networks (see Chapter 3). Exchange of ideas, practical help, and supervision, have always been available through informal contact with colleagues. Support for educational developments in colleges and in practice could benefit, however, from more effective networking and a commitment to the sharing of ideas and initiatives. In this respect, a proposal from the Chief Scientist Office of the Scottish Home and Health Department to support the establishment and co-ordination of local research networks could be valuable.

Opportunities

Much of this chapter has dealt with areas of debate about the planning and provision of teaching and learning about research within courses, but there are many other ways within day-to-day work in which nurses can learn and be taught to develop their awareness of research. A growing body of literature now shows how this can be achieved when nurses at all levels of health care organization become involved in initiating research and translating research findings into practice (Hunt 1987, Lathlean 1988). The ward sister who routinely involves the members of her nursing team in literature searches, the clinical supervisor who questions and analyses care with a student, the health visitor who sets up a journal club in the health centre, all contribute to developing research awareness.

Opportunities for learning outwith formal courses are also improving steadily, for example, through the excellent, innovative series of modules on research awareness produced by the Distance Learning Centre of the South Bank Polytechnic.

Teaching and learning about the research process, when it is geared to practice realities and based on principles of adult learning, can be both lively and interesting. It seems likely, in this as in all other areas of educational development and service provision, that steady, creative development will continue to depend on the effectiveness of partnerships between practitioners, managers, teachers, and researchers.

56 INTRODUCTION TO THE RESEARCH PROCESS IN NURSING

REFERENCES

Armitage S. & Rees C. (1988a) Project supervision. *Nurse Education Today*, **8** (2), 99–104.

Armitage S. & Rees C. (1988b) Student projects: a practical framework. *Nurse Education Today*, **8** (5), 289–95.

Clark E. (1987) Research awareness: its importance in practice. *The Professional Nurse*, **2** (11), 371–3.

Hunt M. (1987) The process of translating research findings into practice. *Journal of Advanced Nursing*, **12** (1), 101–10.

Hunt M. & Hicks J. (1983) Promoting research-awareness in post-basic nursing courses. *Nursing Times* Occasional Papers, **79** (6), 41–2.

Jarvis P. (1988) *Adult and Continuing Education*. Routledge, London.

Lathlean J. (Ed.) (1988) *Research in Action. Developing the Role of the Ward Sister*. King's Fund Centre, London.

Mander R. (1988) Encouraging students to be research minded. *Nurse Education Today*, **8** (1), 30–5.

Nieswiadomy R.M. (1987) *Foundations of Nursing Research*. Appleton & Lange, New York.

Polit D. & Hungler B. (1989) *Essentials of Nursing Research: methods, appraisal and utilization*. Lippincott, Philadelphia.

Sweeney S. (1984) Strategies for teaching nursing research: poster sessions for undergraduate students: a useful tool for learning and communicating nursing research. *Western Journal of Nursing Research*, **6** (1), 135–7.

Weil S. & McGill I. (Eds.) (1989) *Making Sense of Experiential Learning. Diversity in Theory and Practice*. The Society for Research into Higher Education and The Open University Press.

Chapter 7
An Overview of the Research Process
Desmond F. S. Cormack

Irrespective of the discipline in which research is undertaken, the series and sequence of steps are essentially the same. What will differ between disciplines such as nursing and psychology, for example, will be the subject of the research rather than its structure or process. The research process discussed in Part II of this book is a description of what is commonly referred to as 'the scientific method'. The strength of the scientific method as an approach to problem solving is that it optimizes the possibility of arriving at the most 'correct', although rarely perfect, solution. Thus, subjectivity is reduced and objectivity increased in the examination of a particular issue or the asking of a specific question.

It is necessary to recognize that an understanding of the research process is not, in itself, sufficient to enable its application. The topics discussed in the first seven chapters of this book, for example, are each important in the development of research skills. Similarly, the subjects described in the final three chapters are of importance in relation to undertaking, participating in, and using research. Part II cannot be seen in isolation from other parts of this book, it is merely one distinct phase in a number of interrelated parts of understanding the nature, purpose, and structure of research. A knowledge of research principles will not, of itself, make you a skilled researcher. The need for appropriate guidance and supervision during all stages of research experience is of considerable importance. Indeed, it is generally recognized that such guidance and supervision is required even by the most experienced researcher.

As with many activities, including nursing which requires a high level of knowledge skill, the knowledge and skill required to undertake nursing research can be learned. Such knowledge and skill can be learned in a number of ways: being told by others, discussing the subject with others, reading about the subject, and by doing a piece of nursing research. Although all educational methods are of value, the ability to undertake research – like riding a bicycle – is never fully developed until practical experience is obtained.

To some extent, the phases of the research process are sequential, each study tending to follow the same series of steps in a similar order. Part II of this book presents the sequence of steps in the order in which they are normally undertaken. However, as will be demonstrated in this chapter, there is considerable overlap, interrelationship, and possibly some variation, in the sequence of events. Figure 7.1 shows the outline of the research process in terms of each of the phases to be considered and also identifies the chapter(s) dealing with each phase.

The interrelationship of the various phases of research are many and complex. Figure 7.1 is not intended to demonstrate all of these possible relationships; rather it is intended to show the existence of some of them. Although Chapters 8–31 may

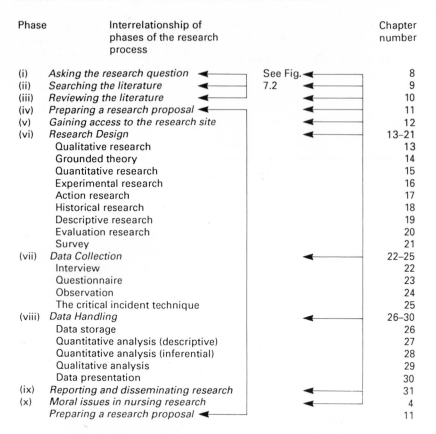

Phase	Interrelationship of phases of the research process		Chapter number
(i)	*Asking the research question*	See Fig.	8
(ii)	*Searching the literature*	7.2	9
(iii)	*Reviewing the literature*		10
(iv)	*Preparing a research proposal*		11
(v)	*Gaining access to the research site*		12
(vi)	*Research Design*		13–21
	Qualitative research		13
	Grounded theory		14
	Quantitative research		15
	Experimental research		16
	Action research		17
	Historical research		18
	Descriptive research		19
	Evaluation research		20
	Survey		21
(vii)	*Data Collection*		22–25
	Interview		22
	Questionnaire		23
	Observation		24
	The critical incident technique		25
(viii)	*Data Handling*		26–30
	Data storage		26
	Quantitative analysis (descriptive)		27
	Quantitative analysis (inferential)		28
	Qualitative analysis		29
	Data presentation		30
(ix)	*Reporting and disseminating research*		31
(x)	*Moral issues in nursing research*		4
	Preparing a research proposal		11

Fig. 7.1 Phases in the research process.

appear to present the process as a series of relatively isolated phases, in practice these overlap.

ASKING THE RESEARCH QUESTION

Although phase (i) is often regarded as the first formal part of the research process, a number of factors and experiences precede it. It is unlikely, for example, that a potential nurse researcher will suddenly decide that a particular subject should become the focus of a research-based study. It is more probable that, in the course of professional experience and activity, a problem area will slowly emerge as a possibility for a research project. For example, a nurse may have suspected for a long time that the design and height of hospital beds prevents nurses from lifting patients 'properly', thus placing the patient and nurse at risk. Similarly, an experienced nurse may suspect that all is not well with the methods used to teach learners how best to develop and use interpersonal skills. These examples, in themselves, are not formal research questions, they need to be developed, refined, and made specific, as described in Chapter 8. Every trained nurse, therefore, has the experience with which to start to participate in the nursing research process, an advantage which is not available to those without a nursing background.

It may well be that the ability to think in this inquiring and constructive manner is one of the most important features of potential nurse researchers. Although such individuals may be considered somewhat strange, difficult, or over-critical by their colleagues, there is no doubt that they are a vital part of the development of research in nursing.

Asking the research question (phase i) will almost certainly overlap with the next two phases of the process, that is, searching and reviewing the literature, and it will do so in the following way. Before having formally identified the research question, and before having undertaken a systematic search and review of the literature, you may dip into published materials in order to help decide exactly what to research. Figure 7.2 demonstrates this relationship.

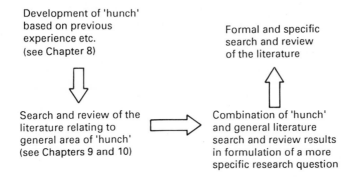

Fig. 7.2   Relationship between research question and literature search and review.

It can be seen that formulation of the research question comes between a general and unstructured literature search and review (from which it is partly derived) and a more structured and specific search and review (to which it gives direction).

SEARCHING THE LITERATURE

The relationship between the literature search and other early stages of the research process has been outlined above. Its relationship between other stages throughout the research is also important, and considerable in that it is related to all stages and continues throughout. Although the intensive and formal search will occur at the early stages of the work, bear in mind that literature continues to be published throughout the time it takes to undertake the study. Similarly, some aspects of the literature may be of particular relevance to the latter part of the study, for example, to data analysis.

Chapter 9 describes and discusses the means of and the facilities available for searching the literature, and shows that a knowledge of this aspect of the research process can make the difference between finding a wealth of appropriate literature and wrongly concluding that 'nothing has been published relating to the subject'. As with all aspects of research, there are rules and guidelines which will make the task easier. There are also an increasingly large range of facilities, aids, organizations and resource personnel who can be of assistance. 'Practice will make perfect' if the potential nurse researcher is motivated to learn and is willing to invest time and effort.

REVIEWING THE LITERATURE

The literature review, although described in a different chapter from that dealing with searching the literature, is closely related to the search in that both occur virtually simultaneously. Indeed, the review of material found early in the search often gives direction to subsequent parts of the search. However, because the search and review require very different skills, these two closely related phases are dealt with in two chapters rather than in one. The major feature of the literature *review*, and one which differentiates it from the literature *search*, is that the review consists of a critical evaluation of the literature obtained as a result of the search.

The value of acquiring the skills required to undertake a literature search and review is by no means restricted to their use in the research process. These skills are also central to the notion of professionalism in nursing in that all nurses have a responsibility to be familiar with the literature in their subject area. Without skills in literature search and review it is difficult, if not impossible, to have a firm understanding of the nursing literature.

PREPARING A RESEARCH PROPOSAL

Figure 7.1 places 'Preparing a research proposal' both towards the beginning *and* at the end of the outline of phases of the research process; this is done for the following reasons. The researcher must have a knowledge of the entire research process before constructing a research proposal. The research proposal, when constructed, will include some detail of all phases of the research process. Finally, having constructed a research plan which is contained in the proposal, you then implement that plan and thereby carry out the piece of research. It is necessary to prepare a research proposal before undertaking a piece of research, but it is only after the first-time researcher is familiar with the research process, that a proposal can be prepared. Thus, you first learn the theory relating to the research process, prepare a practical research proposal, then, if submission of the research proposal is successful, carry out the research.

In Chapter 11, there are general and specific guidelines available to those undertaking a research study and who have to prepare a research proposal. Whatever the local regulations relating to gaining permission, the beginner must be particularly aware that failure to prepare and present the proposal to the appropriate persons and committees may cause long delays or, still worse, destroy an otherwise excellent research project.

GAINING ACCESS TO THE RESEARCH SITE

The research site refers to the place where research data are collected; it can vary in size from a single ward to a sample of hospitals. In some instances you will be part of the organization in which the data are to be collected, and you may consequently find entry to the research site relatively easy. When the nature of the study is more complex and involved, entry into facilities which are not part of the organization in which you are employed, or with which you are associated, may be considerably more difficult. In the absence of guidelines to the means of gaining entry, this part of the research process can present considerable difficulty. Surprisingly, it is a topic which receives very little attention in discussions of the research process, or in many research reports. It is intended that Chapter 12 will provide a number of suggestions which will minimize this potential difficulty.

RESEARCH DESIGN

A considerable range of research designs are available; Chapters 13–21 deal with a *selection* of those which are in relatively common use. The research design should not be confused with the data collection method(s) which are used in a study. The former, research design, is used to describe the overall research approach which is to be used, the latter, data collection method(s), to describe the means by which data for a study will be collected. Thus, the data collection method is part of the research design.

Many data collection methods such as interview or observation can be used as part of a number of different research designs. For example, interviews or observation might be used as part of quantitative, qualitative, experimental, action, descriptive, or evaluation research.

Decisions regarding research design precede selection of data collection methods. First, the design is selected on the grounds that it is the most suitable to answer the research question; the most suitable data collection method(s) is then selected.

Although some research designs are mutually exclusive in that they cannot occur simultaneously, others are less so. For example, experimental and descriptive designs are quite different. Experimental design will include *descriptions* of phenomena before variables are changed and/or introduced as part of the experiment. However, a descriptive research design will not include such a change to, or introduction of, variables. Another example of 'overlap' is the relationship between action research and qualitative and quantitative research designs. For example, action research may include both qualitative and quantitative design.

Grounded theory is both a form of research design *and* a data collection method; discussion of it is equally appropriate in the section entitled Research Design *and* the one entitled Data Collection. Grounded theory is presented in this section as an example of qualitative research design although it is also a method of collecting data.

DATA COLLECTION

Choice of a data collection instrument, followed by actual collection of data, is a phase which offers the researcher considerable scope and choice. Researchers have a wide range of means of collecting data available to them, and they need to consider which of these are best suited to their needs. If you wish to collect respondents' opinions, an interview or questionnaire may be chosen. Alternatively, if you wish to establish what a particular work group does, you may use the observation, or critical incident technique.

The purpose of this book is not to present the entire range of data collection techniques which are available, but to introduce four commonly used ones in Chapters 22–25, and to provide references to suitable publications where more may be learned about the use of each. It is important to realize that, when using an existing method of collecting data, you must judge whether or not it is exactly suitable to your needs and, if not, adapt it to meet personal requirements. Indeed, if no method can be found which will obtain the data required, a new data collection tool may have to be devised.

Finally, bear in mind that no method of collecting data is perfect; each has its own limitations and strengths. The job of the researcher in this respect is to select or adapt a method which is as near perfect as possible, and to discuss fully the strengths and weaknesses of this chosen method.

DATA HANDLING

Having collected data, they then need to be handled in a way which will enable you to meet the aims and objectives of the research. The major elements of data handling are storage, analysis and presentation. Although these three topics have considerable overlap, they do require different skills and considerations.

Data storage

Having collected research data, these are stored in a way which will allow easy access. If very small quantities of data are collected, ten questionnaires, for example, then no special storage techniques may be required. However, if larger quantities of data are collected, 1000 questionnaires, for example, some form of storage which will assist counting and sorting must be used.

At present, nurses store large amounts of data in the form of information about patient care and features of nursing practice. However, the researcher often finds difficulty in retrieving the data in order to examine some aspects of this patient care or nursing practice. This difficulty relates to the means by which information is stored – on charts, graphs and in books – these being the storage techniques with which all nurses are familiar. Chapter 26 describes data storage techniques which are commonly used by researchers and which enable easy retrieval and analysis.

Data analysis

Chapters 27 and 28 describe two approaches to quantitative analysis: the use and manipulation of numbers to describe and make inferences from the data. These chapters introduce two types of data analysis: descriptive and inferential statistics. They are not designed to teach you how to understand fully the statistical techniques but to help you understand what statistics are, what they can and cannot do, and how to further your knowledge of the subject. In dealing with data analysis, the researcher, as in all phases of the research process, must admit to and take full account of personal limitations and seek expert assistance at an early stage.

Data can be analysed by other than statistical techniques; they can also be analysed by means of the researcher's thought processes and the subsequent use of words to describe and discuss the data, that is by using qualitative analysis. Indeed, many perfectly respectable pieces of nursing research have used qualitative, rather than quantiative (statistical), data analysis. Chapter 29 deals with qualitative analysis of data and it demonstrates how conclusions from the data can be arrived at without necessarily applying either descriptive or inferential statistical techniques. However, as with other phases of the research process, the application of quantitative or qualitative data analysis techniques are not necessarily mutually exclusive. For example, in some circumstances, it may be necessary to apply quantitative techniques to qualitative data.

Data presentation

The presentation of data following its analysis and as part of writing a research report, offers a variety of techniques from which to choose. Choice will obviously depend on the nature of the data and what one hopes to achieve with its presentation. Whilst the use of words is a crucial part of data presentation, and one with which nurses are familiar, alternative forms of presentation can add considerably to its impact and meaning.

REPORTING AND DISSEMINATING RESEARCH

Reporting and disseminating findings, including the preparation of a written report, is a feature of all pieces of successfully completed research. There can be no doubt that this phase of the process presents the researcher with real challenges. However, there is also no doubt that, with the help of an experienced supervisor, the beginner can develop the skills required to successfully disseminate research.

While the structure and form of almost all research reports is invariably similar, the same cannot be said of the means chosen to disseminate findings. The word 'disseminate' in this book refers to any means used to present the research findings to others. Examples include the preparation of a research-based thesis, writing articles and books, and speaking at conferences. As will be seen in Chapter 31, researchers must be willing to use any of a range of means available to them for reporting and disseminating both their findings and the research methods used to obtain them.

Throughout this text, the need for full, continuous and complete documentation in relation to all phases of the research process is shown to be absolutely essential. Beginners frequently assume (wrongly) that report writing begins at the stage of the research process entitled 'Reporting and disseminating research'. In reality, nothing could be further from the truth in that the written report will include materials collected during *all* phases of the process. This documentation, appropriate supervision and systematic application of the phases of the research process, will not, of course, guarantee success. However, it will maximize that possibility.

MORAL ISSUES IN NURSING RESEARCH

Although Fig 7.1 concludes with a reference to moral issues in nursing research, it is not being implied here that the subject is either of less importance than the others or that it occurs as an afterthought. Moral issues are an integral part of *all* phases of the research process, as well as to the use and application of nursing research. All phases of the research process, therefore, must include a full consideration of appropriate moral issues. The word 'moral' is used in preference to the more frequently used 'ethical' in the belief that the former term is more comprehensive than, and inclusive of, the latter.

Part II
The Research Process

Although the phases of the research process are presented in sequential and separate chapters, it is essential to see these as being interrelated and, in some circumstances, occurring in a differing sequence. In preparing these chapters, decisions were made about what to include and exclude. Although all major steps in the research process are included, not all research designs, nor all possible means of collecting, storing or handling data, are discussed. However, those topics chosen for inclusion are felt to be in relatively common use in most research studies.

The four major sections of the research process are 'Preparatory Work' (Chapters 8–12), 'Research Design' (Chapters 13–21), 'Data Collection' (Chapters 22–25), and 'Data Handling' (Chapters 26–31).

In this second edition, the opportunity has been taken to revise and update all chapters, and to considerably extend the text by including a number of additional subjects. In particular, aspects of qualitative research have been included, as have a number of additional research designs such as action, historical, and evaluation research.

An understanding of the elements of the research process does not, in itself, equip the beginner to undertake a research study. All beginners must undertake further extensive reading and subsequently work under the supervision of others who have appropriate research skills. Indeed many, if not all, experienced researchers make use of such supervision in order to optimize the quality of their work.

A: Preparatory Work

As with all complex activity, and research is no exception, it is necessary to do a considerable amount of preparatory work prior to undertaking the main task. Time so invested will maximize the possibility of the research being of high quality. The preparatory work described in this section also includes making decisions regarding all of the topics dealt with in Chapters 13 to 31. Thus, a knowledge of the subjects dealt with in those chapters is necessary before the preparatory work can be completed, and decisions regarding research design, data collection, and data handling, made.

This preparatory stage of the research study is more time consuming than is often realized; it may use as much as one third of a total 'time budget'.

The elements of preparatory work, although presented in sequence and separately, are closely related. 'Asking the Research Question', for example (see Chapter 8), is a basis for, and an integral part of, all other aspects of preparatory work, and of the research process generally.

The research question, the subject of this chapter, gives direction to the search and review of the literature (see Chapters 9 and 10) which in turn influences the developing research question.

Once the research question has been finalized, and the preliminary literature search and review has been undertaken, all aspects of the proposed study are encapsulated in the form of a research proposal (see Chapter 11). The proposal has a number of functions, one of which is to enable you to obtain funding, obtain permission to collect data, and gain access to the research site (see Chapter 12).

Chapter 8
Asking the Research Question
Desmond F.S. Cormack and David C. Benton

Excitement and wonder are emotions that are commonly experienced by those who undertake a piece of research. However, we have observed that these emotions are often replaced with feelings of uncertainty when the inexperienced researcher attempts to ask a research question. This uncertainty can be easily rectified if a number of guiding principles are followed.

In this chapter, it is intended to identify and address those issues which often cause inexperienced researchers concern when attempting to formulate a research question. This initial stage of the research process can not only be difficult but is crucial to the success of the remaining parts of the study.

The process of asking a research question is very rarely a once and for all event. It is highly unlikely that, all of a sudden, you will scream 'Eureka!' and be satisfied with the first question that comes into your head. More often the process entails days, weeks, or even months of thought and effort to refine and sharpen a question that you will eventually feel happy and confident about researching.

It has been our experience that attempting to ask a research question generates a large number of associated queries to which the neophyte researcher often finds difficulty in obtaining answers. In this chapter, those questions most frequently expressed about *asking the research question* are identified, and by providing solutions, will assist you in the process of asking your research question.

WHAT IS A RESEARCH QUESTION?

This may seem a rather obvious question, but for those who are embarking upon the research process for the first time, it is often asked.

A research question occurs in one of two forms, that is, either as an *interrogative* or *declarative* statement. A research question in the *interrogative* format is a statement, in question form, which identifies a gap in nursing knowledge. '*What is the relationship between the provision of post-registration education and the retention of staff?*', for example. A *declarative* research question is a statement that defines the purpose of the study by declaring the intention to investigate a particular event, phenomenon, or situation. '*The purpose of this research is to investigate the relationship between the provision of post-registration education and the retention of staff*, for example. The research question (or questions) are often translated into the aims of a study. However, the question comes first.

A 'good' research question is one that is short, sharp, specific, and clearly states or implies a relationship between two or more variables. In the above example, the variables are *post-registration courses* and *staff retention*. The variables identified must be empirical, that is capable of observation and measurement. Furthermore, the phrasing of the question should be free from value judgments and bias since it is the prime objective of any research study to investigate the problem identified from a scientific and objective stance.

DO I NEED A RESEARCH QUESTION?

Research is a scientific and logical process of investigation and requires that you follow a particular direction of inquiry. Unless you have a clearly defined research question you will be unable to progress your study in a planned and efficient manner.

In essence, the research question identifies and describes a gap in nursing's knowledge base which the research study seeks to fill. It helps to focus your thoughts and efforts, assisting you in developing a framework which will guide you through the entire research process. You can *not* undertake a research study without identifying a research question.

Most research studies will have one specific, or primary, research question but some may have a number of secondary, or subsidiary questions. Secondary questions must relate to the primary question. For example, the primary research question, *'What is the relationship between the provision of post-registration education and the retention of staff?'* may have the following secondary questions:

Which post-registration courses are available?

Who provides the funding for post-registration courses?

HOW DO I FIND A RESEARCH QUESTION?

Inexperienced researchers often find difficulty in identifying a research question. Nevertheless, you will find that no sooner have you thought of one topic to investigate when another will come to mind. This experience is often confusing, since with so many valuable topics to investigate how can you decide which is the most important. In addition, you may be unfamiliar with the existing literature, a fact that often compounds uncertainty and confusion. If this is not bad enough, lack of familiarity with the research process may also cause additional perplexity. However, do not let all the initial uncertainty put you off. If you are interested and motivated towards conducting research you will identify, in time, a specific topic which you will find suitable for investigation.

To assist you in the search for a research question, you may wish to consider a number of sources which will help you identify a gap in nursing's existing knowledge base.

Your own experience

Turn to your own experience. How often have you questioned, either in your mind, or with your colleagues, a situation, treatment, or outcome, wondering what has happened, why it should be that way, or how you can improve it.

Professional literature

The professional literature often triggers further research. You may note the findings of a study and consider whether such an approach can be applied in your own area of practice or to the particular client group you work with. The deliberate use of methodology already reported but used in a different setting and with another subject group, is termed replication. Such an approach is extremely valuable since far too few nursing studies have been conducted with more than one client group or in different locations (Chapman 1989). It is perhaps appropriate to note at this point that the research question does not have to be novel to be worthwhile. However, if you choose to repeat a study that has already been carried out, it is important that you examine the previous study carefully and avoid any methodological or conceptual flaws.

Alternatively, if you read a number of research reports about a topic, you may notice inconsistencies in findings which can stimulate further research. You may wonder why the results obtained with one group, or at one location, or using a particular method, are different from those reported elsewhere.

Yet another means by which a research question can be derived from literature is when a gap in the existing knowledge base is observed. For example, increased commitment to the use of computer technology as a means of providing nurse education, has been advocated by a national education body (Procter 1986). Despite the fact that few studies have investigated the effectiveness of this approach to the provision of education, many schools of nursing have allocated considerable resources to the purchase of equipment.

Theoretical frameworks

In the past forty years, a number of theoretical frameworks have been proposed: Peplau's (1952) interpresonal relations model, Roy's (1980) adaption model and Roger's (1970) unitary man model, to name but three. Each of these models can be used as the basis for the development of a research question. The model can be tested to determine whether it can predict the outcome of treatment. To date, few studies have been developed to test the available theoretical models and, as yet, most remain inadequately validated. Theoretical model testing can be seen as an area ripe for investigation.

Conferences and study days

When you attend a conference or a study day it is often the discussion that occurs during coffee and meal breaks that proves to be the most valuable element of the day. Such interactions can result in the discovery of a wide variety of means of treating a particular client, often prompting thoughts which can be developed into a research question.

National directives and Delphi studies

From time to time the government or a national body will identify specific topics which they feel require investigation. Such topics are usually of major national concern and have significant implications for the health of the nation.

Another means of identifying topics of concern to a large number of individuals, is the use of a Delphi survey. A Delphi survey is a technique where subjects are asked to respond to a series of questionnaires. The first questionnaire usually attempts to elicit views on a specific topic. Subsequent questionnaires feed back the original comments made by the subjects who are then asked to rank the statements in order of importance. In the case of a recent study by MacMillan et *al.* (1989), nursing staff in three health boards in Scotland were asked to identify those topics which they felt required to be researched. This approach may yield a number of topics that can then form the basis for further investigation.

HOW CAN I DECIDE WHICH QUESTION TO STUDY?

Often you will have a number of ideas which you may wish to investigate. The tentative questions you have identified may be related or may be on completely different subject areas. The problem facing you is how to decide which one of a number of topics to investigate first. There are a number of guiding principles which will assist you in your choice.

Interest and motivation

The research process can be simultaneously exciting, stimulating, arduous, and depressing. When things are going well, nothing seems to be too much of a problem, but there are those times when you will confront difficulties. Unless the research question focuses on a problem about which *you* feel strongly, it is likely that during difficult times you will be unable to sustain enthusiasm for the study. Any research questions which you may consider for investigation must therefore be of sufficient interest to keep you motivated through the 'bad' as well as the 'good' times.

A researchable question

Not all questions are amenable to investigation. Any question which poses a philosophical or ethical question is not directly answerable by research. For example, 'Should fetal tissue be used for cerebral implantation?' poses an ethical question, and although it is possible to debate this issue, no amount of research will give you an answer. The question is not researchable.

It is often possible to change the focus of a question which addresses an ethical or philosophical dilemma to one that is researchable, 'Does the implantation of fetal tissue alleviate symptoms of Parkinson's disease?', for example. Although it is possible to answer this question by research, it does not address the original ethical question; it may, however, provide evidence which will influence your viewpoint on the issue.

Problem significance

Any problem selected should be of significance to the client group you care for and/or to nursing's knowledge base. The significance of a problem can be best judged by assessing the question's worth in terms of a number of criteria. First, does the question address a problem which affects large numbers of patients? Second, will the outcome of the research significantly improve the quality of life of individuals or groups? Third, does the question address a nursing problem? Finally, will the results be suitable for use in a (non-research) practice environment?

Feasibility

Many potentially interesting and researchable questions have to be discarded because they are not feasible. If you are to assess the feasibility of a research question you must consider a number of issues. These will include time available, researcher expertise, ethical considerations, resources available, subject availability, and the co-operation of others.

Time available

If you are undertaking a piece of research for the first time it is likely that you will have difficulty in trying to assess how much work is involved and how long it will take. You can, however, make a more accurate assessment of the feasibility of undertaking a particular study by drawing up a detailed timetable. It is also important to note, that for certain elements of a study, you will be able to arrange a schedule to suit your own pace but alas some will be determined by those individuals or agencies providing support and information.

A good starting point for attempting to assess the length of time a study will take is to use as a framework the steps in the research process (see Chapter 7). Each step in the process can be broken down into as much detail as possible then time allocated appropriately. The total length of time required can then be calculated and an appropriate decision taken, that is, either to proceed with the study, try and negotiate time from your employer, redefine the study in such a way as to 'fit' the time available, or reject the study as being unfeasible. Remember, if you have a detailed breakdown of time required, you are in a stronger position to argue for the appropriate study time.

If you are aware of anyone who has conducted some research seek their advice. Valuable information about how long literature searches will take and more importantly how long it will take to locate and access literature, can also be obtained from librarians.

If ethical committee approval is required, studies may often be delayed for considerable periods of time. It is not uncommon for such a committee to meet on a bimonthly or quarterly basis. If delays are to be avoided, it is important that you make contact with the committee at an early stage.

Resources available

Closely associated with the requirement for sufficient time, is the need for appropriate and adequate resources. The resource requirements of any study can vary considerably. A study undertaken as part of a course may need only nominal resources, whereas some research will require vast quantities of both material and money.

When attempting to assess feasibility, it is important to clearly identify all those resources you will require to enable you to complete the study. Obviously, the design of your study will influence the amount of resources required. By starting with a detailed timetable you are less likely to omit items. Always consider literature search charges, photocopying, telephone, postage, computer access, any specialized equipment, travel costs, office space (often at a premium), document typing, and report production. The more detailed the list you can produce the better prepared you are to assess the feasibility of the study.

Researcher expertise

It is important that you examine closely the level of expertise required to undertake and successfully complete the study you have identified. Unless such an assessment is undertaken, it is likely that you will end up attempting a study which you are unqualified to carry out. A timetable of events can be particularly useful. If there are a few elements about which you have little or even no knowledge you can seek assistance and support at an early stage. With appropriate advice and supervision, what would have been an unfeasible study can become possible.

Ethical considerations

When assessing the feasibility of a particular study you should always consider the ethics of undertaking the research. Research should cause no harm or distress and it is important that any proposal should be reviewed by an unbiased individual or group. If patients are involved, or if your research involves any invasive procedure, it is normal practice to seek the approval of the hospital's ethics committee.

Research that is undertaken and which does not have the potential to advance our knowledge should not take place. Similarly, any piece of work that does not offer subjects confidentiality and anonymity should on most occasions be considered inappropriate. Only if a study can be shown to be ethically and morally acceptable should it be considered feasible (see Chapter 4).

Subject availability

If you intend to investigate a very rare phenomenon it is likely that either you will be unable to recruit enough subjects to your study, or you will have to travel considerable distances to do so. Consequently, it is important to identify and assess the availability of subjects, for without subjects you have no study. Furthermore, it is important to recognize that potential subjects may not be as enthusiastic about the research study as you are. It is likely that some may refuse to participate and this is a point well worth consideration.

Co-operation of others

When you plan a study, identify those individuals and groups who will come in contact with your work. It is always worth investing time, at an early stage, in gaining their support. Any individuals who will be directly involved should be contacted personally and given the opportunity to discuss issues of concern. Only after obtaining the co-operation of all those involved in the study should the study be undertaken. More specific information on the closely associated issue of gaining access to research sites is provided in Chapter 12.

HOW CAN THE RESEARCH QUESTION BEST BE DESCRIBED?

Research questions, despite being short, clear, and specific, will still require to be explained in some detail to those who read the final report. In addition to being implicit in the title of the study, an explanation of the rationale for undertaking the study should appear very early in any publication. The fact that a gap exists in the knowledge base, and that the research question has relevance to nursing, should be clearly established.

A common difficulty experienced by novice and expert researchers alike is the imprecise nature of language. Words often have more than one meaning, and hence if your research question is to be described in absolute terms there is a need to offer precise definitions for any words, terms, or procedures central to your research. The normal definition which is given in a dictionary is frequently inadequate. It is therefore necessary to state the operational definition of terms, that is, the definition given to words by the researcher, that is by you. For example, a dictionary might define a patient as 'a person who is receiving medical care', whereas you may choose to operationally define the term patient as 'any male, who is hospitalized in a surgical ward, who has undergone surgery in the previous 24 hours, and who is aged between 16 and 65 years'.

DOES THE RESEARCH QUESTION INFLUENCE THE RESEARCH PROCESS?

It should be evident that the research question has total influence on all aspects of the research process. Having asked the research question, all other aspects of the study are designed to answer it. For example, the question determines the scope and content of the literature review. A methodological approach will be selected that is capable of answering the question. All collected data will be destined for analysis and this will provide results. The results will present an answer to the question which when compared and contrasted with previous research will determine any recommendations. The research question is the thread which unifies the entire study.

RELATING THE RESEARCH QUESTION TO THE RESEARCH PROCESS

It is common for inexperienced researchers to have difficulty in defining the exact relationship between the research question and other components of the study.

How does the title of the study and the research question relate?

The research question should be formulated first and subsequently the title of the study should be derived from it. Often there is little difference between the two. A suitable and appropriate title for the research question posed earlier might be:

'A study of the relationship between the provision of post-registration education and the retention of staff?'

Is the aim of the study the same as the research question?

Although they are not identical in expression, they are identical in meaning. Some researchers decide to pose a number of questions which the research seeks to answer. Others convert the question to a series of aims which, when achieved, provide the solution to the research question. In the example used in this chapter the question may generate the following aim:

'To describe the relationship between the provision of post-registration education and the retention of staff.'

Is the research question the same as a hypothesis?

Despite the fact that a hypothesis can be derived from a research question, if that question seeks to establish whether or not there is a relationship between two variables, the research question and the hypothesis are not the same. The hypothesis for the study suggested above might state:

'The retention of staff is increased by the provision of post-registration education.'

It is not always possible to derive a hypothesis from a research question. A hypothesis can only be stated for those studies suitable for investigation at the outset by quantitative methods, and which predict a relationship between two variables. For example, if the research question had asked, 'Which factors influence staff's decision to remain with a health authority for more than five years?', then a hypothesis could not be formulated until the factors had been identified.

How does the research question relate to the literature review?

It has been suggested that the research literature itself may stimulate the formulation of a research question. Irrespective of whether the question was, or was not, stimulated by a publication, the literature review should cover two main domains which support the question formulation. First, the question should be

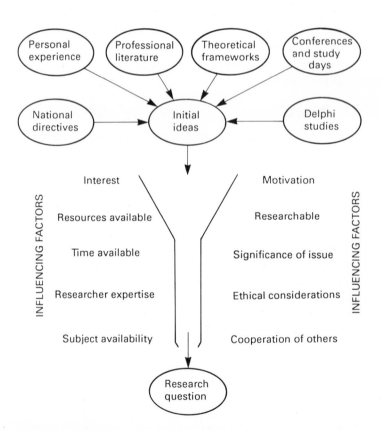

Fig. 8.1 Development of a Research Question.

derived from a specific theoretical perspective so as to ensure that any findings can be appropriately integrated into the knowledge base. Secondly, the literature review should identify any previous research carried out and provide an objective critique of the work. It is common for the literature review to move from a general description of the topic to a more focused evaluation. The move from the general to the specific is a means of identifying surrounding issues so as to place the research question in context.

The literature review should be considered fundamental to the development of any research question. The literature presented to the reader should cogently argue that there is a need for the study to take place and that the findings will have potential significance to nursing or those cared for.

CAN THE ORIGINAL RESEARCH QUESTION BE CHANGED?

Having conducted preliminary work, it is not uncommon for the research question to be modified or even abandoned completely. If it is to be modified, this is done prior to the specific literature review. The research question cannot be changed or modified at a subsequent stage. If this is done, the research process must be restarted.

A change or modification may take place following a pilot study if the pilot study indicates that such a change is necessary. In that case, the pilot study is repeated until the research question is found to be appropriate. Furthermore, it is not uncommon for researchers to be tempted to add secondary questions at the pilot study stage. However, this temptation should be avoided if possible. Any addition will result in extra work and may require further resources which may not be available. If the research question is to be modified or secondary questions added, a full assessment of the implications of such a change requires to be made.

CONCLUSIONS

The process of asking the research question is, in part, simply the logical application of a number of guidelines. However, those questions which identify a significant issue are often the result of inspired curiosity. All professional nurses who take a critical and questioning view of nursing practice, management and education have the ability to identify such issues and generate a research question. Figure 8.1 summarizes the common sources of research ideas and schematically represents the process by which those initial ideas are moulded into a final research question by the influence of various factors. Asking the research question is central to the entire research process. Once you have identified a research question you are well on the way to completing the study. It is now up to you to decide whether you wish to pursue the opportunity.

REFERENCES

Chapman C. (1989) Research for action: the way forward. *Senior Nurse*, **9** (6), 16–18.
MacMillan M.S. *et al.* (1989) *A Delphi Survey Of Priorities For Nursing Research In Scotland*. Edinburgh, University of Edinburgh Department Of Nursing Studies.
Peplau H. (1952) *Interpersonal Relations in Nursing*. Putnam, New York.

Procter P. (1986) *A Framework For The Development Of CAL For Nurses, Midwives And Health Visitors*. English National Board, London.

Rogers M.E. (1970) *An introduction to the theoretical basis of nursing*. F.A. Davis Company, Philadelphia.

Roy C. (1980) The Roy Adaption Model. In *Conceptual Models For Nursing Practice*, (2nd edn.) (Ed. by J.P. Riehl & C. Roy) Appleton-Century-Crofts, New York.

Chapter 9
Searching the Literature
David C. Benton and Desmond F.S. Cormack

The ability to conduct a literature search is central to any type of research. Indeed, it has been argued that the skills associated with literature searching should be considered a fundamental skill requirement of all professional nurses (Department of Health and Social Security 1972; McSweeney 1990). Whether from a research or a professional perspective, the ability to conduct a literature search is essential if nurses are to question their practice, management, or education in a structured and meaningful manner. Without reference to our past, we are unable to learn from our mistakes. The techniques discussed in this chapter help empower the reader with skills that enable the discovery, location, and unlocking of the wealth of material which constitutes our profession's knowledge base.

THE RESEARCH LITERATURE

Every day we come into contact with a wide variety of research literature, the volume of which seems to be ever increasing. By research literature we mean any form of information, either paper or electronic, that relates to nursing research, irrespective of source format or quality. Chapter 10 deals with how to review and evaluate quality.

Research literature can originate from many sources, individuals, groups, academic institutions, professional organizations, government departments, or manufacturers and suppliers of products. Clearly, the volume of material available is unmanageable unless you are selective in the material which you consult. Depending on the research topic, certain types of literature may be of greater value to the inquiring nurse than others. Research literature can come in many forms, each of which have particular characteristics which, if known, can assist you in deciding the likely value of the material prior to obtaining access. Figure 9.1, for example, lists common formats used to convey information to the nursing profession.

Journals
Books
Reports
Theses
Conference proceedings
Government circulars
Computer databases

Fig. 9.1 Common formats used to convey research literature.

Journals

Journals are frequently used by researchers who wish to obtain information on a specific topic. However, not all journals publish original research. Journals such as the *Journal of Advanced Nursing, Nursing Research*, and The *Western Journal of Nursing Research*, which publish original material, are termed 'primary' journals. Invariably, papers published by these journals are refereed, that is, all papers are examined by an independent external expert prior to publication; this tends to ensure that only papers that are of the highest quality are published.

Secondary journals are another valuable source of information and, although they do not usually publish original papers, they do serve an important function. That is, articles published in secondary journals could be described as a means of providing a 'taster' of the full paper. Articles often consist of a brief synopsis of research published in a primary journal, often written in less technical terms so as to appeal to a wider audience. Hence secondary journals are an ideal means of ensuring that a piece of work is disseminated more widely than would be possible otherwise.

There are a number of specific types of secondary journal. First, there is the limited circulation journals which are distributed free to members of an organization or specialist interest group. *Lampada* is an example of a limited circulation journal which is distributed to all Royal College of Nursing (RCN) members. It often contains articles specific to RCN members or gives snippets of information about work that RCN members are undertaking. Second, there are review journals, which provide information on pre-selected topics. The articles are frequently written by subject experts who in the course of the article will debate the findings of a particular piece of research. *Advances in Nursing Science* is an example of such a journal. Third, there are professional journals, for example, *Health Visitor*, which are aimed to cater for the needs of the practitioner as opposed to the academic. This type of secondary journal will often focus on aspects of utilization of research rather than on the pure findings.

Although we have drawn a clear division between primary and secondary journals, the reality is somewhat different. Secondary journals, for instance, will often publish original work – something that can confuse an uninformed researcher and mislead them into discounting an article prematurely simply as a result of its apparently poor 'pedigree'.

Books

Books are a major source of information for researchers. Unlike journal articles, which are limited by space, material published in book form usually has the opportunity to develop arguments in more detail, provide a more extensive literature review, and generally provide a more substantive treatment of the subject. However, books take longer to get into print and are generally published to make money for a publishing company, two factors which *may* detract from their academic value.

Another point to consider is whether a book has single or multiple authors for this can sometimes lead to variations in the quality of individual chapters and problems with the flow and development of arguments. It is fair to say that this should be the exception rather than the rule if the book has an experienced editor.

Reports

Many research studies are published in report form and, unfortunately, as a consequence, only reach a limited audience. Authors can take steps to avoid this by submitting their work to abstracting services such as *Nursing Research Abstracts*. Some regional health authorities also endeavour to increase the availability of reports produced by encouraging authors to submit copies of their work to a regional collection. Despite such undertakings, reports are notoriously difficult to obtain, can be of extremely variable quality, and come in all manner of shapes and format. Nevertheless, it is often useful to obtain original reports as opposed to journal articles since the report will often give fine details which, by necessity of space limitation, are omitted from the published work. It is common to find included within the appendices of reports, copies of data collection instruments, or other such valuable materials.

Theses

Theses, sometimes referred to as dissertations, are usually the product of higher academic study. Accordingly, they can be a veritable gold mine of information since they include in-depth literature reviews, detailed methods sections, as well as findings and learned debate. Usually no more than three or four copies of a theses are produced and this can cause difficulties for those who wish to read them. However, most central institutions and universities send copies of all Doctoral and Master of Philosophy theses to the British Lending Library where they are microfilmed and can then be made available on request. In addition, those nurses who live within travelling distance of London can consult the Steinberg Collection at the RCN library. This collection contains copies of a large number of theses and dissertations, either written by nurses, or of interest to the nursing profession.

Conference proceedings

It is not always possible to attend a conference in person, and although we would argue that there is no real substitute for being there and getting involved in the debate, conference proceeding can provide a valuable source of information. Papers appearing in conference proceedings usually consists of the latest, most up-to-date, state-of-the-art material. Papers are then often rewritten in light of comments made by the audience and then submitted for publication to primary journals. Conference proceedings can thus provide researchers with access to material at an early stage. Although for the more prestigious conference proceedings papers often go through a rigorous review procedure, this is not always the case, hence material gleaned from such sources can be of variable quality.

Government circulars

The Department of Health issues a wide variety of documents each year, many of which can be of interest to the nurse researcher. However, the distribution and access to these documents is often limited in the first instance to senior officers of a health authority or board. Researchers who think that the Department of Health may have published material on a specific topic can peruse the current edition of the *Hospital and Health Services Year Book* (The Institute of Health Services

Management 1989) which, amongst other things, lists all current government circulars.

Computer databases

With the advent of relatively inexpensive computer equipment, increasing amounts of information are being held on computer database. You can often obtain the most up-to-date information from this type of source. Unfortunately, use of these systems is often expensive – you require the correct equipment and you usually have to use a telephone line – and the organization running the service can charge quite high fees for the privilege of access. Another disadvantage of these systems is that the amount of information stored on any one item is often limited to essential details and a brief abstract.

CHOOSING A LIBRARY

Irrespective of your topic of interest, it is highly unlikely that you will have all the literature you require immediately to hand. For most of us, it is necessary to use a library as the main source of our research literature, whether it be in journal, book, or any of the formats previously discussed.

Not all libraries are the same and some offer far more in the way of services than others (Cheung 1988). You should make a point of exploring all local libraries so as to discover their strengths and weaknesses. Some will allow access to all their facilities but some, such as those attached to universities and colleges, may restrict non-students of the institution to reading rights only.

There are a number of features which are particularly useful and will make the task of literature searching far easier. Many of these will be dependent on the size of the library.

First, if the library is large, it may have subject-specialist librarians who will be able to greatly assist you in your search for material. Conversely, in smaller specialist libraries such as those attached to colleges of nursing or institutes of health studies, it is usual for the librarian to have extensive knowledge of healthcare literature. If you are to make the most efficient use of your time, endeavour to contact the librarian at the onset of your search and engage their assistance. Librarians are specialists in literature storage and its retrieval; seek their advice and save yourself some time.

Second, it is important to familiarize yourself with the cataloguing system of the library. Unless you know how material is catalogued you will be unable to retrieve it. Again, seek the assistance of the librarian and read any guides that may be available. Most libraries publish a short guide that will show you the layout of the stock and tell you how it is catalogued. Recently, some libraries have started to employ the use of personal stereos for this purpose and these can be hired or borrowed. These talk you through a guided tour of the layout and give you instructions on how to find material.

There are a number of methods of cataloguing material but the two most commonly used for healthcare literature are, the *Dewey Decimal Classification Scheme* and the *National Library of Medicine Classification Scheme*. The *Dewey Decimal Classification Scheme* uses a series of numeric digits to breakdown subjects from the general to the specific. The *National Library of Medicine*

Classification Scheme uses a combination of letters and numbers. Although manual card index systems are still quite common, larger libraries are now tending to install computer systems for cataloguing their material. Whichever approach is being used, become familiar with the system so as to maximize your chances of finding the material you wish to find when conducting a literature search.

Third, some libraries offer a far more comprehensive range of textbooks and journals than others. If a library is to be of value then a wide variety of stock that covers both major and minor nursing specialities is required. Textbooks should be up-to-date, but, perhaps more important for a researcher, the journal holdings should be extensive and ideally should have been subscribed to for as long a period as possible. Back issues of journals are a valuable literature source and since nursing research often addresses diverse health care themes, access to nursing, medical, general sciences, social sciences, education, and professional journals allied to medicine, is desirable.

Fourth, a range of reference texts, including indices, research abstracts, and bibliographies, is essential. These may be available in a variety of forms. For example, they may exist as books, or they may be accessible by means of on-line or compact disk-based computer systems.

Fifth, even the most comprehensive library will not stock everything that its subscribers could possibly want. Accordingly, access to an inter-library loan service is very important for a researcher who is attempting to achieve an in-depth coverage of a topic. Inter-library loan requests can be expensive but a good library will often offer a subsidized (or even free) service which is prompt to respond to reasonable requests.

Sixth, most researchers will require access to photocopying facilities which are reasonably priced. However, it is essential that copyright laws are not infringed; this does limit the use that can be made of copies and the amount of material which can be reproduced from any one book or journal.

Seventh, micro-fiche and micro-film readers can be useful particularly if you require access to theses. In addition, some libraries stock micro-film of back issues of their journals to save space; if this is the case, some means of obtaining a printed copy of an individual article should be available.

Finally, some libraries will have a special reference collection which can be of great assistance to a researcher. The Royal College of Nursing, for example, holds the Steinberg collection which includes copies of many masters and doctorate theses relating to nursing and conducted both in this country and abroad. The end of this chapter gives details of the Royal College of Nursing and other national libraries.

HOW TO SEARCH THE LITERATURE

Anyone who has attempted to look for literature related to a particular subject, quickly discovers that there is usually a wealth of material available. Of course, not all literature provides exactly what you require, hence it is necessary to systematically identify only those items which related directly to the subject under study. A literature search can be defined as the process of systematically identifying published materials which meet set predetermined criteria. This process, which is a critical component of any research study, can be conducted either manually or with the aid of computer technology.

You will often need to consult the literature at various stages of the research process. First, it will assist you in the definition of the topic to be studied. Second, it will provide substantive material for both the theoretical and methodological frameworks. Third, it will enable you to contrast findings with previously reported studies. The ability to efficiently and accurately search the literature is clearly *central* to the development, conduct, and completion of any research study.

Without a specific strategy, a literature search will not only prove time consuming but will also yield an incomplete coverage of the topic. Try to have a rough idea of an area of interest before you walk into a library. If you simply browse along the shelves, you may or may not, depending on the size of the library, find some material on your topic of interest. Such an approach is clearly unacceptable for it will waste valuable time and is no way of ensuring that you will find all the material available on the subject. Although serendipity is a wonderful and even joyous experience, it is neither scientific nor time-efficient and for these reasons you should make use of tools such as the subject index, author catalogue, classification catalogue, indexes, abstracts, and bibliographies.

Subject index, author and classification catalogues

All libraries will have author and classification catalogues as well as a subject index of their book stock so as to enable you to find material of interest. Author catalogues are simply a listing of all stock organized in alphabetical order by author. Joint authors, series entries, as well as the chairpersons of government committees, are usually included. Classification catalogues list all stock as they appear on the shelves in the library. The order of the stock is determined by the particular classification system in use. By examining the classification catalogue you can identify all books on a particular subject stocked by the library, irrespective of whether they are out on loan. The subject index, for those who are not fully conversant with the classification system, can be considered as a key to enable access to a library's book stock. All major (and minor) subjects are listed along with their corresponding classification codes thus enabling researchers to go to the appropriate part of the classification catalogue and identify the material held.

For libraries that still use manual systems, the index and catalogues often consist of a series of card indexes. If, however, a computerized system is in use, material is stored in a relational database. The term 'relational', although a computer jargon term, effectively emphasizes the fact that although the material on the catalogues and index are separate they are closely related.

Both journal holdings and audiovisual material are usually catalogued and indexed separately from book stock. Although a researcher may consult the audiovisual catalogues and index in the same manner as for books, access to journal articles are usually obtained in the first instance via the indexes, abstracts, and bibliographies.

Indexes, abstracts and bibliographies

The stock held by any one library will be limited by a number of factors such as the needs of the population the library serves, the means by which and by whom new stock is added to the collection, the budget, and the physical space available. The examination of stock held locally on any one topic will on most occasions result in the identification of only a small part of the literature available on the topic. What is required is some means of knowing what material is available not just locally but nationally and internationally if a complete and detailed literature search is required. Examination of indexing, abstracting and bibliographic tools can all be used to achieve far greater coverage of a topic.

Indexes

Indexes are used to list all material published in a specified list of journals. The material is indexed by both subject heading(s) and by author(s). Indexes are generally produced monthly, bimonthly or quarterly and cumulated annually. There are a wide selection of indexes available but not all extensively cover nursing journals. For example, *Index Medicus*, although listing over 3000 journals includes only 20 nursing titles, whereas the *Cumulative Index to Nursing and Allied Health Literature* covers just over 300, the predominant number of which are nursing and allied health periodicals. The *International Nursing Index* and, despite its name, *Nursing Bibliography* are two further examples of indexes commonly available in this country. The choice of index or indexes that should be consulted to achieve optimum coverage of the literature available will be dependent on the specific topic. There is a degree of duplication between the various indexes hence, if time is at a premium, and it usually is, go to the librarian for advice as to which indexes are likely to be the most appropriate.

The amount of detail given in an index about a particular article is limited to that likely to be found in any reference list. That is:

Name of author(s) [but not always all of them]
Date of publication
Title of article
Name of journal
Volume and part numbers
Page numbers of article

The drawbacks of such a brief description are obvious and often what sounds like a valuable reference turns out to be only of peripheral or of no value.

Abstracts

The major drawback with indexes is that no detailed information about the content of an article is given. Only by retrieving the article, often by means of an inter-library loan, can you be sure of the content. Abstracting journals, however, circumvent this problem since, in addition to all the general reference data, a short abstract is also given which gives a succinct synopsis of the article. The quality of the abstract given can, however, vary considerably from, on one hand, a simple outline, to a detailed summary of the entire study giving all the major points.

As with indexes, there are a wide selection of abstracting journals available, all of which have differing criteria for material inclusion. Perhaps the best known abstracting journal in the United Kingdom to deal with nursing research, is *Nursing Research Abstract*; valuable material, however, can often be obtained from those sources that have a wider coverage. These include *Hospital Abstracts*, *Health Service Abstracts*, *Social Service Abstracts*, *Quality Assurance Abstracts*, and *Excerpta Medica*.

Bibliographies

Bibliographies can be a useful starting point for any researcher. They are, essentially, a reference list of books, periodical articles and reports on some particular subject. A number of national libraries, professional organizations, and many college of nursing libraries, produce such bibliographies. For example, the Royal College of Nursing has published *A Bibliography of Nursing Literature* in two series, and the Scottish Health Service Centre Library regularly publishes specialist bibliographies. Furthermore, the Royal College of Midwives, the Health Visitors' Association and in addition many colleges of nursing, produce a 'Current Awareness Service'. This is a particular type of bibliography that regularly covers a (usually preset) number of topics listing all the articles, reports, or newly published books on the topic since the publication of the previous current awareness bulletin.

Citation indexes

Indexes, bibliographies, and abstracts, simply list all the material published irrespective of its quality. However, citation indexes only list those articles that have been cited by other authors in their work. It is assumed that only those articles that are of value or significance will be cited by other authors. The *Nursing Citation Index*, which is a tandem publication of the *International Nursing Index*, records the number of times a particular article has been cited, listing in which publication it was referenced, the volume, part and page numbers, and by whom it was cited. The entries are listed by author.

By examining the number of times an article has been cited, it is possible to speculate as to the quality of the work. Generally speaking, the more frequently cited, the more significant the material. Authors of articles can also use the citation index as a means of identifying colleagues with a similar interest. For example, authors can examine who has cited their work then contact them, thus extending their professional network.

The *Nursing Citation Index* can be used to identify work that is closely related to earlier published material. If you are aware of a particular article that has been written about a specific subject, you can by referring to that article in the index identify more recent work that has cited the original material. Such an approach ensures that you are aware of any debate stimulated by the publication of an author's work.

MANUAL OR COMPUTERIZED SEARCHING

Until the advent of relatively inexpensive compact personal computers, most libraries had only manual systems for accessing literature. Researchers would have to thumb through card after card of the subject index, classification, or author catalogues, until they found the material they sought. This could take considerable time and effort, particularly since there is no way of knowing from a card system whether a book is available or out on loan.

Modern computer-controlled library stock management systems hold their information on a database. A database can be thought of as a form of electronic card index system which is extremely efficient and flexible in the manner in which information can be stored and retrieved. Not only will a database hold all the usual information about a book, it will also record whether that book is in stock, out on loan, or reserved for a subscriber. Users of such systems can, by the use of a limited number of commands, search the library catalogue for books on a subject or subjects, ascertain whether they are in stock, print a list of the books on the topic, and request that those out on loan be reserved on their return to the library, all without leaving the computer terminal.

Similarly, indexes, abstracts, and bibliographies are now available via computer systems. Until two or three years ago the only way to access the databases containing this information was via the telephone line (on-line searching). Databases were located some distance from the library and were maintained by commercial companies (hosts). Although there are a number of databases maintained in the United Kingdom, the most popular and largest host organizations are located in Europe and America. However, the introduction of compact disk read-only memory (CD-ROM) technology, has meant that the entire database for a major index such as *MEDLINE* or *ERIC* can be stored on a single 4½ in. compact disk.

The storage capacity of compact disks is truly phenomenal since the equivalent information contained in the books on twenty feet of library shelving or the entire twelve volumes of the original Oxford English Dictionary can be held on one single-sided disk (Edwards, *et al.* 1989; Green 1990).

Both on-line and CD-ROM systems are more expensive than their manual counterparts. Libraries have to take out a subscription to use the database as well as possess the appropriate computer equipment and, in the case of an on-line system, have to pay telephone line rental and connect charges in addition to a payment for all data accessed. These additional costs have resulted in most libraries not allowing individuals to use on-line systems themselves. Instead, you explain the search that is required to the librarian who then conducts the search on your behalf. Databases held on CD-ROM are, however, usually accessible to the researcher since there is no telephone, connect or access charges. On-line databases are nevertheless more up-to-date (by a month or two) than either the CD-ROM or manual based systems and if this is an important consideration then the additional cost may be justified.

On-line and CD-ROM searching has a number of distinct advantages over manual systems. Specifically, they can save you a tremendous amount of time, are far more flexible in the manner in which literature can be retrieved, and can produce printed lists of references on request. Conversely, there are a few disadvantages: for example, cost and the fact that users do require a degree of computer literacy; keyboard skills, and a knowledge of the commands, are also required.

CONDUCTING A SEARCH

Conducting a literature search, if given detailed thought, is relatively straightforward. The process should be systematic and unhurried if optimum results are to be obtained.

The first step in the process is to think around the research topic. Authors may use different terms for the topic that you are interested in. If you are to successfully retrieve material, time is needed to consider all keywords and their synonyms or associated terms that can be used to describe the topic to be researched. To achieve this, a number of approaches can be used. For example, it is often helpful to 'brainstorm' your thoughts and commit them to paper, all thoughts should be noted and none dismissed prematurely. Having done this, consult a good thesaurus and write down all synonyms. Now start to group them together and form logical links between the topics.

Next, decide whether to conduct a manual of computer search. If a computer system is available, then a considerable amount of time can be saved; a computer will also allow you to use search strategies based upon what are known as logical operators. The two most common logical operators are 'AND' and 'OR'. By use of 'AND' and 'OR' you can search for a combination of keywords simultaneously. For example, if you were interested in finding material on the treatment of alcohol abuse, a search using the word 'treatment' would yield many references as would a search using 'alcohol abuse'. However, by stipulating that you require material that refers to both 'treatment' AND 'alcohol abuse' you would obtain a smaller but more specific result. Use of the logical operator 'OR' will yield a result that includes all those references that include either 'treatment' OR 'alcohol abuse' (or both).

Irrespective of whether a computer or manual search is to be conducted, great care should be taken on deciding which catalogues, indexes, abstracting journals, and bibliographies should be consulted. An inappropriate choice may result in few references being found (Fox and Ventura 1984; Schoones 1990).

Throughout the literature search, the help and assistance of a subject-specialist librarian, or an experienced researcher, can be invaluable. Both can often help to focus thinking, offer advice, and assist in the selection of appropriate sources. Having selected the sources, it is now necessary to examine the subject and keyword headings, those used by the index, for example, so as to enable you to finalize the search strategy. Computer systems will allow entries to be searched word on word but often this will result in references that are inappropriate to the research topic. The use of keyword fields will increase the number of usable references. Bear in mind that the more specifically defined and exacting your search criteria, the fewer references you will retrieve. Figure 9.2 illustrates how a seemingly unmanageable number of references on research can be searched to produce a useful bibliography. The search was conducted using a CD-ROM-based version of the ERIC (Educational Resources Information Centre) database. As can be seen, the commands issued (in block capitals) are easy to use and simple to recall.

Command	References found
FIND Research	101222
FIND Utilization	4839
FIND Nursing	1661
FIND Research AND Utilization AND Nursing	41

Fig. 9.2 Sample dialogue of CD-ROM-based literature search.

The complete list of 41 references, including abstracts, can be reviewed on screen before deciding whether to widen or restrict the search further or to print the entire list for future use.

Literature searching is a simple process but it does take time. Even when computer technology is used it is not always possible to be absolutely sure if a reference is exactly what is required. Only once an article is read can you be sure of its value and significance to the study. The process of accessing articles is invariably the most time consuming. Often, articles are not available locally and it is necessary to request them on inter-library loan. The process of requesting an inter-library loan for material can add considerably to the time required to conduct a literature search. However, when the literature search and retrieval is complete, it is then necessary to read and critically appraise the articles obtained. These and subsequent steps, such as the coherent synthesis of material, are dealt with in the following chapter (Chapter 10).

REFERENCES

Cheung P. (1988) Library and information services in a Health Authority. *Nurse Education Today*, **8**: 6, 364–5.

Department of Health and Social Security (1972) *Report of the Committee on Nursing [Briggs Report]*. Cmmd. 5115 London, HMSO.

Edwards A., Heap N., Loxton R. & Pim D. (1989) *Information Technology In Education and Training, DT200 Block 4 Part B, Satellites and Optical Storage*. The Open University Press, Milton Keynes.

Fox R.N. & Ventura M.R. (1984) Efficiency of automated literature search mechanisms. *Nursing Research*. **33**: 3, 174–7.

Green T. (1990) CD-ROM going for a song *What Personal Computer?* **1** (7), 78–80.

McSweeney P. (1990) How to conduct a literature search. *Nursing*. **4**: 3, 19; 22.

Schoones J.W. (1990) Searching Publication Data Bases *The Lancet*. **335**: 8687, 481.

The Institute Of Health Services Management (1989) *The Hospital And Health Services Year Book 1989*. (Ed. by N.W. Chaplin) The Institute of Health Services Management, London.

LIST OF NATIONAL LIBRARIES

Users and material available

Department of Health
Alexander Fleming House
Elephant and Castle
London   SE1 6BY
Tel: 071 407 5522
Ext 6363/6415

Open to all NHS Employees but appointment is required. Holds an extensive international collection of material relating to health services. Photocopying available.

Health Education Authority Health
Promotion and Information Service
78 New Oxford Street
London   WC1A 1AH
Tel: 071 631 0930

Open to the public. Wide selection of health education material. Photocopying and selective literature searching service available.

King's Fund Centre
Library
126 Albert Street
London   NW1 7NF
Tel: 071 267 6111

Open to the public without appointment. Extensive collection of material on health care, equipment and practice. Photocopying and literature search service.

Northern Ireland Health and Social
Services Library
Queen's University
Institute of Clinical Science
Grosvenor Road
Belfast   BT12 6BJ
Tel: 0232 322043

Open to students and staff of Queen's
University and all health and social services
staff throughout Northern Ireland.
Comprehensive collection of material on all
aspects of health and social sciences.

Royal College of Midwives
Library
15 Mansfield Street
London   W1M 0BE
Tel: 071 580 6523

Open to RCM members, open to the public
on request to the librarian. Extensive
collection of material on midwifery and
computerised literature search services
available.

Royal College of Nursing
Library
20 Cavendish Square
London   W1M 0AB
Tel: 071 409 3333
Ext 345

Open to RCN members, non members
should contact the librarian. Holds the
Steinberg collection of nursing research, and
material on nursing and allied health
subjects. Photocopying and bibliography
service available.

Scottish Health Service
Centre Library
Crewe Road South
Edinburgh   EH4 2LF
Tel: 031 332 2335

Open to all Scottish Health Service
employees. Comprehensive collection of
material relating to all areas of health care
and practice.

Welsh National School of Medicine
Library
University of Wales
School of Medicine
Heathpark
Cardiff   CF4 4XN
Tel: 0222 755944

Open to all students and staff of the
University and for reference to all nurses.
Collects material mainly on medicine,
dentistry and nursing.

Wellcome Institute for the History of
Medicine
Library
183 Euston Road
London   NW1 2BP
Tel: 071 387 4477

Open to the public for research and
reference only. Collection of material relating
to the history of medicine and allied subjects.

Chapter 10
Reviewing and Evaluating the Literature
David C. Benton and Desmond F.S. Cormack

Reviewing and evaluating the literature is central to the research process. However, many neophyte researchers have great difficulty in mastering the skills required to systematically read, critically appraise, then synthesize their view into a coherent, structured, and logical review of the literature. Unfortunately, not all published articles are of the same quality or scientific integrity, and all research papers have both strengths and weaknesses. By being able to identify these strengths and weaknesses, the researcher is able to make sound judgments regarding the adequacy, appropriateness, and reliability of the material presented, the validity of the conclusions drawn, and the applicability of the recommendations made.

While this chapter cannot hope to teach these skills, it does set out to identify a number of pointers as to how they can best be developed.

A PLACE TO READ

How often have you sat down to read an article only to be interrupted by the phone or a request for assistance? Although this may be acceptable when reading material for pleasure, such interruptions can cause the researcher to waste a great deal of time reading and re-reading the same article unproductively. If you are going to conduct a critique of a research paper, or, more commonly, papers, find a quiet, comfortable, well lit spot with plenty of room to spread out the material. Try and choose an area which you can, over time, associate as the place where you go to work on your research study. Ensure, at the outset, that you have at hand adequate supplies of pencils, highlighting pens, and papers for taking notes. One final point: set yourself a time limit or, better still, decide to complete certain tasks before you stop for a break. Many researchers, and we ourselves are no exception, will spend their time drinking cup after cup of coffee when work is to be done.

IDENTIFYING THE STRUCTURE OF A RESEARCH PUBLICATION

Most research publications, whether qualitative or quantitative, follow a recognized structure. A knowledge of the structure of research reports gives clues as to where to look for certain facts or details and thus enables the researcher to scan an article rapidly so as to assess whether the article is of value and worth the investment of time in detailed reading.

The process of scanning an article should be systematic and thorough. Examine a full page at a time with a left to right movement of the eyes while simultaneously 'panning' down the page. Inspect the start of each paragraph for clues to its content. Pick out headings, enlarged, bold, underlined, or italic prints, as well as perusing all illustrations, graphs, and tables. For books, monographs, theses, or longer research reports, use the contents list or index for initial clues as to the content. Always stop and read any phrases that signal conclusions or recommendations, for example, 'it has been demonstrated . . .', 'the outcome of the investigations is . . .', 'it is suggested . . .', 'in conclusion . . .', 'therefore . . .', 'hence . . .', and 'it is recommended . . .'.

Certain types of article, for example, the research report, consistently follow a standard format. By being aware of the format, you can turn, in the first instance, to those parts of the report that are most likely to yield valuable information. Furthermore, by being aware of the form and function of the various parts of a research article, readers are in a position to evaluate the worth of the material presented.

Title

Research article titles should be both concise and informative. A title should clearly indicate the content and, preferably, the research approach used. Unfortunately, some authors have a tendency to use cryptic titles which can create certain problems. Accordingly, researchers may discount a valuable piece of work as being irrelevant if the only information available is contained in a vague title. Worse still, researchers may spend a considerable amount of time and effort trying to track down what they feel is a promising article, only to discover that their interpretation of the title is at odds with the author's intent.

Author(s)

The author of an article is often neglected as a source of information in the review process. However, by examining the author's professional and academic credentials, the researcher can often judge whether the author has an appropriate background to enable them to successfully conduct the study. Additionally, the author's place of employment can, if known to be a centre of excellence, indicate that the quality of the published research is likely to be high. Neophyte researchers will often publish work that names a distinguished experienced researcher, who has contributed or edited the article, as the second author. Multiple authors may indicate that there was a need for specialist input at various stages of the study or, conversely, the principle author is simply attempting to acknowledge the assistance of individuals in the conduct of the study.

Abstract

If one is present, a research abstract can be of considerable value and should be read in its entirety. By reading the abstract, the researcher should be able to determine an article's relevance to the topic under review. It should identify the research problem, state any hypothesis (if appropriate), outline the methodology, give details of the sample subjects and the manner in which they were selected, specify data collection approaches, and report all significant results, as well as the principal conclusions.

Introduction

Authors should, within the introduction, clearly identify the problem to be addressed. Details of the rationale for conducting the study should also be specified. Readers can then judge whether the problem is significant and the purposes of the study worthwhile. Any limitations or delimiting factors should also be addressed within the introduction. In the absence of any abstract, closely examine the introduction as a means of assessing an article's potential relevance to the review topic.

Literature review

Journal publishers often place stringent conditions on the length of literature reviews that can be included within an article. As a result, literature reviews often appear superficial and incomplete. However, a good indicator of whether this is a function of the journal, or is a result of a poorly written article, is to compare the length of the literature review with others appearing in the same journal. If all reviews are short, then it is likely that the journal editors are imposing strict limitations.

In the case of research reports, books, monographs, and dissertations, literature reviews should be complete and detailed. They should present information on the conceptual framework(s) appropriate to the subject under study as well as including reviews of those articles previously published on the topic. Literature reviews should, generally speaking, move from a general discussion of the subject to the specific topic under investigation. Both the strengths and weaknesses of previous studies should be highlighted; the absence of either could indicate that the author has reviewed the material from a biased perspective.

The absence of up-to-date references may indicate that the research was carried out some time ago. Consequently, findings may be dated. Fortunately, most research journals will quote the date when the article was accepted for publication. The omission of relevant findings subsequent to that date is then understandable.

Finally, the omission of any references that are central to the development of the research topic must always be treated with suspicion. The absence of such material could indicate that the original review of the literature was incomplete or biased, or worse still, that the author was unable to conceptualize how the information could be meaningfully integrated into the review.

The hypothesis

A hypothesis is only appropriate if the researcher is conducting experimental research. In some cases there may be sub-hypotheses, and on such occasions, these must be clearly linked to the main hypothesis. Hypotheses must be unambiguous and must be phrased in a manner that is capable of being tested.

Operational definitions

Closely linked to the literature review is the operational definition of terms. Often words in everyday use may be poorly defined and require to be given unique unambiguous definitions for the purpose of research. The absence of operational definitions may result in the collection of data of questionable relevance to the study, and hence invalidate findings. Readers are also left in the position of having to place a personal interpretation upon terms. For example, the word 'patient' may mean a child, an adult, or an individual with physical or psychological problems.

Such ambiguity is unacceptable in a research study, therefore the 'patient' is usually defined and you might read: 'For the purposes of this study a patient is any male, aged between 25 and 65, who has been admitted to the district general hospital with an initial diagnosis of myocardial infarction'.

Methodology

The methodology section of a research article will consist of several sub-sections. However, these will be dependent upon the research approach chosen. Authors should clearly state the research approach, adopted and this should be consistent with the problem stated and the theoretical framework identified.

Subjects

The subjects of any study, that is, those individuals or situations that are being examined, must be clearly defined. The author should provide as much detailed information as possible so as to enable readers to judge whether the findings of the study may be applicable or relevant to their needs.

Sample selection

The manner in which individuals or situations are selected for study must be clearly specified. For example, random selection of subjects may enable the author to conclude that the findings of the study are applicable to a larger population. The size of the sample will be dependent on many factors, but authors should clearly identify the rationale, and specify any criteria for subject selection.

In reviewing literature, sample selection must be closely scrutinized to ensure that the results obtained are representative. For example, the results obtained from a self-selected volunteer group may not be applicable to the general population. Similarly, the results obtained from a single in-depth study of a patient suffering from a terminal disease may have little relevance to patients with the same diagnosis in another setting.

Data collection

There are a vast number of ways that data can be obtained: questionnaire, interview, observation, and direct measurement, are but a few examples. When considering the data collection section of a paper, care must be taken to ensure that the method selected is compatible and appropriate to both the aims and the theoretical framework being used by the study.

If questionnaires or other instruments are designed for or being used with a group of subjects, there should be clear evidence that these instruments have been piloted and that their reliability and validity has been established. Unfortunately, it is common to read in the literature of researchers using instruments that have had their reliability and validity previously established with one particular group of subjects. It is then assumed, quite wrongly, that these instruments are then a valid and reliable measure for a completely disparate group.

Ethical considerations

All studies should at some point address the ethical issues and consequences of conducting the research. If human subjects are involved there should be some evidence that the approval of an ethics committee has been obtained. Specific points that require to be considered relate to confidentiality and anonymity of subjects, as well as any difficulties that may arise from role conflict when a researcher is also a care provider.

Results

Results should be presented in a clear, concise, precise, and logical manner. The reader of a research report should examine whether the results presented are sufficiently complete and detailed to answer all the research questions posed. Furthermore, if any form of statistical tests are used, are these appropriate to the design of the study? If various approaches – tables, graphs, and text – have been used to present data, do they adequately summarize the information and enhance the clarity of presentation (see Chapter 30).

The results section should be considered as the evidence upon which subsequent sections – that is, discussion, conclusions, and recommendations – are based. A complete, detailed examination and understanding of the results section is necessary if critical appraisal of the remaining sections of the report are to be achieved.

Discussion

In this section, all results should be discussed in relation to their implications to the original research question. The discussion should be balanced, objective, and draw upon previous research findings (if they exist) to explain, compare and contrast the results obtained. Any limitation or weaknesses in the research study should be identified and, if possible, suggestions as to how they may be overcome in the future documented.

Conclusions

Any conclusions presented must be supported by both the results, and the discussion. More importantly, conclusions should only be reported if flaws or weaknesses in the study have been adequately addressed. Any researcher who reports unsubstantiated conclusions is committing a grave and unethical impropriety.

Recommendations

Researchers will often make recommendations for further study. Like the conclusions, these should be closely examined so as to ensure they are supported by the evidence presented. Some researchers will, in addition, also report what they see as the implications of their findings for practice. This can be extremely useful, but care must be taken to assure that the interpretation being made is accurate and appropriate.

RECORDING A CRITICAL EVALUATION

Having conducted a detailed appraisal of an article, it is essential that all relevant information gleaned is recorded in a manner that will facilitate recall at a later date.

Without such documentation, it would be necessary to read, re-read, and perhaps ˄ even search for articles time and time again.

There are several approaches that can be used to store the information necessary to recall the essential facts. Emerson and Jackson (1982) argue that the use of a 'marginal punch card system' is particularly useful since such a system is inexpensive, readily available, and it is possible to devise quite flexible means of recalling the information stored. These cards are approximately 4 in. by 6 in. and have a series of holes cut into the margins. Each hole represents a specified subject. By extracting all the cards on a particular topic, for example, care of the elderly, then extracting those relating to the treatment of incontinence, all articles relating to the treatment of incontinence in elderly patients can be identified.

Tyznik (1983) suggests that by using the International Classification of Diseases, 9th revision, Clinical Modification (ICD–9–CM), literature can be indexed in such a way as to facilitate recall on a disease-orientated basis. While this may provide a well established, international framework, we would suggest that the use of the subject classification systems used by indexes such as the *Cumulative Index to Nursing and Allied Health Literature* or the *International Nursing Index*, is more applicable to those conducting nursing research. In addition, using one of the nursing index classification systems has the advantage that references identified from these sources will be already classified. The use of the existing subject classification will accordingly save the researcher time and will also ensure that personally held references will be consistent with their internationally classified source.

With the advent of inexpensive and powerful micro-computers, reference material can be stored by means of database software packages (Cormack & Benton 1990). A database package enables references to be recalled in a fast, efficient, and flexible manner. References can be searched simultaneously by a number of criteria, and those identified can be displayed on a screen or printed for subsequent use.

Irrespective of the type of approach chosen to store the information, it is necessary to ensure that a minimum amount of data in addition to the critique are recorded. For example, in the case of journal articles, it is necessary to record author(s), publication date, article title, journal title, volume and part number, and page numbers. In the case of books, additional information such as book title, editor(s), publication place, and publisher is required. This information can be recorded, on the front, in the case of card-based systems, on the back for the critique. For computer-based systems, two screens can be used, the first equating to the front of the card, the second to the back.

WRITING A LITERATURE REVIEW

The ability to critique an individual article is essential to the writing of a literature review. However, it is the manner in which these individual reviews are integrated that often presents the greatest challenge to both the experienced and inexperienced researcher.

A review of the literature should be written objectively with all criticism being based on factual material and supported by appropriate evidence and argument. In addition, any review should be balanced with both the positive and negative aspects of material being discussed. Furthermore, the implications of any flaws identified in previous work must be highlighted. A well written review will provide far more than a critical appraisal of a series of articles, it should create a structure upon which further research can be based. The issue of structure is central to the production of sound scholarly work and warrants detailed discussion.

THE STRUCTURE OF A LITERATURE REVIEW

Having spent hours, days, or even months reviewing individual articles, it is essential that equal emphasis be placed on how these individual appraisals will be woven into a structured, coherent review. Just as with all other component parts of the research process, unless this activity is planned, then time and effort is likely to be wasted. By spending some time on the development of an outline, the researcher will have a guiding framework for the production of the review. Figure 10.1 identifies the component parts of such an outline.

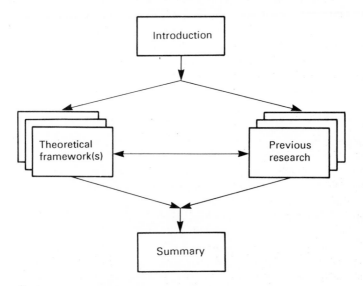

Fig. 10.1   Literature review outline.

As can be seen from Fig. 10.1, the literature review should start with an introduction. The introduction should contain some reference to the sources consulted as well as an indication of the amount of previous work published. In addition, the introduction should (briefly) describe the structure and purpose of the review so as to guide the reader and help place all elements in context.

The main body of the review will consist of the critique of previous work addressing both the theoretical and previous research dimensions. The author should paraphrase previous work whenever possible. Direct quotes can be used to emphasize central issues, but when these are taken out of context from a document, their significance may be lost, or worse still, they may be interpreted differently by the reader. Furthermore, long quotes may interrupt the flow in the development of an argument.

Figure 10.1 attempts to convey that when reviewing the literature on any topic, a number of competing theoretical frameworks may exist, as well as any number of previous research articles that provide conflicting research results. A well organized review will clearly identify the various theoretical perspectives, identify the strengths and weaknesses of each, and compare similarities and differences between them. Research findings should be related to the appropriate framework and any anomalies explored and explained (if possible) in terms of the theoretical models available. Any gaps in the research or inconsistencies should be clearly identified. Articles central to the development of arguments should be dealt with in depth.

The review should conclude with a summary of the synthesized findings of previous work which should clearly describe the extent of the current knowledge base. Gaps in the knowledge base or inconsistencies in the theoretical frameworks should be re-stated succinctly, thus forming the rationale for conducting further research.

Unless the literature is analysed in detail and the inter-relationships between previous publications identified, the quality of the review will be poor. Inadequate analysis and synthesis of literature results in a review that merely presents a series of disjointed paragraphs that echo the findings of previous studies. By planning the review, a logical, structured and coherent argument for further research, or an appraisal of the current state of our knowledge can be presented.

IDENTIFYING THE ANATOMY OF A PUBLISHED REVIEW

To conclude this chapter and to reinforce the various points made, a published review of the literature on 'learning to care' by Smith (1985) is examined.

First, the title of this work clearly informs the reader of its content. Specifically, it states that the article is a literature review and that the topic is learning to care. The author is identified as being a 'Senior Nurse (Research)' and is both academically and professionally well qualified.

Second, an abstract is provided. Although it has no title, it is enclosed in a box, at the start of the article, and separated from the main text. It clearly outlines the content of the article, identifying that the author intends to review the literature on the relationship between the provision of care and learning to nurse. Furthermore, it is identified that the principle means of evaluating this relationship is by examining the quality of care, and this is identified by use of reference to dependency studies, quality assurance instruments, and the nursing process.

Third, the introduction informs the reader of the extent and nature of the literature review conducted as well as providing a succinct statement of the purpose of the article.

Fourth, major headings are used throughout the publication and these conform with the principle elements reported in the abstract. This consistency assists the reader in comprehending the logical progression of the arguments presented. Various themes are well integrated throughout the article with the relevance of material being frequently stated in terms of the relationship between learning to nurse and the giving of patient care.

Fifth, throughout the article, the author does not simply report the findings of previous studies, but examines and critiques the material in terms of content, method, and theoretical perspective.

Finally, although the author does not include a heading in the article, a summary is presented. This final paragraph draws together all the various threads presented, but, unfortunately, an additional element is also introduced. The introduction of Donabedian's (1966) 'structure process outcome' model at this late stage, without the inclusion of appropriate debate, detracts from what is otherwise a well written critique of the literature.

CONCLUSION

The article by Smith (1985) demonstrates many of the points that have been discussed in this chapter. Writing a critical review of the literature is a skill that requires to be learned. If you are to become a nurse researcher, or you are to practice from a research base, it is essential that you are able to proficiently conduct a critical review of the literature. By learning from the past you can change the future and increase the quality of care delivered. However, the initiation of change must be supported by research that stands up to critical evaluation and review.

REFERENCES

Cormack D.F.S. & Benton D.C. (1990) Reading the professional literature. In *Developing your career in nursing*, (Ed. by D.F.S. Cormack) Chapman and Hall, London.

Donabedian A. (1966) Evaluating the quality of medical care. *Millbank Memorial Fund Quarterly*, **44** (2), 166–206.

Emerson S.C. & Jackson M.M. (1982) Organize your references. *Nursing Administration*, **13**: 6, 33–7.

Smith P. (1985) Learning to care: a review of the literature. *Nurse Education Today*, **5**, 178–82.

Tyznik J.W. (1983) Taming the medical literature 'monster'. *Postgraduate Medicine*, **74**: 1, 77–80.

Chapter 11
Preparing a Research Proposal
Senga Bond

Research proposals may be written for a number of reasons: to obtain funding, to present to a higher degrees committee in a University or Polytechnic, for ethical approval, or as an academic exercise as part of a research course. This chapter focuses on the first of these since this is the most frequent and in some ways the most important reason for writing a proposal. However, features of proposal writing apply to all of the situations mentioned.

The preparation of a research proposal will be addressed in two ways. The purpose of the first is to provide researchers with some straightforward guidance about possible structure and content. The second is to suggest some ways of making a proposal more appealing and thus more likely to be funded.

The most important function of research proposals is to make explicit a reasoned argument about the need for the proposed study on practical and theoretical grounds and how it will be carried out. The very act of writing a proposal assists in identifying the strengths and weaknesses of a study. This is achieved through the process of setting down a clear statement of the question that the study proposes to answer, the methods that will be used to find the answer, and the resources required to do it. The particular form that a proposal takes will depend on the requirements of the organization to which it is being submitted, and some produce special forms giving guidance about the different sections within which information should be provided. However, what follows is general guidance about the preparation of a proposal which should be amended to suit the requirements of a particular case.

THE CONTENT OF A RESEARCH PROPOSAL

It is useful to have a checklist of the main topics to be included. Such a list would contain the following:

(1) Title of project
(2) Summary
(3) Justification for the study
(4) Related research
(5) Aims and objectives
(6) Plan of investigation
(7) Ethical considerations
(8) Resources
(9) Budget
(10) Curriculum vitae

Let us consider each of these headings in turn and give some pointers to the kind of information within each one.

Title of project

Research projects become known by their title so it is important to make the title explicit and, while describing the proposed study, relatively brief. Sometimes studies change direction during their evolution while the subject matter remains essentially the same. An experiment may collapse or the nature of the variables being considered in a survey may be altered on the basis of pilot work. The title should be able to override these changes while still conveying the essence of the study. The use of words like 'evaluation' and 'survey' in titles are helpful in alerting readers to the approach the study will take. It is more informative to call a study 'Evaluation of a counselling scheme for patients who have undergone mastectomy', even if the design of counselling methods change over time, than to call it 'Caring for mastectomy patients'.

Summary

Most research award applications ask for a brief summary. In practice this is usually written after the main body of the proposal has been put together since it requires to be a succinct yet clear statement of the objectives of the study and how it will be carried out. It should contain only the most relevant information. The space allocated to it or the word length specified means that every word is important and it is an art to describe a major project in less than 50 words.

Because it appears early, the summary again alerts the reader to what to expect in the subsequent text. The summary is an important indication of the quality of the remainder of the proposal and so it requires careful consideration and probably several drafts.

Justification for the study

The statement of the problem which opens the main body of the proposal must convince the reader that the proposed study is important. It must introduce the research questions and put them into a context which indicates the importance of the problem and the generalizability of the research. It should identify how the proposed study will add to previous work and build on theory. In nursing studies, any research is likely to have practical implications, so that, as well as having value in contributing to knowledge, its utility value needs to be stressed. These may be methodological gains, for example, in developing a new research instrument which would have future applications, as well as gains in education or practice. It is not always obvious what the practical gains of a study may be, but it is worth giving consideration to this if the funding body is likely to be more interested in practical rather than theoretical findings.

In developing the problem statement, the researcher needs to keep a careful balance between putting forward claims for the study which are either too grandiose or too general, or that imply that the study is no more than the whim of the researcher, based on some closely held belief. Novices often express research as setting out to prove something, for example, that parents prefer booked visits from health visitors, rather than as an open question of their response to different systems of visiting. There is also a tendency to be over ambitious, and this applies even to quite experienced research workers when the enthusiasm for the topic overrides their judgment about delivering the goods. A key piece of advice, therefore, is to *focus on the manageable*.

When writing this section, it is sometimes helpful to underline or type in a bold face a succinct statement of the problem to catch the reviewer's attention and to foreshadow the remainder of the proposal. Sketch out in a couple of sentences the broad approach that the study proposes to take.

Related research

Next, it is important for the researcher to demonstrate a command of the current state of the field and how the planned study would move it forward. To achieve this, those few key studies which provide the basis for the proposed project should be included. Indicate, in language for non-specialists, how they are relevant to the proposed study and how this study moves beyond them. This review should relate both to substantive concerns and methods, and be provided in sufficient detail to inform the reader of its relevance. It may also be useful to include any knowledge of studies under way as a reflection of the author's competence in keeping abreast of developments.

At this point, competence can also be demonstrated in appreciating the theoretical aspects of the study and the firmness of the theoretical base. This information can be extremely influential in demonstrating the researcher's grasp of complex issues.

The development of the literature base is a major feature of the research process described in Chapters 9 and 10 and, equally, it is an important feature of the research proposal. If the literature search and the writing of the literature section of the proposal is thought of as an afterthought, it will shine through by virtue of its unrelatedness to the remainder of the proposal.

Aims and objectives

Any reviewer of proposals likes to see clear, specific, and concrete objectives which are achievable. List and number them in order of importance in a clear sequence, taking only a sentence or two for each.

The remainder of the proposal will be judged in relation to what you have told the reader about what this study aims to do. To achieve this, avoid vague terminology and generalities; define criteria as specifically as possible. Do not leave it up to the reader to have to do the guesswork about what the objectives are or their order of priority. You will stand more chance of being clearly understood if you list them than if you leave it to the reader to abstract objectives out of a prosaic statement.

The objectives of the study may take the form of questions, when research is exploratory, or of a survey, where specific facts are being sought. It may be possible to state objectives in the form of testable hypotheses where there is a basis for predicting results, such as in an experiment. It is more enlightening, as well as more convincing, if hypotheses are stated whenever possible. However, these need to be precise and relationships clearly specified.

Plan of investigation

This section could be called *Plan of Investigation*, *Procedure*, or *Method*, and is likely to be the section most carefully read by both funding and ethical committees. Up to this point, the researcher has been able to present a picture of the positive implications of the research and what it hopes to achieve. It is when procedures for this achievement are spelled out that those reading the proposal gauge the researcher's capacity both to undertake and complete the proposed work.

The specific format of this section will depend on the methods adopted. Different emphases will be required depending on whether the study takes a survey, experimental, or field study approach. Irrespective of method, there are several important matters to convey to reviewers and these are best written in discrete sections.

Population and sample

As well as giving a clue to the generalizability of the study findings, this section will include the researcher's understanding of the 'numbers' problem in relation to the amount of variability likely within the measures employed. It is better not to cut corners by suggesting smaller numbers than statistical analysis would demand but, at the same time, limit numbers reasonably since more does not necessarily mean better.

Questions of sample size are dealt with elsewhere in this book. What reviewers will be looking for are indications that the sample size will be big enough to detect differences or allow other appropriate statistical manipulations to be carried out, especially if these are complex and include a large number of variables. It is helpful to include a statement of the acceptable size of difference, and the sample size required to detect it. Equally, reviewers will be concerned that the sample type is suitable to make appropriate generalizations. When particular sampling techniques are used as described in Chapter 21, this choice should be justified. Randomization, or the absence of it, requires explanation. Should a whole population be used, rather than a sample, the reader will want to know why this is so. The sample is not only a matter of size but also of accessibility and likelihood of availability. Convincing information should be provided that there is an available sampling frame, criteria for inclusion and exclusion are appreciated, that they can be easily recruited, and that consideration is given to how non-respondents would be managed.

Design

Design will be a greater feature of experimental and survey research than of other types since it is clearly specifiable in advance. For exploratory studies, case studies, or ethnographic research, this section will require appropriate adaptation and Sandelowski *et al.* (1989) offer such guidance. However, details of the initial steps to be taken, and their sequence, could be given, together with whatever information is available that will guide theoretical sampling or justify the selection of particular cases.

For experimental studies, details will be required about which variables are controlled and how control is to be achieved. In some instances, there may be complete randomization while in others subjects may be either matched on known relevant variables or included in a factorial design. What is important here is to show awareness of as many relevant variables as possible and how control can be realistically managed. In health services research, control of all variables is virtually impossible and the challenge is to make the best use of available situations and adapt methods to the closest approximation to experimental proof.

When compromises have to be made to facilitate experimental design in the 'real world' of patient care, then the reasons for such compromises should be made clear. For example, if patients are to be allowed some degree of choice of treatment, or nurses are to manage control of particular kinds of work, alternatives to randomized control trials will be necessary. It would be virtually impossible in the current climate to conduct randomized controlled trials of the effectiveness of resettlement of people from long-stay hospital care to community care. Equally, in some studies, a control group does not exist and reasons for the adoption of other designs are required.

Specification of design in survey research will include details about sample recruitment. It may also include details of how a large survey will be managed to avoid a flood of mail going out or being received at one time.

Data collection

In this section, measures and procedures to be used in data collection are described. These should reflect back to the variables to be measured and show that the measures to be used represent acceptable operational definitions of them, and that they have appropriate measurement characteristics. In many topics of relevance to nursing research, well-validated scales already exist and it would be foolish to develop a new scale. Where proposed measurements have been used in other relevant studies, it is helpful to indicate this. When methods of measurements do not already exist and new methods are proposed, it would be worthwhile to include details in an appendix to the proposal. In some cases reviewers wish to see copies of instrumentation, test items, questionnaires, or interview guides. It makes sense to find out in advance if this is required. However, for some studies, a substantial part of the work entails such methodological developments.

While data collection techniques may involve conventional methods using questionnaires and interviews, they may also involve more invasive biochemical or physical measures, or assessment of observed behaviour. Mention should be made of the apparatus to be used to obtain these data and whether any special conditions are required for their use. If the data to be collected, or the methods used to collect them, are likely to be sensitive or controversial, then plans indicating how the researcher has anticipated problems and how they would deal with them sensitively would be reassuring to reviewers.

Pilot study

Once the proposed methods of data collection have been spelled out, the obvious next stage is to tell reviewers what steps will be taken to ensure that they are workable and are both acceptable to subjects and manageable by researchers. This is usually carried out using a pilot study and it is worth specifying this in some detail. To conduct a postal sample survey from first principles, for example, would involve going through several stages to arrive at a suitable questionnaire before going on to a postal pilot study to gauge its acceptability and response rate. If an already validated instrument was to be used then obviously the amount of development and pilot work would be that much less. When new methods are to be used, for example, lap-top computers to collect interview data, or if new scales have to be developed, then the pilot work will be time-consuming but nevertheless important to the eventual quality of the study. It is always worth investing time and effort to ensure that the development work or pilot work for a study is thorough, and to stress this in the proposal.

Analysis

It is prudent to have considered the question of analysis in the development of any study even although it may be some way off from becoming actuality. Most important is to show that the methods of analysis are consistent with the objectives and design of the study. Again, this is easier to specify in advance in the case of experimental studies.

In non-experimental studies, it is somewhat less easy to anticipate the complete nature of the data and hence the analysis. This is especially so when qualitative research is being carried out but it is also true for statistical analysis of complex survey data. In cases where complete specification is not possible, the stages of data analysis can be outlined indicating an appreciation of the kinds of methods likely to be used. If studies rely on multivariate or discriminant techniques or longitudinal analyses, then this should be specified even if it has to be done so at a general level. It should be indicated that sufficient statistical expertise is available to inform, and, if necessary, to carry out statistical analysis. If a statistical package such as SPSSx or MINITAB is to be used (Chapter 27), then say so.

When the analysis is qualitative, an indication of the hardware and computer software to be used will alert reviewers to the fact that some thought had gone into at least the mechanics if not the conceptual work of analysis.

Work plan

Details of the timescale and plan of work should be included to show the anticipated duration of each stage of the study. The complexity of the plan of work will reflect the complexity of the study. You need give no more than an indication of the time allocated to each major stage of the study – for example, pilot study, main data collection, data analysis, and report writing. When the study is more complex, and different activities are happening simultaneously, then more sophisticated flow charts or critical paths may be necessary to identify the anticipated progress of work. Often a diagram will say more than words.

Generally, the time taken to complete each part of a study is underestimated. This is particularly true in the case of data collection, which depends on a prospective series. The tendency is to be over-optimistic. This can also apply to the time it takes to negotiate entry and gain ethical approval to collect data. Software like InstaPlan may be used in the case of a complex study to assist in considering the timescale required in relation to critical events and resources.

The compilation of a clear and realistic time schedule is further indication of the researcher's competence and the likelihood of a successful project.

Expected end-products

The end-product of most research studies is a final report. However, products may also include new research instruments or methods of data collection as well as teaching or clinical aids. Furthermore, reports are not the only way to present results: videos, presentations, and the like, may be equally if not more relevant in some instances as a means of disseminating findings.

There is now increasing emphasis on adequate dissemination and utilization of research. It may be appropriate to make specific suggestions about how this is to be achieved, especially through executive summaries of findings which are oriented to specific target audiences, and to take account of it in both the timescale and the budget. Some grant-awarding bodies are more interested than others in funding further dissemination over and above the traditional academic articles.

Ethical considerations

The reviewer of a research proposal will have been alerted to any ethical problems while reading the methods section. The proposal may be reviewed by a committee whose primary objective is to assess the scientific methods of a study but they will not be unaware of ethical issues and they are likely to assess whether 'the ends justify the means'. A proposal that is viewed by an ethics committee, however, will take an entirely different perspective and will be at pains to protect human and animal subjects from undue distress. Before going ahead, it is wise to obtain written consent from adults, or from parents, guardians, or advocates, when the subjects themselves cannot give approval. Ethical matters may also be relevant to protecting subjects from any negative consequences of a study, and protection of staff can equally apply when they may be involved in handling noxious substances or administering procedures, as, for example, with nurses carrying out skin tests. It is also a matter of ethics when staff themselves may be the subject of research.

At some point in the proposal it is necessary to clearly indicate what the research regards as the major ethical issues and to clearly state how these will be handled. Some funding bodies require evidence that ethical approval has been obtained before a funding decision is made.

Resources

It is important that the resources required to carry out the study are realistically appraised. Resources, whether human, material, or financial, fall into different categories.

Personnel

The person who will direct the project should be clearly identified together with the amount of time they intend to devote to the project. It may be that this is a proposal for a full-time commitment or, alternatively, for only a few hours in a week: spell out the time implicated. The relationship of others to the project, and their responsibilities, must be stated. Where a team effort is involved, the mix of available expertise may be an important element.

It can be especially important for inexperienced researchers to obtain the support of established research workers. In this respect, it can be useful to show that active consultation has taken place in the development stages of a proposal. Indicate the kind of assistance offered by those experienced in research, or who have a particular technical competence. When collaborative efforts are involved, spell these out.

Other resources

A description of particular services or back-up facilities can also strengthen a proposal. Good computer and library facilities fall into this category, as do sufficient space and secretarial support. Where established networks are integral to a project or co-operation has been obtained from particular agencies or institutions, some indication of this, such as a letter of agreement, may be included as a helpful appendix.

Budget

The preparation of a research budget requires as much skill as preparing other parts of the proposal. Part of the skill lies in locating people who know the cost of necessary commodities – staff salaries, as well as equipment and other consumables. Preparing a budget means translating the timescale and plan of work into financial terms.

Novice writers have a tendency to want to skimp the budget because they earnestly believe that if a project costs less, it improves the chance of its being funded. Undercutting the budget, however, simply reflects inexperience. Sharp-eyed critics will quickly notice where there has been undue trimming and equally where excesses are included. Sometimes, if they are thought to be too high by virtue of over-elaborate sampling or extended timescales, budgets can be a matter of negotiation. However, to be caught short of cash and time can be disastrous, and funding bodies do not take kindly to requests for extensions of time or increased budgets. In preparing a budget, use a checklist to include main headings, such as:

Research staff salaries
Secretarial staff salaries
Data collection costs, e.g. purchase of equipment and other materials,
                    printing, travelling expenses, stationery, and postage
Data processing costs
Book purchases
Conference attendance
Dissemination

It is sometimes useful to separate costs into capital costs, to include the purchase of equipment, and recurrent costs. It may be possible to obtain funds for books as well as for travel to conferences. Put them in; there is no harm in trying! Some organizations, especially universities, ask for reimbursement of overheads. Check whether this is so, and the current rate. Parent organizations will also wish to check a budget statement before it is submitted, and salaries, etc. usually have to be countersigned by someone with specific expertise in this matter. An appropriate budget is always a matter of careful specification rather than of just pulling some notional figure out of the air.

Curriculum vitae

Attach an appropriate curriculum vitae. This is not always essential but it is usually asked for and it does no harm to include one. Its contents should be appropriate and include details of:

Name
Age
Qualifications
Education
Work experience
Research experience
Recent relevant publications

A curriculum vitae should be included for each applicant.

FINAL REVIEW

It is likely that a research proposal will go through several drafts. Indeed, there would be major cause for concern if it did not! There are a number of things to be achieved in reviewing proposals. Not least is to consider its physical presentation. Nicely spaced typescript with a major emphasis on legibility, lucidity, and clarity of presentation, are all important. While readers of a proposal will not consciously evaluate it on how it is presented, nevertheless, the relatively small amount of time it takes to ensure a pleasant layout which can be easily followed, will be time well spent. Using devices like a bold typeface, underlining, spacing, and the inclusion of diagrams, flow charts, and tables, are useful to attract the reader's eye. The latter are often more useful in terms of presenting detailed information than are reams of text.

It is also useful to ask someone who has experience of submitting proposals successfully to check over your efforts. Most people are pleased to assist here, so long as there is evidence that you have made proper attempts to produce a good piece of work.

SOME GENERAL COMMENTS

This chapter has discussed developing a research proposal primarily from the point of view of having it approved for funding. It should have demonstrated also the need to write down a clear statement of proposed research that will assist the researchers themselves. Matters such as making explicit a proposed time schedule can be fundamental to the successful execution of a project.

Some funding bodies offer the opportunity to submit an outline proposal for approval before submitting the full proposal. This permits a degree of negotiation about the focus, content, methods, and so on. Recent data have shown that while 30% of applications to a funding body were funded, 38% of those which had been submitted for informal advice and comment were successful compared with 19% which had been submitted without prior notice (Watt 1990).

The different bodies who consider a proposal will be looking at quite different things, and it is important to identify a particular body's primary concerns and to give special consideration to this. Check whether the funding body has any special requests in terms of the subject matter they are likely to fund, or whether there is any specific geographical area or limits to funding. Some bodies may prefer a particular kind of proposal – for example, they may look more kindly on proposals asking for capital equipment rather than those asking for staff costs. In Chapter 3, some sources of research funding were identified. Check if these sources have any particular requirements in the manner in which a proposal is presented. This may involve no more than a telephone call to the appropriate secretary. Some organizations issue a check list or a specific form on which proposals must be made. Notes of guidance may be available and it is wise to adhere to these as strictly as possible. Other organizations regard the form of the proposal as a measure of the worth of the researcher and offer no guidance on its preparation.

It is also helpful to know how proposals are to be viewed. Sometimes they are sent to external referees who have particular expertise for comment; others are dealt with completely 'in house'. As well as scientific referees, government bodies may also have 'customer' referees who are looking for the utility of the research in practical or policy terms rather than at the science involved. Knowledge of the membership of a review committee can be useful in anticipating areas to which special attention should be given. When a committee of mixed expertise reviews proposals, it is important that all members should be able to understand the nature of the study. At times there could be a problem of orientation – when biological or physical scientists, for example, are asked to review a proposal that has a social science orientation. In instances like these, it is important to try to avoid jargon since this can only add to the chances of your proposal being dismissed as 'unscientific'.

There is a skill involved in achieving a balance between identifying every single possibility, and spelling out every detail, and providing sufficient detail to convince reviewers that the proposer has the ability to complete a worthwhile study. To some extent the degree of specificity is related to the state of knowledge in a particular field and to the extent to which the study is exploratory or explanatory. Writers of proposals must rely on their judgment to some extent, but, as a general principle, it is better to include more information rather than to leave out something others may regard as important.

The length of the proposal can be a matter of some concern. Sometimes the length and number of pages or words will be specified. This is usually meant not to be taken rigidly but to serve as a guideline to help prevent over-excesses. If more lengthy details of specific steps are required, these can be included as appendices so as to avoid crowding to much information into the main text. The purpose of appendices is to provide additional supportive information for reviewers who feel that the main text is not sufficiently detailed but it should not be necessary to read such information to obtain a clear impression of the study.

This book is intended primarily for people who are new to research and this chapter may be used to assist some who have never before either developed a proposal or developed a successful one. Some funding bodies are keen to support new research workers but, on the other hand, are not likely to want to risk large sums of money or invest in potentially unmanageable studies. It is wise then to begin in a relatively small way or to ask for funding for only the first stage of the project. This safeguards both the funding body and the research worker should something go drastically wrong. Better still would be to ensure that you have an experienced researcher as a co-applicant.

Finally, do not be dismayed if a first attempt is rejected. One can always learn from this. Unfortunately, not all grant awarding bodies provide information detailing why a proposal is rejected and this is singularly unhelpful to the recipient of the rejection slip. However, increasingly, referees' comments (in an anonymous form) are given. In some cases they may refer the project, that is, suggest that the researcher re-work it under guidance. In some cases it seems almost as if referral is the rule and few proposals are accepted the first time round. It is always helpful to obtain copies of proposals which have been accepted by the body to which you are applying. This does not imply the need for slavish adherence to that particular format but it does give some indication of the type of proposal more likely to be welcomed and hence succeed in being funded.

Other useful hints on writing research proposals can be found in many general research texts (Burns & Grove 1987; Polit & Hungler 1987; Woods & Catazara 1988) as well as Parahoo (1989) and Hodgson (1989). Sandelowski *et al.* (1989) provide guiance for writing a grant proposal in qualitative research while Watt (1990) describes the submission of proposals for health services research in a government agency.

REFERENCES

Burns N. & Grove S.K. (1987) *The Practice of Nursing Research*. W.B. Saunders Philadelphia.

Hodgson C. (1989) Tips on writing successful grant proposals. *Nurse Practitioner*, **14** (2), 44; 46; 49.

InstaPlan. InstaPlan Corporation, Mill Valley, California.

Parahoo K. (1989) Writing a research proposal. *Nursing Times*, **84** (41), 49–52.

Polit D.E. & Hungler B.P. (1987) *Nursing Research Principles and Methods*. 3 Ed. Lippincott, Philadelphia.

Sandelowski M., Davis D.H. & Harris B.G. (1989) Artful research. Writing the proposal for research in the naturalist paradigm. *Research in Nursing and Health*, **12** (2), 77–84.

Watt G.C.M. (1990) Development of health services research applications. *Health Bulletin*, **48** (1), 41–9.

Woods N.F. & Catazara M. (1988) *Nursing Research Theory and Practice*. C.V. Mosby, St. Louis.

Chapter 12
Gaining Access to the Research Site

Jenifer Wilson-Barnett

Any researcher needs several attributes: intellectual, professional, and personal. All may be put to the test when attempting to gain access to the research site, that is, obtaining permission to conduct data collection. This is a complex, essential, but often frustrating stage of research where any apparent progress is often delayed. However, this stage should be seen as a vital element of any study, and must be anticipated, planned carefully, and viewed as a learning experience. Accessing the research site offers the opportunity to contact and meet many members of staff, several of whom will be able to provide comments and insights on the proposed research. These discussions may also help the researcher, that is you, to gain confidence as well as more understanding of the topic.

Few people realize that there are quite so many individuals and groups that nurse-researchers must convince before gaining access, or that this process may take as long as the data collection phase. Yet, ultimately, it is by this means that those staff who have this responsibility are able to protect subjects against unnecessary and intensive studies. Researchers must never forget that they are being invited into health care settings, and that it is the staff in these settings who must judge whether those who are potentially vulnerable; in their care, should be exposed to an additional person seeking yet more information. As a researcher, you have few automatic rights but several duties and obligations. The provision of a full account of your study to all those who may ask for it is but one of these.

BEFORE CONTACTING THE SITE

It is necessary to gain confidence and knowledge in the subject of the research before seeking access to the research site. To avoid the potential embarrassment of appearing nervous and diffident when meeting staff, certain preparatory measures should be taken. Peers are probably the most sympathetic allies at this time and should be used for rehearsals in the form of role play. You may need to practise replies to their questions and think through issues before perhaps later being put on the spot by someone in a key position. Colleagues may already have been through the access hurdle and can ask the awkward questions such as 'what will you do if someone refuses', or 'asks for the results'. As with all stressful situations, planning and rehearsal reduces anxiety.

You should also try to talk to as many experts in their own field of research as possible before contacting those in the chosen site. This is invaluable, not only for thinking through methodological difficulties, but obviously also for gaining knowledge and further reference sources. An open mind, at all times, helps you to recognize new perspectives on the study and predict any criticisms which may be met in the early stages of work.

KEY CONTACTS

When seeking access to a hospital or other health care institution for research, it is essential in the initial stage to contact the most senior officials. An up-to-date *Hospitals and Health Services Year Book* will contain details of all the key post-holders in every NHS organization. (Institute of Health Services Management 1989.) When unsure, it is wise to first telephone the institution concerned to confirm the names of these officials. Conventionally, a written form of introduction and request for access should be sent. The most senior persons may be contacted simultaneously if the study involves many groups of staff but usually the most senior nurse in the organization is the most appropriate initial contact for nursing studies. The request may then be 'sent down the line' to supporting staff, or the respondent may suggest a meeting to discuss the project. However, for clinical studies, many sets of staff will need to approve the project and these are shown in Fig. 12.1.

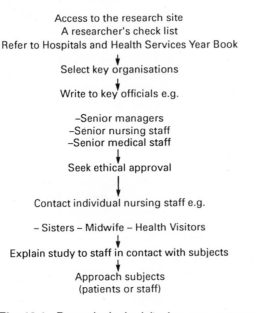

Fig. 12.1   Researcher's check list for access to research site.

It is useful to prepare several copies of your proposal for meetings with senior staff. On several occasions this author has been surprised by how many senior personnel have participated in these early meetings. Not only is it efficient to supply them with these papers, but the very act of distributing them may give the researcher time to calm their 'nerves' at such meetings. Clearly, it is also useful to have a pre-prepared opening explanation of the study because there may be a request from the general manager or chief nurse to 'talk them through the proposal'.

Other meetings may then be set up with other staff. Researchers should write down all the names of contacts suggested or, better still, ask those at the meeting to supply a list, and to suggest in which order contacts should be approached. At this time it is also important to establish whether the proposal should be sent to the Ethics Committee (or the Research Committee if one exists, or both), and to gather details of its membership, chairmanship, and secretary.

This initial meeting with key contacts – if it is a wide-scale study that is proposed – may have to be conducted in several districts, and should achieve specific objectives, each of these should be listed in the form of an aide-memoire. Of primary importance is a decision on whether these staff will support the research and whether you have convinced or even given them enthusiasm that it is worthwhile. Secondly, a clear plan of who will be contacted for access must be clarified. At the end of this meeting the researcher should know who to approach next and whether this should be done by letter or meeting. Thirdly, a commitment by these staff to support the researcher in subsequent negotiations will be helpful. It may be that they would be prepared to write a short letter or statement to this effect. Certainly it was such a letter (by the Chief Nursing Officer for Scotland) which, nearly twenty years ago, helped this author to gain access for an observation study on nursing officers. Clearly, this should not be seen as forcing others to comply, but at times it can help to provide added authority to your efforts in time of need.

ESSENTIAL QUESTIONS ON THE STUDY

Several questions may be anticipated from senior officers as they are responsible for protecting patients and relatives, and their staff, as well as running an efficient organization. They can be expected to ask some obvious and searching questions. Clearly you must be able to give confident and meaningful explanations.

First and foremost will be questions on the benefits and purposes of the study. Justifications for the worth of the research study must be made and these should be thoroughly convincing. It is perhaps easier to 'sell' a study which may lead to improvement in the quality of care or to cost containment. More difficult are those which aim to explore methods, or describe 'what is' with the possibility of finding that many things could be improved. However, most recently, attitudes towards research have become really quite positive, with even the realization that some unforeseen advantages may result. Obviously, throughout, you must maintain your integrity, and avoid exaggerated and unrealistic claims for the study.

Senior officers may be favourably impressed if the researcher offers to provide detailed feedback on the study both to them and to the staff. Seminars and workshops may be appropriate, as well as written summary reports for all interested parties. However, more continuous involvement by staff in the research process can be seen as an educational opportunity and this should be maximized. Those projects which involve investigations of clinical work are usually of great interest to nurses and they tend to be quite enthusiastic participants, especially if they receive either direct training sessions or feedback on their performance. Because of the rapid turnover of staff, it is extremely beneficial, design permitting, if regular sessions with researcher and staff involved can be set up. This type of professional reciprocity has been found to be most beneficial to researchers and nursing staff alike (Wilson-Barnett et al. 1990).

Managers will also require detailed explanation of the study before the researcher is permitted to ask other staff for access. The type of data collection process must be described carefully, with a clear account of any instruments, recordings, or analysis of records. Subjects involved will need to be told how long they would be needed for data collection and whether or not this data collection exercise would need to be repeated. Ethical issues of informed written consent, anonymity, and confidentiality need to be reinforced at this time. Senior staff will obviously be concerned that their organization could be identified, possibly with adverse consequences. You must be confident that you have fully considered the rights of individuals and the reputation of the organization. In short, research should harm no one.

Staff time is an exceedingly precious resource. It should not be squandered on useless activities. Research interviews or observation may affect a staff member's availability to give care, and the applicant must be aware that senior officials will need to think very carefully if staff are required to spend 'on-duty time' with the researcher. In general, it is obvious that most senior staff are exceedingly generous, as are the research subjects themselves.

NURSING STAFF

The primary concern of all nurses should be the welfare of the patient (or those they care for). (United Kingdom Central Council for Nursing, Midwifery and Health Visiting 1989.) When requesting access to do research involving clients, nurses must often consider the effects on what are rather vulnerable people. If they have doubts about the costs versus the benefits when weighing up their decision, they should perhaps reject the research. In the case of nursing research, such rejection is unlikely to occur. Nurses tend to be generally helpful and have thus far responded very positively to most research in progress.

When seeking consent from nurses for their co-operation in research, clear and full explanations should be given. Ward sisters, or those of similar status in non-institutional settings, may need to give permission for researchers to invite patients and relatives to provide research data. They therefore need to feel confident that the researcher is sensitive to the needs of individuals and aware of factors in the general health care environment. Researchers must demonstrate that they realize that other people and treatment activities take priority over data collection. Many researchers, for example, are quite used to merging into the background during emergencies or waiting for long periods until the subject is available. It is useful to be able to demonstrate this awareness during initial meetings with senior staff.

Although Sisters or Charge Nurses can be approached quite conveniently during their regular sisters' meetings, it may be more appropriate or less stressful for you to meet them individually. If one member of a group opposes the research or raises objections, others may be negatively influenced whereas you may be able to encourage individuals more easily. Another advantage of a one-to-one meeting comes from the opportunity to establish rapport and trust between you as the researcher and those who will be caring for patients.

Research workers in the community should also consider several factors when requesting access. It seems to be quite difficult to make definite appointments with community nurses as they are quite independent and extremely mobile. However, once more, the researcher must be willing to meet them at their convenience. Before such meetings, it is also helpful to discuss the project with colleagues or friends in the community, to ensure that most likely questions are anticipated.

Once the data collection has commenced, a continued good relationship with members of staff is necessary. Nurses in particular have responsibility for the day-to-day welfare of those they care for and are in a position to judge whether the research is affecting their work. Observation studies can be particularly difficult in this respect, if it is the researcher's intent to try to merge into the background and not interact with staff or others. Once more it is the initial and, if necessary, repeated explanations of the aims of the study and the role of the resercher which must be provided.

If nurses themselves are the subjects for study, their seniors or tutors should be contacted in the first instance and care should be taken not to impose authority on groups which may feel that they have little option but to oblige. Access must always depend on the freedom of individuals to withdraw or decline to participate if they so wish. However, students tend to enjoy helping with studies and this enthusiasm can be reinforced by careful feedback.

OTHER HEALTH CARE STAFF

Nursing research, like any other health care work, cannot be undertaken without the co-operation of many other people. Those involved in health care may be particularly interested in research affecting clients or patients, and may also feel responsible for assessing whether this research is beneficial and worthwhile. For research involving patients, senior medical staff should be contacted initially and their collaboration requested. This may be done either in writing or in face-to-face meetings depending on the extent to which the people they care for are to be subjects of the research. If a particular medical speciality is concerned it is likely that the appropriate consultant should be seen in order for the researcher to introduce themselves, and for the consultant to ask questions if they so wish.

Not surprisingly, some doctors feel rather protective of patients in their care and may ask their junior staff to meet and work with researchers and even to monitor the effects of the research. It is important that the researcher is not offended by this attitude. In the experience of this writer it is those who take the most cautious approach who are the most interested and subsequently the most helpful. However, if an individual refuses access to patients in their care there is really little one can do except use rational and persuasive powers to change their mind or perhaps enlist the help of other medical colleagues who are more supportive of the researcher and the research. In any case, those patients under the care of other consultants who have agreed, may of course still be included.

Junior doctors and other health professionals in the hospital setting need to know about the study on the grounds of courtesy and consideration but also in order to avoid any confusion or extraneous events which could affect the research. Physiotherapists, for example, may be most interested to learn of work closely related to their area of practice. The future may well provide many opportunities for collaborative work if nurse researchers make an effort to explain and interest such staff in this research.

Daily contacts with hospital and/or community staff can provide quite valuable support for the researcher. Good relationships not only help to maintain easy access but they can add satisfaction to a stage in the research where activities can be very repetitive and tiring. Many staff and patients alike show genuine interest in nursing studies and, through informal conversations, can be encouraged to consider doing research themselves, and helped to appreciate the value of such work.

ETHICS COMMITTEE APPLICATION

Several fundamental ethical issues have been discussed in Chapter 4 but, as this stage of approval for the project is vital, a few points will be reiterated. Initial interviews with key officials can pave the way through to the process of ethics committee approval. The chairman and secretary should be contacted personally by the researcher in order to gather specific information and in order to introduce herself as a credible professional. Ethics committees as constituted run in varying ways, although the Department of Health is to issue guidelines in their role and membership. Most committees will tend to review any scientists' or medical proposals which concern patients as subjects. They therefore tend to be most familiar with drug trials and treatment evaluations and it is wise to gain the support of either the chairman or another member who may be useful in providing additional explanation to the other members on the different types of research proposed.

Researchers should consider that it is both the research proposal and the researcher that are being judged by this committee. The proposal should therefore document in detail professional qualifications and experience (see Chapter 11). A personal appearance at the meeting may be considered but this should only be agreed to if the researcher feels confident in such an arena and the committee feel this is necessary.

Any research proposal should contain details of how and when subjects will be approached and how they will be identified as part of the sample. It should also mention whether staff will be involved in selection. This committee should be able to picture the chain of events in the particular research process and identify what checks or safeguards will be possible. If nursing staff, for example, are always asked if patients are well enough to participate, this may reassure the members. In the community, this sort of process may not be so feasible and the researcher must convince members that she will always ensure that they assess whether the subject feels able to participate.

Anonymity of data can usually be assured, and this may be quite essential if particular staff are involved and their work assessed in some way. Repeated reassurances and an open and honest attitude in the researcher may help to gain acceptance and over time trust should build up. Indeed in most nursing research reports discussion of such points tends to confirm the fact that professionals are helpful and grateful for the experience of knowing and working with a nurse researcher.

All ethics committees concentrate on the manner in which individual research subjects will be asked for their consent. Clear details of how the study is to be explained and whether there will be a witness to this should always be given.

ACCESS AND INFORMATION FOR SUBJECTS

Very few people refuse to participate either in nursing research or in research conducted by other health care staff. This fact alone should alert all researchers to the 'captive' nature of their respondents and therefore to the need for extra care when seeking to gain access or consent for research. Full and careful explanation for potential subjects is rightfully required prior to seeking access. However, this should not deter researchers; rather it should encourage them. People are much more likely to willingly participate in studies when approached in the respectful and correct spirit of partnership that is now acceptable. The fuller the explanation, the fuller the participation tends to be!

Access to subjects thus comes at the end of a number of negotiations and the final stage involves the researcher establishing her presence and the right to make *requests* to staff and possibly patients. This may involve gaining consent for interviews, for systematic observation, or for access to records. In each case it is up to subjects to choose whether they participate. It is wise for you to clarify the fact that as the respondent may refuse or withdraw from the study at any time, you need to consider this carefully in the first place. It may be wise for you to explain that subjects who are unsure of their commitment to the study should think very carefully before agreeing initially. (It is often they who withdraw later.)

It is quite apparent that the confidence and skill of the researcher can influence the level of collaboration that is forthcoming. Quiet, polite, and assertive negotiating styles are usually most successful. One should never forget that impatience or tactlessness on the part of the researcher may alienate staff and prohibit access to subjects. On the whole, subjects are only too willing to help but this can never be assumed. The good name of nursing has also aided this aspect of research progress!

CONCLUSION

Gaining access can be time-consuming and difficult to co-ordinate. Once negotiated, it is unlikely that staff will object or obstruct the data collection but you should never forget that you are present in an invited capacity and should, as a nurse researcher, uphold the principles of good research and be bound by the code of conduct which applies to nurses. In the research role, you are frequently benefiting more than the people you involve in data collection: any outcomes from the research may not give direct benefit to the subjects but only to those who receive related care in the future. 'Public relations' are rather important; polite greetings and offers of help, as and when possible, may be appreciated. Gradually, researchers normally do become accepted and this can make data collection more enjoyable. We owe it, as researchers, to respect the generosity of those (of foremost importance) who permit access. We should always remember that we must all first preserve the rights of human beings before the potential advances from new information or research-based insights.

REFERENCES

Institute of Health Services Management (1989). *The Hospitals and Health Services Year Book*. Institute of Health Services Management, London.
Wilson-Barnett J., Corner J. & de Carle B. (1990). Integrating Nursing Research and Practice: The Role of the Researcher as Teacher. *Journal of Advanced Nursing*, **15** (5), 621–5.
United Kingdom Central Council for Nursing, Midwifery and Health Visiting (1989). *Exercising Accountability: Advisory Document*. United Kingdom Central Council for Nursing, Midwifery and Health Visiting, London.

B: Research Design

The research design represents the major methodological thrust of the study, being the distinctive and specific research approach which is best suited to answering the research question/s. As will be seen in chapters 13 to 21, the major research designs – not always entirely mutually exclusive – each have individual advantages which make them appropriate in particular circumstances.

Selection of the research design is influenced both by the research question and the aim and objectives of the research. Selection of a research design is always preceded by clearly identifying the purpose of the research. In selecting an appropriate design, it is useful to have a general knowledge of a variety of designs and thereby be able to consider a range of possibilities, eliminate those which are not appropriate, and select the one which is best suited to your particular study. As with many aspects of the research process, it is rarely possible to achieve perfection. In selecting a research design, bear in mind that whichever one is chosen, it will be imperfect and have some limitations with regard to your particular needs. However, careful consideration and selection of research designs will enable you to select the one which has the 'best fit' for your particular study.

The chapters in this section are intended to give readers of research reports an insight into a few selected research designs. They are also intended to give researchers, working under supervision, an introduction to the major research methodologies, and to provide the basis for selecting a specific design which can then be studied in detail by making use of the references provided at the end of each chapter.

Chapter 13
Qualitative Research
Maura Hunt

'Over the past three decades, the majority of nurse researchers have been strongly socialized to value and use quantitative types of research as the only legitimate method for "scientific" nursing research.'

Although the above quotation (Leininger 1985, p. 5) refers to nursing research in the United States of America, it could just as easily describe the development of nursing research in Britain. Literature on the research process for nurses has reflected this position and concentrated largely on methods represented as rational, objective, and quantitative. Until recently there has been little debate on the processes involved in knowledge creation or the different philosophical positions that underpin the choice of quantitative and qualitative research methods.

DIFFERENCES BETWEEN QUANTITATIVE AND QUALITATIVE METHODS

The primary purpose of both qualitative and quantitative research is the same in that both aim to contribute to knowledge about a particular subject. The essential differences between them are, amongst other things, that quantitative methods rely heavily, as their title implies, on acquiring data that is numerical and can be statistically interpreted. Qualitative methods are primarily concerned with in-depth study of human phenomena in order to understand their nature and the meanings they have for individuals involved. Field and Morse (1985) point out that the basic distinction between qualitative and quantitative approaches are that the former aims to develop theory inductively from the data while the latter's intention is to generate and test theories deductively from existing knowledge through developing hypothesized relationships and proposed outcomes for study. Not all quantitative research involves hypothesis testing since data from the widely used large scale statistical survey only describes opinions, feelings and aspects of people's lives. More fundamental differences between the two methods stem from the development of the quantitative approach as the 'scientific' method, derived from the physical sciences, while qualitative methods were created to represent different views of human beings. These underpinning assumptions will be discussed in more detail later.

Questionnaires and surveys seem to have been the most widely used data collection methods adopted by nurses, especially in course projects designed to teach nurse learners the rudiments of research. Possibly because of this orientation, research which did not produce numerical data and widely applicable results, has tended to be presented in nursing literature as of lower status and less 'scientific' than experimental or evaluative quantitative methods. It has been implied that in-depth, non-statistical studies are merely springboards for generating hypotheses and measuring nursing practice and are not capable in their own right of contributing to knowledge development.

Couchman and Dawson (1990, p. 112) encapsulate these views when they represent quantitative and qualitative techniques as a continuum with standardized questionnaires generating 'hard' data and facts, and 'depth interviews', at the qualitative extreme, producing 'soft' data and theory suggesting implicit evaluative connotations. They further describe the differences as:

'Qualitative methods are generally regarded as being less "scientific" less concerned with establishing causality, descriptive rather than explanatory, exploratory rather than testing. Qualitative methods work from the particular to the general (inductive logic) whereas quantiative methods, with their hypothesis testing and high dependence on statistical significance of findings, work from the general to the particular (deductive logic).'

The focus on techniques as representing the differences between the two approaches rather than the views of mankind they reflect, has arisen because, initially, nursing research developed using knowledge and methods designed to study the natural or physical world. From this perspective, research as a tool of science derived from assumptions about the universe, which was regarded as orderly, while human reality was assumed to consist of subjective, private dimensions, and outer observable, objective aspects. Thus it was thought they could be studied separately and that cause–effect relationships could be identified. To understand qualitative research and its development in nursing, it is necessary to contrast the assumptions on which it is based with those generated from the physical sciences that form the basis of quantitative research. The discussion of differences is not to imply that one approach is superior or inferior to the other. The discussion is designed to provide a basis from which choices of research approaches and data collection methods can be made appropriate for the questions asked, while studies that use different approaches can be read with understanding.

Two published nursing studies illustrate the assumptions uderlying qualitative and quantitative research as represented by inductive and deductive thinking. One study (Baker 1983) of 'care' in a geriatric ward, sought to gain some understanding of how nurses in a variety of settings in one hospital perceived their work of looking after old people. Although Baker was aware of nursing literature which proposed how old people should be cared for, no hypothesis or propositions for testing were formulated. The part of the study published focused on two identified divergent styles of nursing that co-existed in one ward. Through participant observation over a period of two months, Baker describes and explains the differences and processes utilized in the two styles of nursing, generating theories that one style had the components of what was propounded to be 'individualized' care while the other approximated more to that defined as 'routine' orientated. The styles of care were interpreted in relation to the organizational contexts in which they were carried out, thereby identifying divergent priorities, values and perceptions of care between ward sisters, staff nurses, learners, nurse managers, and medical staff. The conclusions of that study were reached by inductive reasoning and represent a qualitative approach.

In contrast, an investigation by Metcalfe (1983) utilized a deductive approach in formulating a hypothesis that midwifery care, delivered through the organization of patient allocation, and representing 'individualized' care, was preferable to task allocation methods associated with alleged ritualistic and routine care. A quasi-experiment was instituted in a midwifery ward to test these assumptions. The results of that study were inconclusive, as were previously similar cited studies, and the researcher questioned the suitability of an experimental design for such studies. Though some data collection methods used by Metcalfe could be termed as qualitative in nature in that observations were made and nurses were interviewed, the presentation of results (mainly in statistical form), with the design of the study and the thinking generating it, classifies it as a quantitative study.

The problems associated with generating theories deductively and testing them are recognized by Metcalfe in that she points out that although patient allocation organization of nursing care was being presented to nurses as a better form of care for patients, no evidence existed to support this assumption. Yet Metcalfe's hypothesis was formulated on that basis. It has been pointed out that researchers tend to create and test hypotheses consistent with established theories which can be tested as statistically significant and thereby support current thought. Field and Morse (1985, pp 2–3) have made the following suggestion:

> 'extensive and important theories may continue to be used for prolonged periods of time (and be "confirmed" by research), yet, in essence be totally and completely wrong . . . Theory, derived inductively because it is derived from reality, is unlikely to be a product of the researcher's cultural reality or a distortion of the "truth" although present day values or personal biases are always a threat to validity'.

The above supposition that the use of qualitative approaches reduces the possibility of distortions by the researcher needs qualification. Field and Morse (1985) later advocate caution by recommending that an acute self-awareness needs to be developed and made explicit by anyone undertaking research of perspectives, values, and biases held, and the influences they are likely to exert on the study methodology. If a qualitative approach is fully understood and adopted, the alleged 'objectivity' of the researcher should be regarded as problematic, this being invariably unquestioned in quantative studies reflecting its 'rational' orientation.

QUALITATIVE RESEARCH ASSUMPTIONS

As quantiative research methods and assumptions about the world have emerged from the physical sciences, qualitative approaches have been generated from 'humanistic' disciplines such as history, philosophy, anthropology, sociology, and psychology. In the early stages of their development, social sciences research also tended to adopt the assumptions and research methods developed by and for the physical sciences.

This resulted in an emphasis on surveys in sociology and laboratory experiments in psychology. As social science research developed, dissatisfaction emerged with the concentration on traditional, natural science approaches. Sociologists, in particular, focused their discontent on the influences that the natural science traditions had had on sociological theories. These, it was alleged by Filmer, Phillipson, Silverman and Walsh (1972, p. 4), had:

> 'minimised the differences between social and physical worlds and sought to impose upon sociology a way of defining problems and of studying relationships which follows the canons of what its proponents take to be the "scientific" method.'

One of the deficiencies of many of the books written for nurses which give information on the research process and methods of data collection, has been that they are presented in mechanistic ways without consideration of the different views of human beings and their behaviour that the methods implicitly reflect. The quantitative research debate raises the fundamental question, 'can human beings and their social endeavours be studied in the same way as rats, plants and planets'? If the latter stance is taken by researchers, human beings can be regarded merely as reacting and responding to the environment. Predictable responses and behaviour can therefore be determined and prescribed while objective and subjective realities can be studied separately, viewed as static, controlled, and held constant.

In contrast, different views of the human world produced dissatisfaction with the physical sciences' research assumptions and the methods which led to the development of qualitative approaches. Underpinning the latter are the assumptions that human beings not only react but act upon and create the meaning of their experiences so that inner and external 'realities' interact and cannot be separated.

Because of this, the social world is considered dynamic and it can be interpreted in many ways. In addition, human language is a powerful, symbolic means of communicating perceptions of 'realities' but can be understood only in the contexts within which it is used (Munhall & Olier 1986; Silverman 1985).

Contexts are taken to mean not only the circumstances and situations in which specified events take place but what leads up to and follows them. From this stance, aiming to produce research findings from the study of a particular context may not be generalized to predict human behaviour in all circumstances. However, theories can be generated and, taken with results of studies done in similar contexts, used for comparative analysis.

An example, in nursing research, of the tendency to disassociate communications between nurses and patients from the circumstances in which they occur, results in criticism of all nurses' interpersonal skills. In hospitals, much of patients' contacts can be with learner nurses and nursing assistants. In such a context, the use of evasive tactics by such staff in response to patients' requests for information, can be explained not only as poor communication skills, but as a rational means of dealing with situations in which the nurse learners and assistants have neither the appropriate knowledge nor the authority to do otherwise.

In the different context of patients' homes, with experienced, specialist nurses providing consultative services for the terminally ill, Hunt (1990) found that such staff were not evasive in talking about and providing information about cancer. The patients in the latter study had a lengthy history of medical consultations, investigations, and hospitalization before being referred to the specialist home care nurses. Not only did the patients and relatives have many opportunities to obtain direct and indirect information about their illnesses, but the nurses gave them time over a number of visits to openly acknowledge the 'truth' about their illnesses. More importantly, these nurses had appropriate knowledge of the patients' background through access to their previous medical records, and the formal authority to 'tell the truth'. These nurses accepted referrals to them on the understanding that they would not tell 'lies' to patients. Such differing circumstances can, regardless of the communication skills training received by individuals, produce very different forms of interactions, as pointed out by Fielding and Llewelyn (1987).

The desire to render research results context-free and transpose them into recommendations for all nurses, seems, however, to be strongly ingrained, as reflected in an editorial directive attached to, and extrapolated from, a published article by Hunt (1990). Because the specialist nurses in Hunt's studies used the taking of illness histories as a means of finding out what patients and relatives knew about the diagnosis and prognosis, the editor of the journal publishing the article (Hunt 1990, p. 24) added:

> 'Nurses *must* (my emphasis) compile new records on the history of the patient's illness so that they are able to clarify what the doctor has told the patient about his or her illness.'

No such recommendation was made by Hunt since the outcomes achieved by the nurses in her study might possibly not be achieved by different nurses in other working situations. The editorial licence taken represents the 'natural science' ethos in that the recommendation assumes that all nurses, patients, and their interactional circumstances, are similar so that a sweeping generalization that includes all of them can be made. Further, it is believed that study methods used in one context can be replicated in dissimilar nursing contexts with the aim of finding out if the same results are achieved so that 'the truth' can thus be found.

QUALITATIVE METHODOLOGIES

Qualitative research methodologies represent more than the use of particular methods of collecting information which do not involve numerical processes, as Leininger (1985, p. 5) points out:

> 'the goal of qualitative research is to document and interpret as fully as possible the totality of whatever is being studied in particular contexts from the people's viewpoint or frame of reference. This includes identification, study and analysis of subjective and objective data in order to understand the internal and external worlds of people'.

The achievement of this goal requires the use of in-depth observations, participation by researchers, interviews, and informants' explanations and interpretations of their views. Because of the in-depth nature of such studies and the analysis of the data required, samples of people included usually have to be small and selective. Theories and propositions are generated in qualitative studies mainly from the data collected during, and at the end of the research, rather than before the study starts, as in quantitative approaches. As in Baker's 1983 study already discussed, though qualitative research is carried out within broad theoretical notions about the phenomena under study, inductive reasoning, moving from the particular to the general, is utilized to derive knowledge from the data collected. In contrast, as in Metcalfe's (1983) study, deductive reasoning, moving from the general to the particular, is generally employed in quantitative research where theories and hypotheses constructed from another data source are applied or used as criteria for interpreting and evaluating the phenomena being studied.

The inductive approach in qualitative research is evident in the grounded theory strategies (Glaser & Strauss (1967) discussed in Chapter 14 and as used in Baker's study (1983) presented earlier. Other conceptual qualitative research methodologies, such as ethnomethodology, historical analysis, and participatory and co-operative inquiry, have also been developed and are being used in nursing research.

Ethnomethodology

The origins of ethnographic methods for doing qualitative research are akin to those used in anthropology and have been described by Leininger (1987, p. 14) as:

'the systematic process of observing, detailing, describing, documenting and analysing the lifeways or particular patterns of culture (or subculture) in order to grasp the life ways or patterns of people in their familiar environment.'

The purpose of ethnographic studies are to find ways of describing the following:

(a) How people know, understand, and give meaning to experiences of their world;
(b) through inductive analysis, to develop theories about the use of language, values, beliefs, and actions of specified groups of people in their familiar environmental contexts.

Ethnographic data collection methods are not regarded merely as a given set of research techniques to be manipulated, but as the processes through which the researcher generates and constructs abstract views of the situations studied. Thus theory and research are inextricably linked. It is assumed that a commonsense view of the world is shared by people in particular cultures and sub-cultures. These commonsense views are shared also by researchers and constitute taken-for-granted assumptions about the worlds they inhabit. The aim of the ethnographer is to explain the meaning of the commonsense, taken-for-granted aspects of the world being studied. This is more difficult to do than to focus on unusual or dramatic phenomena or to study unknown or 'strange' cultures as is done traditionally by anthropologists. To get to know how members of a culture perceive and give meaning to their experiences require of the researchers that they become part of that world while attempting to view it as 'anthropologically strange'. For nurses studying nursing situations, this process can be difficult but can be helped by having access to non-nurse ethnographers as sounding boards.

This approach to taking commonsense or mundane views of the world as problematic, is absent in much quantitative research. This can be seen in the use of standardized questionnaires when it is assumed that all respondents will attach identical meanings to each of the questions asked and that these will coincide with the researcher's intentions in creating the questions (Cicourel 1964). That the questions selected, how they are expressed, and the assumptions underlying them, are reflections of implicit and unexplained 'commonsense' views of the world held by researchers, are rarely recognized, nor that the ways they use of interpreting such data spring from similar sources. Thus for social scientists to assume that they can take peoples' accounts of their acts or social situations and transform them into allegedly objective statements of what they think actually happened, or to uncover 'real' underlying patterns of events, is, it is suggested, to give no credence to the above concepts.

The research interview

Silverman (1985) has argued that data derived from research interviews do not simply reflect the 'real' world of the respondents. He cites a study by Baruch (1981) where interviewing of parents of sick or handicapped children took place. In first accounts given of their experiences, parents frequently told 'atrocity' stories which presented some health care professional (GPs, health visitors, or school medical officers) as being neglectful or slow in identifying the nature of the children's problems, or were unsympathetic in dealing with them. There was no way of determining the accuracy of these stories, but Baruch took them seriously because of the regularity with which they were presented. He noted, however, that such stories were told far less frequently at second and third interviews with parents held several months apart.

The explanation suggested was that at the beginning, parents were dealing with the guilt and responsibility of having sick children. By identifying health professionals as appropriate sources of 'blame' they shifted the possibility that they might be regarded as 'irresponsible' parents in failing to obtain the best possible treatment for their children. Thus, the parents presented to Baruch 'moral' historical accounts but, at later interviews, they felt less helpless about their situations and were able to display their 'moral' worth through accounts of their successful actions rather than attributing blame to others. Time was identified as constituting the key factor in understanding the moral 'careers' of the parents interviewed rather than presenting the accounts as 'true' representations of what occurred.

Deviant cases

In quantitative research, the analysis of results focuses on the presentation of numerical data and attempts, when possible, to demonstrate levels of statistical significance. Data not displaying significance are often neglected or sometimes attention is centred on 'substantial minorities' of respondents (representing 18% to 20% of the total sample) because they present 'problems' for which recommendations for change can be made as the traditional research formula suggests. Why 80% of respondents are not displaying the identified 'problems' is then left unexplored. In ethnographic studies, 'deviant' cases should be constantly identified and accounted for. As Silverman (1985, p. 21) proposes, such an approach can make research critical and 'serve to increase the reliability and inclusiveness of analytic schemes'.

An example of this method is demonstrated by Hunt (1989) who analysed conversations between symptom control team nurses, terminally ill cancer patients and their relatives in their own homes. It was concluded that the nurses adopted a morally neutral stance in avoiding making critical judgments of colleagues, patients, or relatives. One nurse appeared 'deviant' in that she agreed with a patient who was expressing criticism of a hospital doctor because no indication had been given that the patient had cancer. But because the nurse, after being critical, stated she was, 'being a bit disloyal here in a way', she indicated awareness that she knew she was breaking an accepted rule, thus confirming the theory that there was such a value shared by all the nurses in the study.

Conversational analysis

Central to ethnographic studies are conversational interactions through which people achieve common cultural understandings. The analysis of 'talk' has developed at two levels, both of which are trans-situational and context-related. The trans-situational approach has attempted to determine universal rules of the social organisation of talk. It has been identified that generally in conversation, attempts are made by participants to take turns at talking and to avoid gaps and overlaps. The matter of how such organization is achieved has been addressed. Other studies of conversations are based on the assumption that language only has meaning in relation to the contexts in which it is used. An example of context-related talk could be where a doctor in his consulting room asks a patient to go behind a screen and remove his/her clothing. If a solicitor in his office made the same request of his client, the same words would be given very different meanings. These situations display the common, culturally shared understandings that underpin them. The request made by the doctor may be considered acceptable and unremarkable because it is regarded in Western cultures as legitimate for intimate examinations to be done to make a diagnosis. In contrast, it has not been considered necessary for a solicitor to act similarly to accomplish his work.

Conversation analysis, in contrast to interaction analysis, is not done through breaking down verbal behaviour into pre-determined categories. Instead, theoretical assumptions about social life inform and shape conversation analysis. It is assumed that conversations are not random, disorderly, irrelevant or accidental, but are socially organized and contextually orientated. Neither are there pre-determined criteria for evaluating the interactions as 'good' or 'poor'. Such idealization distances the researcher from the data while the aim of the analysis is to determine how interactants display their competencies in organizing and giving meanings to their social life. Some British nurses are engaging in such studies and are discussed by Hunt and Robinson (1987) and demonstrated in their own studies (Robinson 1988; Hunt 1989).

Participatory research

The traditional, natural science-based research processes present the researcher as one who defines a problem for investigation, formulates propositions about the issues to be investigated and the data collection methods, gains entry to the appropriate research site, collects and analyses results, and makes recommendations. In the interest, supposedly, of maintaining objectivity and reducing bias, the persons to be studied are usually kept naive about the study's propositions and methodology. They are often left untouched by the research yet are expected to translate the study findings into practice. This approach tends to treat those being studied as 'objects' and mere sources of data, with minimal interactions between them and the researchers.

Action research (see Chapter 17) is research methodology that promotes maximum interaction between researchers and subjects: the latter are co-researchers and the researcher participates in making any identified required changes in practice. As Hunt (1987) demonstrates, quantitative methods can be used within an action research framework but the concepts underlying the action research approach are those of qualitative research. Greenwood (1984) has argued that action research is the most appropriate approach for nursing in that it is situational, collaborative, and participatory, while effecting change in the functioning of the 'real' world. Reason and Rowan (1981) and Reason (1988) present co-operative inquiry as 'a genuine new paradigm for human research' in that it honours individual experience and attempts to transform it into a 'critical subjectivity' through reflecting on, and making sense of, such experiences. Schön (1983) proposes similar approaches in suggesting 'reflection-in-action' as an appropriate form of research for practitioners.

Mehan (1979) further makes a case for revising the traditional researchers' 'authority' in claiming to be experts who make recommendations for changes. His objections are that it assumes that research information is a static commodity, to be transferred between people, which treats the recipients as passive receivers of research findings. Furthermore, such research separates researchers from practice, giving them a privileged position as possessing allegedly superior 'scientific' knowledge. In action research, the continuing dialogue, participation of all concerned, and co-operative inquiries, overcome such obstacles. The issues identified for investigation are determined by practitioners as of relevance and importance in practice; at the same time critical and reflective thinking develops in the process of exploring practical problems. Because solutions to problems are sought, research approaches are perceived as of practical value. Research is seen not as a compartmentalized academic activity nor merely as course work for examination purposes. This lack of relevance to practice, on the other hand, seems to be the impression given to nurses by compartmentalized, poorly supervised and critiqued quantitative 'projects', primarily using badly designed questionnaires, which have formed the research component of many short nursing courses (Hunt & Hicks 1983). Equally, the non-participation of practising nurses in the creation of knowledge through research suggests that practical competencies and professional experiences are of little value since theoretical 'models' of how nursing should be done are created by nurses who are usually not directly involved in giving day-to-day services. The implication is that practising nurses have developed no useful 'models', while much nursing research produces findings suggesting that nursing practice is rule and ritual ridden, with deficient communications and an unsound knowledge basis. This is unlikely to promote self-esteem and professional confidence among nurses directly involved in giving the services and on whom rests the responsibility for justifying research and theory development through demonstrating its usefulness in practice.

SUGGESTED LIMITATIONS OF QUALITATIVE APPROACH

It is recognized that all research methodologies have limitations. The limitations of quantitative research have been discussed while those of qualitative studies are considered to be primarily their situational, in-depth nature, precluding duplication and generalization of results to other contexts. In attempting to take the viewpoint of those studied over time, Denzen (1970) suggests also that a participant observer stance may not take account of relevant issues occurring before the researcher's entry into the situation. The participant researcher may change the situation by his presence, his informants may be unrepresentative of less responsive people in the social setting, and the observer may 'go native' by identifying so much with participants that what is being studied is similarly taken-for-granted.

To counteract the limitations of all research methodologies, it has become fashionable in nursing to suggest the compromise of 'triangulation' proposed by Denzen (1970). It is suggested that through 'triangulation' multiple research methods can be used in a variety of settings in order to gain a 'total' picture of some phenomenon. Silverman (1985) points out that the proposed 'triangulation' methods reflect the natural science, positivist frame of reference. It assumes that one 'truth', or a single, undefined reality, can be found, and various accounts can be treated as multiple mappings of such a reality which can be fitted together like pieces of a jig-saw to gain a 'complete' picture. But according to Silverman (1985, p. 21) 'What goes on in one setting is not a simple corrective to what happens elsewhere – each must be understood in its own terms'. Equally, if competing versions of a situation are provided, the researcher's role is not to adjudicate as to which is the 'true' account but to attempt to understand the situation.

UTILIZATION OF NURSING PRACTICE DATA

Because of these reservations, reflecting the differing and opposing concepts that underpin quantitative and qualitative methodologies, correlating data derived from both methods used in one study present problems. However, it is possible to utilize some quantitative methods within a qualitative framework. Silverman (1984) demonstrates this combination in a qualitative study by counting and timing consultations by a doctor, first in his private clinic, then in a National Health Service one, and then using the data for comparative analysis. In conversation analysis, it may be appropriate also to count units of interaction. In the final analysis, methodologies used may be judged, as Silverman (1985, p. 20) suggests below, by:

'the increasingly accepted view of science that work becomes scientific by adopting methods of study appropriate to the data at hand'.

If nurses were to consider what methods are appropriate for using data they have to hand, more efforts could be made to draw on the volume of information available which nurses giving direct day-to-day services 'know' and collect. Proponents of the nursing process who advocate the use of blank paper for recording patient assessments, mitigate against the systematic exploitation of such data. In addition to co-operative inquiries, the utilization of individual case study analysis and clinical ethnographies (Benner 1985; Watson 1990) could contribute, not only to understanding what constitutes the 'know-how' of clinical nurses, but also to the accumulation longitudinally, over time, of information about specified patient 'careers'. Their analysis could reveal trends, and patterns of care and their outcomes, over time in relation to the contexts in which they occur. This would require the recording of assessment processes and care planning in more structured and systematic formats. These developments might make recordings easier, improve their quality, save nurses' time and motivate them to increase the accuracy of records because the information generated could be seen to be used. In addition, the process could also be a vehicle for integrating research methods into practice while demonstrating that value is being given to clinical experience and expertise. The development could also further quality assurance initiatives which advocate the creation of standards, and auditing systems which require precise, explicit, and measurable objectives. Unless qualitative research approaches are incorporated into these developments, knowledge we gain from them is likely to be impoverished. Such study methods, it should be added require them to be no less rigorous or systematic than those of quantitative research.

REFERENCES

Baker D.E. (1983) '"Care" in a Geriatric Ward: An Account of Two Styles of Nursing' In *Nursing Research – Studies in Patient Care*. (Ed. by J. Wilson-Barnett). John Wiley, Chichester.

Baruch G. (1981) Moral Tales: Parents' Stories of Encounters with The Health Profession. *Sociology of Health and Illness* **3**, 3, 275–96.

Benner P. (1985) The Oncology clinical nurse specialist: An expert coach. *Oncology Nursing Forum*, **Vol 12**, No. 2, 40–4.

Cicourel A. (1964) *Method and Measurement in Sociology*. Free Press, New York.

Couchman W. & Dawson J. (1990) *Nursing and Health Care Research: A Practical Guide*. Scutari Press, London.

Denzen N. (1970) *The Research Act in Sociology*. Butterworth, London.

Field P.A. & Morse J.M. (1985) *Nursing Research: The application of qualitative approaches*, Croom Helm, London.

Fielding R.G. & Llewelyn S.P. (1987) Communication Training in Nursing May Damage Your Health and Enthusiasm: Some Warnings. *Journal of Advanced Nursing*, **12**, 281–90.

Filmer P., Phillipson M., Silverman D. & Walsh D. (1972) *New Directions in Sociological Theory*, Collier-MacMillan, London.

Glaser B.G. & Strauss A.L. (1967) *The Discovery of Grounded Theory: Strategies for Qualitative Research*. Aldine Press, Chicago.

Greenwood J. (1984) Nursing Research: A Position Paper. *Journal of Advanced Nursing*, **9**, 77–82.

Hunt M. & Hicks J. (1983) Prommoting Research Awareness in Post-Basic Nursing Courses. *Nursing Times* Occasional Papers **Vol 79**, No. 6, 41–2.

Hunt M. & Robinson K.M. (1987) 'Analysis of Conversational Interactions' In *Research Methodology* (Ed. By M. Cahoon). Churchill Livingstone, Edinburgh 150–68.

Hunt M. (1987) The Process of Translating Research Findings into Nursing Practice. *Journal of Advanced Nursing* **12**, 101–10.

Hunt M. (1989) *Dying at Home: Its Basic 'Ordinariness' displayed in Nurses' patients' and relatives' "talk"'. Unpublished PhD Thesis, Dept. of Sociology, Goldsmith's College, University of London*.

Hunt M. (1990) Caring for the Terminally Ill at Home. Nursing Standard **Vol 4**, No. 39, 23–5.

Leininger M.M. (1985) *Qualitative Research Methods in Nursing*. Grune and Stratton, Orlando.

Leininger M. (1987) 'Importance and Uses of Ethnomethods: Ethonography and Ethno-nursing Research' in *Research Methodology*, (Ed. by M. Cahoon). Churchill Livingstone, Edinburgh.

Mehan H. (1979) *Learning Lessons: Social Organisation in the Classroom*. Harvard University Press, Cambridge, MA.

Metcalfe C. (1983) 'A Study of Change in the Method of Organising the Delivery of Nursing Care in a Ward of a Maternity Hospital' In *Nursing Research – Studies in Patient Care*, (Ed. by J. Wilson-Barnett). John Wiley, Chichester.

Munhall P.L. & Oiler C.J. (1986) *Nursing Research – A Qualitative Perspective*. Appleton Century-Crofts, Connecticut.

Reason P. & Rowan J. (Editors) (1981) *Human Inquiry*. John Wiley, Chichester.

Reason P. (Editor) (1988) *Human Inquiry in Action*. Sage, London.

Robinson K.M. (1988) *The Social Organisation of Health Visiting*. Unpublished PhD Thesis, Polytechnic of the South Bank.

Schön D.A. (1983) *The Reflective Practitioner*. Basic Books, New York.

Silverman D. (1984) Going Private: Ceremonial Forms in a Private Oncology Clinic. *Sociology* **Vol 18**, No. 2, 191–202.

Silverman D. (1985) *Qualitative Methodology and Sociology*. Gower, Aldershot.

Watson R. (1990) 'Research on the elderly'. *Nursing Times*, **Vol 86**, No. 16, 43–5.

Chapter 14
Grounded Theory
David C. Benton

In the past ten years there has been a noticeable increase in the number of published studies which employ the use of qualitative techniques (Chapman 1989). Omery (1987) suggests that this increase can be attributed to the fact that nurses now feel confident enough as researchers to select the most appropriate methods to meet the needs of the topic under study.

Aamodt (1982) has argued that any method which facilitates the discovery of variables associated with the provision of care can contribute to the development of nursing knowledge and the associated theory base. Furthermore, Aamodt (1982) suggests that inductive approaches to the development of theory can be readily employed by nurses who wish to undertake research into practice-related topics.

One means of inductive theory generation which has been consistently utilized by nurses since its development by Glaser and Strauss (1967), is that of the *grounded theory* method. This method has been used by nurse researchers to develop inductive theories on topics as diverse as the dying patient, the referral process in health visiting, and the informed consent process (Benoliel 1967; Luker & Chalmers 1989; Nusbaum & Chenitz, 1990).

Field and Morse (1985) have identified that there is a need for nurses to develop their own theories of health care, theories which have been developed directly from the everyday practice of members of the profession. Since grounded theory entails the development of theory from data which have been methodically obtained from the real life setting, it is ideally suited to the needs of nurses who wish to investigate topics about which little has been previously known.

Many aspects of nursing are qualitative in nature and as yet under-researched (Chapman 1989). This fact, along with the need to develop the nursing knowledge base, has resulted in the utilization of the grounded theory method. It is the intention of this chapter to clearly identify the processes involved in undertaking a grounded theory study and provide guidance which will assist you should you wish to conduct research using this method.

THE GROUNDED THEORY METHOD

The grounded theory method is ideally suited to the investigation of those topics about which there is little prior knowledge. The method developed by Glaser and Strauss (1967) requires that you approach data collection without a preconceived framework. Without an open-minded approach, there is a danger that significant material will be ignored since data are seen as not fitting the existing model.

The use of a grounded theory approach will enable you to develop theories based in the reality of the topic under study. This process will encourage you to explore data so as to discover the basic social and psychological processes operating within the area of inquiry.

Unlike quantitative methods, the grounded theory approach does not proceed in a linear fashion. Grounded theory is typified by the concurrent activities of data collection, organization, and analysis. This process continues until a theory is developed which is of sufficient detail and at a sufficient level of abstraction to explain the variation in the data observed. The process by which the grounded theory is generated is known as the constant comparative method, a method by which every element of data is compared with every other element.

DATA SOURCES AND METHODS OF COLLECTION

Data are commonly generated through field observation or by examination of documentary evidence. Field observation is a process where data are generated by observation, interview, or video or audio taping. This entails close interpersonal contact with the subjects of the study. To help you understand the role you play in this process, it is advisable to keep a daily journal or diary. Thoughts, impressions, or emotional reactions experienced, can all be recorded and may assist you in understanding the material gathered.

Data collection initially starts with an attempt to examine the wider issues surrounding the topic under study. Only when you have established the wider context, should more focused investigation begin. Luker and Chalmers (1989), for example, describe the process of referral as it emerged from an in-depth study of health visiting practice.

Interviews and observation are two techniques frequently used to generate data for a study utilizing the grounded theory method. These techniques are not unique to grounded theory and are described in detail in Chapters 22 and 24 respectively. Nevertheless, Strauss (1987) has suggested that data obtained from these sources can be confusing at first. However, since organization and analysis of the data begins at an early stage, this should enable you to identify areas which can be clarified in subsequent interviews or observations.

RELIABILITY AND VALIDITY OF DATA

Goodwin and Goodwin (1984) have reported that there is a tendency to ignore the issues of reliability and validity, or to consider them irrelevant, when undertaking research based in the qualitative paradigm.

If research is to be of value, then it must address the issues of reliability and validity. Glaser and Strauss (1967) and Stern (1985) have argued that reliability is established by taking findings back to those respondents who provided the original data from which you generated the theory. Respondents can then confirm or refute the theory developed. Stern (1985) points out that if this process is used on an ongoing basis, then it is similar to the test-retest approach of establishing reliability that is used in quantitative research.

Validity of the theory can be established on the same basis as that advocated for reliability. By taking developing theory back to the original informants, you can receive feedback which can be used to establish validity.

Grounded theory does address the issues of reliability and validity. More general issues concerning reliability and validity as applied to qualitative research are addressed in Chapter 13. However, Hinds *et al.* (1990) identify a specific approach for examining a completed piece of work for both reliability and validity. By using independent experts, it is possible to examine various aspects of the process of developing grounded theory for reliability and validity. It is suggested that not only can the method provide data on the reliability and validity of a study, but it is also capable of identifying investigator bias and conceptual clarity.

DATA RECORDING

The grounded theory approach is integrally dependent upon the accuracy of source data; thus, data recording is a vital step in the entire process. Data are most frequently recorded by use of audio tape or/and written notes. Alternatively, you may choose to use video tape which, in addition to a verbal record, can also provide data on non-verbal behaviour. If audio tape is used then it is necessary to add non-verbal data at the stage of transcription. Transcription is the process where the audio record is typed ready for coding and analysis.

The choice of audio, video, or written data recording, will be dependent upon a number of issues. The recording and transcription of audio or video tape requires access to equipment and possibly secretarial resources. Written methods of recording are less expensive, but the data may not be as accurate or complete unless you are able to use shorthand. Consequently, since completeness and accuracy is important, and if adequate resources are available, tape should be used. However, dependent on the location and preferences of the respondents, it

---

Interview: **John Brown, Director of Standards**

Date and Time: **10/05/1990   10.30AM**

Location: **Bigtown Health Authority**

Researcher: **Alan Smith**   Page **3** of **28**

INTERVIEWER
What were your hopes for the post?

INTERVIEWEE
While there might have been more lofty aims to do with integrating research into practice and all of that sort of thing, it was much more about safeguarding or, it was about getting influence, it was felt that nursing had lost influence when general management came in, because of the kind of work that was put forward and it was very much a feeling that we're worth a lot, but we are not seeing this, you know having this credibility and it was about taking the initiative and getting that back again. . .

Fig. 14.1   Excerpt from interview illustrating a suitable layout.

may not be possible or appropriate to use recording devices. Informants may refuse to participate if tape is used, or they may be working in areas where background noise would result in a poor quality recording incapable of transcription.

If you are unable to use any form of data recording technique during the interview or observation, then it is important that a permanent record is made as soon after the event as possible. Go somewhere quiet and either write or dictate notes, identifying and recording as much detail as possible.

Whichever approach is used, it is important that certain information always appears on the data record. First, the name of the interviewer/observer and the date, time, and place where the interview/observation occurred. Second, the individual, group or subject being interviewed/observed. For clarity, all pages should be typed double spaced and with ample margins. Ideally, the interviewer data should appear on one side of the page and the interviewee data on the other. All pages should also be numbered and referenced so as to ensure that data do not go missing or appear out of context. Figure 14.1 illustrates an example of how a transcribed interview should appear. Please note that the name and source of data would not normally appear in published material: in this case, all identifying characteristics are fictitious.

EXPLAINING TERMINOLOGY

There are a number of terms that have particular meaning when applied to the grounded theory approach. These include substantive codes, categories, properties, theoretical constructs, core categories, and saturation. An understanding of the meaning of these terms and the relationships between them is vital if you are to undertake a study using a grounded theory design.

Substantive codes

When data are collected, you require to examine the various incidents so as to label those items or words which you feel contribute to the comprehension of the underlying processes. Coding of the actual substance of the data is referred to as substantive coding. At this early stage of coding, individual words or short phrases are highlighted in the text and codes written in the margin. To ensure detailed theoretical coverage, each sentence and incident should be coded into as many substantive codes as possible – a process known as open coding. This may result in some data being coded into more than one substantive code.

Categories and properties

Glaser and Strauss (1967) suggest that categories can be thought of as analogous to variables in quantitative research. Categories are produced when a number of substantive codes are condensed into a higher level of abstraction. Categories are commonly used to describe a class of individuals, events, situations, or phenomena that have certain characteristics in common. To have meaning, a category must be capable of being uniquely identified. For example, when examining data about the help-seeking behaviour of alcohol abusers, the category 'support person behaviour' emerged, which referred to 'nurses', 'doctors' 'psychologists', 'social workers', 'family', and 'friends' who exhibited certain characteristics.

In grounded theory, the characteristics of a cateogry are referred to as the 'properties' of the category. By studying the properties exhibited in different occurences of the category throughout the text, similarities and differences can be identified, thus refining the definition of a specific category or, conversely, leading to the generation of new ones. Furthermore, such examination will allow you to identify the situations or conditions under which the categories occur.

Theoretical constructs

Having identified the substantive codes and then derived categories, there is a need to interweave the component parts into a coherent entity which has meaning both to you as a researcher and to those who contributed to the data. Theoretical constructs are the means by which the various categories are linked. However, it is important not to attempt to develop theoretical constructs at too early a stage as there is a danger that vital codes, categories and properties will not yet have been discovered (Corbin 1986).

Corbin (1986) suggests that one means of identifying theoretical constructs is by asking questions of the categories so as to attempt to move categories from lower to higher levels of abstraction. Specifically, 'What is the category conveying?'. Alternatively, you can hypothesize about the relationships that may exist and test them back in the field.

Glaser (1978) suggests that by posing a series of six questions it is easier to identify relationships amongst categories. The six questions should address cause, context, contingency, consequence, covariance, and conditions. Table 14.1 illustrates how these questions can be posed in general terms, and, in addition, a supplementary question is identified that can assist in theoretical construct formation.

Table 14.1   Questions to assist the development of theoretical constructs.

(1) 'What is/are the cause(s) of the behaviour manifest in a particular category?'

(2) 'Under what context does the category manifest itself?'

(3) 'Is the category contingent upon any circumstances?'

(4) 'What are the consequences of the existence of this category?'

(5) 'Does a change in this category result in a change in another category – do two or more categories co-vary one with another?'

(6) 'What are the conditions for the existence of this category?'

(7) 'How does cause, context, contingency, consequence, covariance, and conditions, interrelate.

Core category

By linking categories together, one, and occasionally more, core categories will evolve. When you generate a theory, the core category should be at its centre and should be capable of explaining much of the variation in behaviour discovered in the data. Most other categories and their properties should relate to the core category, integrating in such a way as to produce theory that is capable of explaining the maximum amount of variation in behaviour.

Strauss (1987) identifies a number of criteria which can be used to assist you in the identification of the core category in study data. Table 14.2 summarizes criteria for a core category.

Table 14.2   Criteria for a core category.

(1) It is central to the theory.

(2) It is capable of accounting for a large percentage of variation in the pattern of behaviour.

(3) It must appear frequently in the data.

(4) It is clearly related to the majority of other categories.

(5) It takes longer to define the precise nature of the core category and its properties than other less central ones.

(6) A core category has clear implications for more general theory.

(7) As the core category is developed and its properties discovered theory formation as a whole will move forward.

Saturation

A category is said to be 'saturated' when examination of data reveals no further properties and the category is completely developed. In other words, examination of data yields only recurrences of material that has already been discovered, coded, and integrated. Despite attempting to identify new data from diverse sources, nothing new is found and only at this stage can a category be termed saturated. This implicitly implies that a category developed by studying only one data source can not be considered saturated. Glaser and Strauss (1967) suggest that single sources can at best yield only a few categories and some of their properties. If you therefore intend to undertake a piece of research which uses the grounded theory method, you will require access to diverse data sources if you are to achieve saturation of categories.

CONSTANT COMPARATIVE METHOD

The constant comparative method lies at the heart of the grounded theory approach and is the principle method of data analysis used in theory generation. This method of analysis entails the comparison of incidents with incidents, allowing the generation of categories. Incidents are then compared with categories, a strategy which allows you to identify the properties of the categories. In the early stages of category development, the comparison of incidents with categories will generate anomalies and it is at this point that you should stop coding and record a memorandum on your thoughts on the matter (such memos are discussed in detail later in this chapter). This process then progresses to the comparison of category with category, category with construct, and construct with construct.

Comparison of similar incidents will assist you in defining the basic properties of categories; it will also help you identify the context under which the category exists or operates. Specific differences between incidents aids the clarification of boundaries and the relationships or links that exist between categories.

As this process proceeds you will eventually discover that you no longer are identifying new properties or categories and that the relationship between categories begins to crystallize – saturation has been reached. No longer are you discovering major anomalies in your categories, and modifications are more in terms of clarifying the relationships which link the categories and constructs together. When you have reached this stage, it is likely that you will be able to write a theory that is dense and capable of describing the basic social processes involved in the area under study. However, it is important to compare the various categories for underlying similarities which will allow you to reduce any duplication of properties or categories before you write the theory.

THEORETICAL SAMPLING

Theoretical sampling is the term used to describe the manner in which data sources are identified and selected for inclusion in a study and is integrally linked with the constant comparative method of data analysis. Initial decisions about sampling are based upon general understanding of the area under investigation. This initial decision is the only decision that you can pre-plan, since the selection of all other data sources is controlled by the emerging theory. Unlike other forms of research, such as the experimental or survey design, you are unable to identify the size and characteristics of the sample at the outset of the study. In a grounded theory design, you are only able to identify the sample, retrospectively, once the theory has been generated.

Individuals, groups, or situations, are selected to provide comparison data. Theoretical sampling can either attempt to minimize or maximize the differences between the comparisons being made. By minimizing differences, you can collect data which can assist you in identifying the basic properties of categories and the specific conditions under which they exist. Furthermore, minimizing differences can also assist you in identifying those fundamental ways in which categories vary. Maximizing differences between data sources increases the chance of identifying different properties of the categories and finding those properties which are most stable.

MEMOS AND MEMO WRITING

Memos and memo writing when undertaking grounded theory research is the means by which you facilitate and record the analytical process. Memo writing is at the very centre of the grounded theory method. By recording thoughts, questions, and hypotheses in a permanent form you will find it is easier to track the development of categories, properties, theoretical constructs, the core category, and ultimately the theory. However, memo writing is much more than simple note taking.

Memo writing should start soon after the first data have been gathered and you have started to code and analyse the content. At first, memos may be rather superficial in nature but they will become more abstract as increasing amounts of codes, categories, and properties are discovered. The memos should be thought of as a tool to assist you in exploring the developing categories and the relationships between them. Memos are written by you and are intended for you. Unfortunately, this process can be time consuming and monotonous but it is essential to the development of theory.

For clarity, memos should be recorded on separate cards and not on the data source. Index cards are ideal, facilitate cross-referencing, are inexpensive, and easy to store. Furthermore, when recording memos, it is important that in addition to the memo, certain other information is noted so as to allow you to identify what prompted your thoughts, views, questions, or hypotheses. For example, the memo should be dated, titled by the categories to which it refers, and referenced to the point that initiated your thinking. Figure 14.2 illustrates these points and gives an example of a memo written at an early stage of analysis based on the data contained in Fig. 14.1.

12/05/90   Professional Empowerment

Source: John Brown Interview 10/05/90 page 3

A number of words and phrases seem to link together these include *getting influence, credibility, taking the initiative*. I wonder how other professions see nursing research. Is nursing research seen as a way of winning back power lost as a result of organisational change?

Fig. 14.2 Index card illustrating memo writing.

Figure 14.2 illustrates that memos need not be long. However, it is important that they are recorded immediately, when thoughts are still clear. Hence always keep some index cards near at hand and record memos as and when thoughts occur. You will often find that this can be at unexpected times and not just when you are working with data.

SORTING

Having accumulated a large number of memos, it is then necessary to sort them so as to facilitate the development of your theory. Initial memos, which focus on substantive codes, can be sorted so as to enable you to identify categories and their properties within the data. When adequate numbers of memos relating to categories have been written and are sorted, it is likely that a core category and basic social processes can be identified. Hence, sorting is seen as a means of achieving higher levels of abstraction.

When sorting, it is advisable to start by ordering memo cards by category. All memos relating to one category can then be compared for the existence of consistency. When reading through the sorted memos, frequent cross-reference to other categories may indicate that it is possible to reduce these into one category at a higher level of abstraction. Any anomalies discovered may suggest the need to develop another category or at least gather further data so as to explain the differences.

USING LITERATURE

When conducting research which attempts to test existing theory, literature is used to place the research in context, describe its significance, identify variables and address issues of method, instrumentation, subjects, and setting. Literature is consulted prior to the study so as to identify the hypotheses under examination. Although previous published research may be used to compare or contrast findings in the 'discussion' section, the literature is predominantly accessed, reviewed, and critiqued prior to commencement of the study.

A research study that uses a grounded theory design uses literature in a significantly different way. First, an initial literature search can provide evidence that little is known about the subject under study, thus supporting the need for research and, more specifically, the appropriateness of a grounded theory approach. Second, an in-depth critique of literature prior to data collection and analysis should *not* be undertaken since this may provide you with a framework which includes categories that are inappropriate or incomplete. Third, literature should be treated simply as another data source. That is, it should be examined, coded, analysed, and have memos written about it. Finally, access to literature should be ongoing. Concepts reported in published material can be examined at various stages throughout the duration of the study and compared with those developing in your theory. Such an approach is particularly useful when addressing issues of reliability, validity, and generalization. The existing literature can thus be used to support the developing theory.

THEORY WRITING

Theory writing is an integral part of the grounded theory method and can be thought of as a natural extension of the memo writing process. As categories are discovered then saturated, and theoretical constructs are proposed and evaluated, memos will concurrently become more abstract. By examining these abstract memos, the developing theory can be identified. Hence, writing the theory is not a deliberate and separate act but an ongoing process. Nevertheless, when writing the theory, a number of points must be considered.

First, the theory should describe the underlying basic social-psychological process which accounts for the majority of variation in the data gathered.

Second, you will have been working with the data for a considerable period of time. What seems perfectly clear to you may not be as easily comprehended by colleagues. To a certain extent, this is guarded against by constantly taking your developing theory back to those who are providing data. However, peer review is a useful way of checking that the theory is understandable and not open to misinterpretation.

Third, is the theory dense? It is essential that you examine your theory and assure yourself that all categories are saturated and that they are all connected via constructs in a meaningful way. Furthermore, it is necessary that conditions under which categories exist or operate are well defined, described, and supported by sufficient evidence from the data.

Fourth, the theory presented must be linked to existing knowledge. If you have used existing literature and documentary sources during the process of theory development this should not present a problem. However, if discrepancies between the existing literature and the newly developed theory remain, they must be explored and explained.

Finally, a well written grounded theory must be testable. That is, hypotheses (sometimes referred to as propositions) should be clearly stated. By stating hypotheses you will provide direction for subsequent investigation. However, more importantly to those who provided the data, hypotheses should offer new insight into the practice, situation, or event under study.

CONCLUSIONS

The grounded theory approach is a means of identifying the basic social psychological processes involved in the situation under study and as a result can be considered as a powerful means of developing nursing's knowledge base. By using this method, theory evolves from nursing practice, consequently it is likely that it is directly relevant to the clinician thus offering greater understanding of everyday care. In conclusion, if you believe, as does the author, that understanding is necessary for the provision of high quality care, then research using the grounded theory approach has much to offer the nursing profession.

REFERENCES

Aamodt A.M. (1982) Examining Ethnography for Nurse Researchers. *Western Journal Of Nursing Research*, **4**: 2, 209–21.

Benoliel J.Q. (1967) *The nurse and the dying patient*. Macmillan, New York.

Chapman C. (1989) Research for actions: the way forward, *Senior Nurse*, **9** (6), 16–18.

Corbin J. (1986) Qualitative data analysis for grounded theory. In *From practice to grounded theory – qualitative research in nursing*, (Eds. W.C. Chenitz & J.M. Swanson). Addison-Wesley, Menlo Park, CA.

Field P.A. & Morse J.M. (1985) *Nursing Research the application of qualitative approaches*. Chapman and Hall, London.

Glaser B.G. & Strauss A.L. (1967) *The discovery of grounded theory*. Aldine Publishing Company, New York.

Glaser B.G. (1978) *Theoretical Sensitivity*. Sociology Press, Mill Valley, CA.

Goodwin L.D. & Goodwin W.L. (1984) Qualitative vs Quantitative Research or Qualitative and Quantitative Research? *Nursing Research*. **33**: 6, 378–80.

Hinds P.S., Scandrett-Hibden S. & McAulay L.S. (1990) Further assessment of a method to estimate reliability and validity of qualitative research findings. *Journal of Advanced Nursing*. **15**: 4, 430–5.

Luker K.A. & Chalmers K.I. (1989) The referral process in health visiting. *International Journal of Nursing Studies*. **26**: 2, 173–85.

Nusbaum J.G. & Chenitz W.C. (1990) A grounded theory study of the informed consent process for pharmacologic research. *Western Journal of Nursing Research*. **12**: 2, 215–28.

Omery A. (1987) Qualitative research designs in the critical care setting: Review and application. *Heart & Lung*. **16**: 4, 432–6.

Stern P.N. (1985) Using grounded theory method in nursing research. In *Qualitative Research Methods In Nursing*. (Ed. by M.M. Leininger). Grune & Stratton, Orlando.

Strauss A.L. (1987) *Qualitative analysis for social scientists*. Cambridge University Press, Cambridge.

Chapter 15
Quantitative Research
Diana E. Carter

INTRODUCTION

For many years the quantitative approach was the predominantly used method of scientific investigation in nursing, and proponents of this approach argue that it provides a more objective knowledge base to guide practice than does the qualitative approach. However, given the complexity of many of the phenomena of interest to nurses, this aspect of the quantitative–qualitative debate has waned in recent years and there is now a general recognition that each approach can make a valuable contribution to the investigation of phenomena significant to nursing.

Clearly, the precise research approach adopted depends on several factors including the nature of the phenomena to be investigated, the aim of the research, and the state of existing knowledge. For the researcher who is trying to achieve understanding of life experiences and give them meaning, a qualitative approach is appropriate (see Chapter 13). Dewis (1989), for example, used a qualitative approach in her study of spinal cord injured adolescents and young adults. She argued that such an approach was necessary because of the degree of absence of specific previous research related to the research questions and because it allowed the examination of the meaning of the body changes resulting from spinal cord injury from the perspective of the young people who had themselves sustained the injury.

Where the collection of more numerically and measurable information is a priority, a quantitative approach is called for. Such an approach can be seen in the comparative analysis of patients' and nurses' perceptions about nursing activities in a postpartum unit carried out by Morales-Mann (1989). Questionnaires in which patients and nurses were asked to rate the importance of nursing activities on a scale of 1 to 5 (not at all important to very important) provided numerical data and facilitated measurement of the importance assigned to various activities by these two groups.

Today, many studies use a combination of approaches and the area of nurse–patient interaction is just one example of this. Many of the early studies of nurse–patient interaction involved activity analyses which were produced on quantitative data – that is, the amount of time nurses spent carrying out various tasks or activities. The qualitative aspects of the interactions were ignored. However, it is now recognized that as communication is central to nursing then it is likely that the quality of the interactions will in some way be related to the overall quality of the care given to patients.

This type of combined approach was employed by Macleod Clark (1983) in an investigation of nurse-patient verbal interaction on surgical wards. Data were collected using audio- and video-tape recordings, observation schedules, and field notes. As a result, Macleod Clark was able to measure (quantify) the length of interactions between nurses and patients, and the total time nurses spent interacting with patients during two-hour sessions. She also analysed the interactions in terms of whether the nurses used encouraging or discouraging verbal strategies, thereby describing some qualitative aspects of nurse–patient interactions.

WHAT IS QUANTITATIVE RESEARCH?

Burns and Grove (1987) define quantitative research as 'a formal, objective, systematic process in which numerical data are utilized to obtain information about the world'. They point out that it is a research method which is used to 'describe, test relationships and examine cause-and-effect relationships', and that sometimes referred to as the traditional research process, it is regarded as being the acceptable method for developing a science.

These sentiments are echoed by Haase and Myers (1988) who associate the quantitative approach with the empirical–analytic paradigm and an approach which has laid claim to the term 'the' scientific method. The purpose of science is to describe, explain and to predict natural and social phenomena. Empirical knowledge, which is objective, verifiable, and quantifiable has, for many years, been regarded as being synonymous with science.

The quantitative approach emerged from the branch of philosophy known as *logical positivism*, which was founded on the belief that the world could be viewed as a machine, and that the task of science was to discover the laws by which the machine operated. Having discovered these laws and learned about them, the achievement of perfect predictability was seen as a natural follow-on. The means of understanding the world can be seen in the emphasis that was placed on the measurement and quantification of observable data.

TYPES OF QUANTITATIVE RESEARCH

Quantitative research includes descriptive, correlational, quasi-experimental, and experimental research.

Descriptive research

Descriptive research – as the name implies – is intended to describe the characteristics of particular individuals, groups, or situations. You can use this type of quantitative research to determine the frequency with which a particular variable occurs or is associated with another variable. Instruments used to obtain data in descriptive studies include interviews, questionnaires, and observation schedules.

Interviews

Interviews vary in the degree to which they are structured. Quantitative research calls for what is known as a 'structured interview' in which an interview schedule is used, each respondent being asked the same questions in the same order. The schedule can consist either of open-ended questions or closed-ended (fixed alternative) questions. For example, as part of a study you might be interested in finding out why ex-smokers gave up the habit, and decide to ask an open-ended question: 'Why did you decide to stop smoking?'. Once you had collected all your data it would then be necessary to develop categories and assign the open-ended responses to those categories so that tabulations could then be made. Alternatively, a closed-ended question could be used so that each respondent has to choose the most appropriate answer from a limited number of alternatives. For example: 'What was the main reason why you stopped smoking? Was it: (a) because you were worried about the effects of smoking on your health; (b) for financial reasons: (c) because you were advised by your doctor to stop; (d) because of pressure to do so by family members and/or friends?' It is then an easy matter to tabulate the number of responses to each alternative in order to gain some understanding of why the sample as a whole decided to stop smoking. (Interviews as a method of data collection are discussed more fully in Chapter 22.)

Questionnaires

Questionnaires are designed to elicit information through the written responses of subjects. As with the structured interview, questions can be either open-ended, requiring a written response from subjects, or closed-ended, where the response options have been previously selected by the researcher. The data collected are handled in the same way as interview data, with the number of responses in each category being tabulated. (Further discussion on the use of questionnaires can be found in Chapter 23.)

Observation

Observation is most commonly used in qualitative research, but quantitative research also makes use of observation techniques to produce numerical data. Structured observation uses a previously developed mutually exclusive category system so that behaviours or events being observed can be organized and structured. Observers may also make use of *checklists* and *rating scales*. Checklists are used to indicate whether or not a particular behaviour or event occurred and the number of times it was observed to occur, while rating scales allow the observer to rate the behaviour or event on a scale, thus providing more information than the dichotomous data from checklists which simply indicate whether or not it occurred. (Chapter 24 gives more information on observation as a method of data collection.)

Correlational research

In this type of quantitative research, the aim is to systematically investigate and explain the nature of relationships between variables in the real world.

Experimental research and quasi-experimental research

Experimental research is the most appropriate for testing cause-and-effect relationships, and it is considered to be the most powerful quantitative method because of the rigorous control of variables. Quasi-experimental studies are not quite so powerful in that they lack the intensity of control which is an inherent feature of experiments. (Experimental research is further discussed in Chapter 16.)

REALITY AND ITS MEASUREMENT

From the quantitative perspective, the world is seen as stable and predictable, and the researcher believes that 'truth' is absolute and that there is one single reality that one can define by careful measurement. Hence, as Leddy and Pepper (1989) explain, numbers (for example, amount, position, time, location, etc.) are used to describe both humans and the universe in such a way as to quantify their properties. In order to achieve such quantification, precise measurement tools that will generate numerical data are called for. These data can then be subjected to statistical analysis (see Chapters 27 and 28) in order to reduce and organize them and determine significant relationships. As with logical positivism, 'truth' – according to the quantitative researcher – is to be discovered in common laws, principles and norms, and having discovered these it will then be possible to achieve the goal of quantitative research, which is generalizability. Generalization involves the application of trends or general tendencies (identified by studying a sample) to the population from which the research sample was drawn. However, caution must be exercised when making generalizations in that sound generalization requires the support of many studies (Burns & Grove 1987).

REDUCTIONISM

In quantitative research, the process for discovering reality is reductionistic – it is believed that knowledge of the whole can be gained through knowledge of the parts. The researcher aims to break the whole into parts that can be carefully examined, as can the relationships among the parts. The underlying assumption is that the whole is the sum of the parts and the parts organize the whole. For example, Stanton et al. (1984) investigated adjustments made by patients during the first six months after cardiac surgery. 'Adjustments' were broken down into 12 components and patients were asked to indicate on a four-point scale the extent of their adjustment (from 'a great extent' to 'not at all') in each instance. In this way, the researchers were able to examine and quantify the various areas of life-style adjustment made by the patients.

OBJECTIVITY

The quantitative researcher objectively distinguishes self from the subjects of the investigation, believing that boundaries must exist between them in order to ensure objectivity. Objectivity is achieved by the researcher endeavouring to remain detached from the study and trying to avoid influencing the study (including the subjects) with his own perceptions and values. Avoiding researcher involvement will help to guard against biasing the study towards these perceptions and values. (The qualitative researcher also strives to achieve objectivity but some of the methods of data collection used [for example, participant observation] can, by their very nature, sometimes allow subjectivity to enter into the research situation.) In quantitative research, the position is held that subjectivity (for example, values and feelings) cannot enter into the measurement of reality – human behaviour is held to be objective, purposeful and, providing a valid and reliable tool is used, measurable.

CONTROL

In order to increase the probability that findings accurately reflect the reality of the situation being studied, the study needs to be designed in such a way as to maximize the amount of control over the research situation and variables. Through control, the influence of extraneous variables, variables which are not being studied but which could influence the results of the study by interfering with the action of the ones being studied, is reduced.

The remainder of this chapter will discuss some of the mechanisms of control at the quantitative researcher's disposal.

Sampling

It has been suggested (Polit & Hungler 1987) that the characteristics of the participants in a study are the most common extraneous variables. Let us take the example of a study investigating the effect of a ward-based teaching programme on newly diagnosed diabetic patients' knowledge of their condition and its management. Such variables as age and educational level could function as extraneous variables. Both variables might be related to the outcome of interest, the patients' knowledge of their condition and its management, quite independently of the teaching programme. Thus their effects are extraneous.

What you would have to try to do here is to select a sample of subjects that is as representative as possible of the population being studied in terms of, among other things, age and educational level.

By using random sampling techniques, you can ensure the representativeness of the sample in that such techniques ensure that each member of the population has an equal chance of being included in the study. (More detail of sampling techniques can be found in Chapter 21.)

Randomization

According to Brink and Wood (1983), randomization is the only method of controlling all possible extraneous variables. Randomization is 'the process of assigning objects (subjects, treatments, etc.) to a group or condition in such a way that every object has an equal probability of being assigned to any particular condition' (Polit & Hungler 1987).

It is often thought (erroneously so), that randomization is relevant only in respect of experimental research where subjects are randomly assigned to various treatment and control groups. However, it is also very relevant in non-experimental research. For example, to investigate patients' attitudes towards information given to them during hospital stay, you might decide to use a series of written statements with which subjects are asked to agree or disagree. Ideally, you should ensure that the order of these statements is randomized so that, for example, there is no pre-determined pattern in terms of positive and negative statements which could unwittingly interfere with subjects' responses.

The Hawthorne effect

This is a psychological response in which subjects alter their behaviour because they are aware of their participation in a study. As the quantitative researcher is trying to measure reality, every effort must be made to avoid influencing subjects' responses. This can be achieved in a number of ways. For example, you may decide to give the subjects a simple explanation of the study but omit to advise them of the actual relationships you are interested in. Alternatively, where an experimental study is being conducted, provided their rights are not infringed, you might decide not to inform subjects as to whether they have been assigned to the treatment or the control group. (Chapter 4 contains a discussion on informed consent.)

Constancy of conditions

When conducting quantitative research, you need to ensure that the study design is such that the conditions inherent in the research are the same for all participants. This section will look briefly at three aspects – the research setting, control of input, and time factors.

The research setting

In the interest of achieving constancy, consideration needs to be given to the degree of control exerted over the actual research setting.

Let us return to the earlier example of an investigation into the effects of a teaching programme for newly diagnosed diabetic patients. If one subject were to be taught in a quiet side-room away from the main ward area while another underwent the same teaching programme at his bedside in the middle of a busy medical ward, although both may have been given the same information presented in the same manner, the environment in which this took place would be very different for each patient. A similar discrepancy could exist when their knowledge of their condition and its management was subsequently tested. If the environment in which this is carried out is not held constant then the outcome (that is, the patients' measured knowledge level) may not be so much a reflection of the actual teaching programme but more a reflection of the effects of the environmental conditions in which the teaching and testing were carried out.

In this particular example, it would not be too difficult to partially control the research setting by ensuring that the teaching and testing were carried out using the same environmental conditions for all – in a quiet side-room, for example.

Clearly, the more the research setting can be controlled, the more effective you will be in reducing the influence of extraneous environmental variables, and the more accurate will be the examination of the cause-and-effect relationships of the variables studied.

Control of input

Much nursing research is concerned with measuring the effects of specific nursing interventions and it is therefore important that control over these interventions is exercised. However, during the course of a study, many members of the health care team are likely to come into contact with the subjects who form the sample, and their uncontrolled, unmeasured input is likely to be different for each subject.

In some instances, the role of the subject's family and friends may influence the situation the researcher is trying to control. These types of input are often difficult to control. Input in the form of information given to the subjects about the study *is* within the researcher's control, and one should ensure that each subject receives identical information about, for example, the purpose of the study and the use that will be made of the data.

Time factors

Depending on the time of day, the subject may be more or less attentive to information being given. Responses to testing will also be influenced by whether this is carried out in the morning or in the afternoon. The timing of research activities, that is, data collection, in relation to other events may also be important. In all these examples you need to ensure constancy among the subjects.

CONCLUSION

Both the qualitative and quantitative approaches are concerned with the development of knowledge and there is a place for both as nursing strives to develop its own body of scientific knowledge. The qualitative approach is invaluable for the exploration of the subjective experiences of patients and nurses, while the quantitative approach facilitates the development of quantifiable information.

It is now recognized that there are many situations in nursing where both the qualitative and quantitative approaches can be used to advantage within a single study, each approach serving to complement the other and each generating different kinds of knowledge that will be useful in practice.

REFERENCES

Brink P.J. & Wood M.J. (1983) *Basic Steps in Planning Nursing Research, from Question to Proposal.* Wadsworth, California.

Burns N. & Grove S.K. (1987) *The Practice of Nursing Research: Conduct, Critique and Utilization.* W.B. Saunders, Philadelphia.

Dewis M.E. (1989) Spinal cord injured adolescents and young adults: the meaning of body changes. *Journal of Advanced Nursing* **4** (5), 389–96.

Haase J.E. & Myers S.T. (1988) Reconciling paradigm assumptions of qualitative and quantitative research. *Western Journal of Nursing Research* **10**: 128–37.

Leddy S. & Pepper J.M. (1989) *Conceptual Bases of Professional Nursing.* Lippincott, Philadelphia.

Macleod Clark J. (1983) An analysis of nurse-patient conversation on surgical wards. In *Nursing Research, Ten Studies in Patient Care* (Ed. by J.C. Wilson-Barnett) John Wiley, Chichester.

Morales-Mann E.T. (1989) Comparative analysis of the perceptions of patients and nurses about the importance of nursing activities in a postpartum unit. *Journal of Advanced Nursing,* **14**, 478–84.

Polit D. & Hungler B. (1987) *Nursing Research: Principles and Methods.* Lippincott, Philadelphia.

Stanton B.A., Jenkins C.D., Savageau J.A., Harken D.E. & Aucoin R. (1984) Perceived adequacy of patient education and fears and adjustments after cardiac surgery. *Heart and Lung,* **13** (5), 525–31.

Chapter 16
Experimental Research
Allan S. Presly

This chapter is not designed to enable you to carry out experimental research unaided, but is intended to familiarize you with the more common types of experimental design, so that accounts of research can be read more critically and with greater understanding. As the name implies, experimental design refers to the overall plan of any experimental research project. It is important to note the term design, as it emphasizes that all good research should have been planned or worked out in advance. This is to ensure, as far as possible, that the researcher, at the end of an experimental research project, can make a statement of the kind: 'The introduction of, or change in variable A (the independent variable) caused the change in B (the dependent variable)'. This will only be possible if the experimental design has ruled out the possibility that a variety of things other than A could have caused the change in B. That is, if it is claimed that it has been proved that drug A causes improvement in condition B, the research design has to be such that other possibilities such as better nursing care, bedrest, or better diet in hospital, have not caused the improvement. There is no single all-purpose experimental design. Many different ones have been proposed to tackle different sorts of problems, but they all have in common the fact that they are intended to help eliminate explanations of research findings other than the one in which the researcher is interested.

Three main types of design will be discussed. In the first of these, a comparison is made of two or more independent groups of subjects treated under different conditions. In the second type of design, repeated measurements are carried out on the same group of subjects, but under different conditions. In the third design, a single subject only is used, and the subject's response studied under different conditions.

COMPARISON OF INDEPENDENT GROUPS

Suppose that the researcher is interested in what causes the birth weight of babies to vary. Obviously, human beings vary naturally among themselves in all sorts of ways even when they come from very similar backgrounds. Birth weight is no exception to this. That is to say, most characteristics of human beings show a range of variation which, within certain limits, is considered normal. This could be said not only of physical factors such as height and weight, but also for psychological and social factors such as intelligence or sociability.

Sample averages

Suppose then that all the babies born in a large city in one year are examined and their birth weight recorded. The average birth weight of babies in that city might be calculated and found to be 3.2 kg. Checking all the babies' weights, or assessing all the members of any research population of interest, is often an impossible task. More often one would select a sample of the population and try to generalize on the basis of that. Thus, a random sample (see Chapter 5) of 50 babies born in the city in a given year could be selected and the average birth weight calculated again. A result very close to the result which would have been obtained from the whole population is likely to be obtained. If this exercise was to be repeated with a second random sample of 50, an average weight close to (but probably not identical to) the true average would be obtained. If this sampling of sets of 50 were repeated over and over again, the averages would not be exactly the same. If, however, the samples are truly random, the sample averages will tend to cluster, or be distributed, around the true average, some lower and some higher. This variation will be accepted as normal variation in average birth weights.

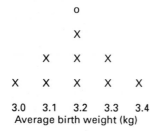

Fig. 16.1 Normal birth weight variation (example).

Figure 16.1 shows this normal variation in diagrammatic form. 'O' represents the true average birth weight of all the babies in the city. Each 'X' represents the average obtained from a random sample of 50 babies. It can be seen that in three cases the average was the same as in the total population; in three cases it was slightly above and in three cases slightly below. This is taken as a normal, acceptable variation in average birth weights. Any one of the random samples will give an average which will adequately represent the average of the whole population.

Forming an experimental hypothesis

If these findings were made public, it might be the case that one general practitioner might indicate that he and his health visitor colleagues have kept records of birth weights of babies in his practice. The average he gets is considerably lower (2.8 kg) than that found by the researcher and it looks as if it is outside the range of normal variation which has been established by the researcher's sampling procedure. What might be the explanation of this? A first step would be to compare the GP's sample with the one used by the researcher. Only if his sample could be considered a random sample from the total population can it be directly compared. It might then be discovered that this GP works in a rundown city area with poor housing conditions and amenities. If so, his sample must be regarded as a biased one and not properly representative of the whole population; thus, his average cannot be directly compared with that in the original research. Something other than normal variation due to sampling must be found to explain the difference.

There are a number of factors which might account for such a situation in a poor area; less money, poorer attendance for antenatal care, poorer nutrition, higher rates of smoking and alcohol use, and so on. Any of these variables might be the reason for the lower average birth weight, but from this information alone there is no way of knowing which. It could be any one of them or a combination of several (see Dowding 1982). One way to find out would be to design an experiment. Suppose it is hypothesized that poor nutrition in the mothers is the most likely cause of low birth weight. How can this be tested separately from the effects of all the other possible factors? One suggestion is a comparison of two groups of babies who are similar in all respects except for the nutritional state of their mothers. That is, by comparing two groups in this way, one can control for, or eliminate from consideration, all the variables except the ones of interest; birth weight, the dependent variable, and the nutritional state of the mothers, the independent variable. The research can then set out to discover what effect planned variation in the one (nutritional state) causes in the other (birth weight). More technically, the hypothesis is that if the nutritional state of pregnant mothers is improved, then the average birth weight of their babies will increase.

A comparison of two independent groups

A typical experimental design to test this hypothesis could be a comparison of independent groups.

(1)   A large group of pregnant mothers from a defined area would be selected. Ideally, it would be selected to be representative of all such mothers from that area. In practise, however, it is more likely to be drawn from a population readily available, such as those attending one large hospital rather than from several hospitals scattered across the area. The group would thus not be as representative as might be desirable. Members of the group would then be randomly allocated to two equal sub-groups, an experimental group and a control group.

(2)   The independent variable, the nutritional state of the mothers, must now be manipulated in one group and not in the other. That is, one new factor, and only one, is introduced into one group (the experimental group) which is not present in the other (the control group). It could be argued that the nutritional state of mothers might be improved through dietary advice and supervision by health visitors, and a programme of such advice to be given to only one group of mothers could be arranged. The details of the dietary advice programme would then be worked out: where, how often and in what form, and by whom the advice would be given. This will ensure that the procedure of the experiment will be the same for all subjects and that the experiment can, if necessary, be replicated exactly by someone else.

(3)   Birth weights would be recorded in the same way for each group, preferably by someone who is not aware of which group the mother falls into. The birth weights provide the experimental data and from them the average birth weight for each group can be calculated.

(4)   The question in this experiment is whether the average birth weight of the experimental group is greater than the average of the control group. However, suppose it is established that this is the case but only by a very small amount. It would be difficult to conclude with any certainty that the experiment has been a success since it is known (see Fig. 16.1) that average birth weights of different samples vary slightly anyway. Therefore the real question then becomes: 'Is the difference between the average birth weight of the experimental and control groups greater than would be expected if any two random samples from the same population are compared?' That is, is the difference apparently produced via the independent variable greater than would be expected by chance?

(5) It could clearly be difficult to reach agreement on this simply by inspecting the average weights, especially where differences were small. It is to help reach such agreement that some inferential statistical methods have been developed (see Chapter 28). These are specifically designed to assess what the normal variation in birth weight is likely to be and whether the experimental group average is outside this range.

(6) Suppose that the application of such statistics allows us to conclude that there is a significant difference between the experimental and control group averages, with the average weight of the experimental group being significantly higher. It can then reasonably be concluded that better nutrition in pregnant mothers will result in an increase in the average birth weight of babies.

The foregoing example is only one of many possible types of experimental design although it is probably the simplest and most commonly used. It is widely used to evaluate new drugs and new treatment procedures, and numerous examples can be found in almost any medical journal (see Rimer *et al.* 1987).

No-treatment and placebo control groups

In a typical drug trial, the experimental group might receive the new drug and the control group no treatment. This use of a no-treatment control, however, has been shown to be not entirely satisfactory. There is an ethical problem in withholding treatment, even temporarily, from those patients who might benefit from it, but there is also a scientific problem. The belief that one is being appropriately treated for a given condition even when one is not, has been shown in itself to produce some improvement. This alone might account for the difference between a group receiving genuine treatment and a group receiving none. This is commonly referred to as the 'placebo' effect. It has become the usual procedure in treatment research, therefore, to include a placebo control group rather than a no-treatment control group to compare with the experimental group. In drug research, a placebo might be a tablet made up in exactly the same form as the treatment tablet but containing a substance known to have no effect on the condition concerned. This would then have the effect of making the procedure much more similar between treatment and control groups than a treatment/no-treatment comparison.

Referring back to the previous example, it could be argued that the difference produced in the birth weights might not have been due to the dietary advice. It could be, for example, that through more regular contact with the health visitors, mothers were more likely to attend clinics, and that this factor, rather than improved nutrition, made the difference. It would, therefore, have been a better-designed experiment if, for example, the control group mothers received the same number of visits from health visitors but during these visits no dietary advice was given. This would then be a form of placebo rather than no-treatment control. It would be a better test of the value of dietary advice since it would eliminate another possible explanation of our result. An example of this type of design can be found in the study by Creason *et al.* (1989) on reducing levels of incontinence. One group (experimental) received regular reminders about toileting; the second group (placebo) received the same amount of additional social contact, but no such reminder; the third group (no treatment) continued under the same conditions as before.

'Blind' assessment

In this and other types of research design, it has also proved to be the case that those assessing the effects of treatment can be influenced by knowing whether a patient was receiving the real treatment as opposed to the placebo. There will naturally be a greater inclination to see improvement in those in the experimental (treatment) group and so possibly to exaggerate the overall differences between the groups. It has thus become common practice that the assessors are not made aware of which group a patient belongs to, a procedure known as a 'blind'.

Theoretically, there is no limit to the number of groups which can be included in an experiment. One might perhaps have three randomly selected groups in a drug evaluation experiment, one treated with a new drug, one with a placebo, and one with a drug previously found to be helpful for the condition being studied. In this case, the new treatment must prove itself superior not only to the placebo, the 'expectation-of-treatment' effect, but also to the existing remedy. Again, there is no reason why two new procedures or treatments cannot be evaluated at once, for example, two new teaching methods versus an existing one, two different types of dietary advice, or two or more doses of a new drug against a placebo. Provided that groups are selected at random and the only procedural difference among the groups is in the level of the independent variable, type or dose of drug, type of dietary advice or teaching method, any number of groups can be included in this research design.

REPEATED MEASURES

The comparison of independent, randomly selected groups does have one major disadvantage. It may require a larger number of possible subjects than are readily available in the time required. One alternative, therefore, is to use what is known as a 'repeated measures' design. In this design, both procedures or treatments are given to the same sample in succession rather than separately to two different samples. At first sight this design appears to have considerable advantages: there is an obvious saving in the number of subjects required since the same group is used twice, or more often if necessary. Also, random sampling of independent groups will result in some, usually slight, differences between the samples which might affect the outcome of the experiment. This is obviously ruled out in a repeated measures design, as the sample used for each treatment is identical. However, this design has one major disadvantage. The effect of the second treatment or procedure may be influenced by the fact that the subjects have already undergone the first. There may be a carry-over effect in that by the time they received the second treatment, the sample of subjects is not exactly the same as the one which received the first.

Cross-over design

Another design which was developed to try to cancel out the effects of any carry-over is known as a 'cross-over' design where half the subjects, Group A, will receive Treatment I followed by Treatment II, and the other half, Group B, Treatment II followed by Treatment I. This does not eliminate the carry-over effect, but it may be reduced. It can be argued that any difference that may then be found between Group A and Group B cannot be put down to the fact that Treatment II always follows Treatment I or vice versa. Although this design is still commonly used, it is now known that it does not reduce the effects of carry-over as much as was once thought. Considerable caution should thus be used in interpreting any results from such an experiment.

An example of a repeated-measures design with cross-over is to be found in the article by Campbell (1989) where a comparison was made of the effectiveness of two types of milk in treating infant colic. Figure 16.2 shows the design of this experiment.

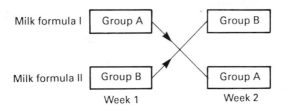

Fig. 16.2 Repeated-measures design with cross-over.

A group of babies with severe colic was selected. They were randomly allocated to two groups, A and B. Before the experiment began, an initial assessment of the degree of colic was made over a one-week period. This is called a baseline. It is an essential element in any experimental design as it represents accurately the situation existing before any change is introduced. Group A then received milk formula I for 1 week followed by milk formula II for a further week. Group B received formula II followed by formula I. The degree and frequency of colic was assessed by the mothers at regular intervals.

If all the babies had received formula I followed by formula II, and if formula I had apparently proved to be superior, that conclusion would have been open to the criticism that it was simply the fact that formula I was tried first which explained the outcome. By giving half the babies formula I first and the others formula II first, this criticism is apparently overcome. This supposed solution to the problem of order and carry-over effects is known as counterbalancing. Even with counterbalancing, however, the repeated measures design still has problems concerning the applicability of conventional statistical methods. Also, as noted earlier, the capacity of the cross-over variation to eliminate carry-over effects remains in some doubt.

This experiment by Campbell (1989) also provides an example of 'blind' assessment, referred to earlier. The milks were packaged in identical coded tins, and the code was not made known until the end of the experiment. Thus the mother's assessment could not have been influenced by knowing which formula her baby was receiving at any given time.

SINGLE-SUBJECT DESIGN

The third type of experimental research design is usually referred to as 'single-subject' or 'single-case' design. As the name implies, this design uses only one subject who is exposed to the different treatments or experimental conditions in sequence. One of the arguments put forward in favour of this design is that the traditional method of comparing average scores of independently selected groups may give little useful information about how any individual in those groups may respond or how any similar individual, as opposed to a similar group, will respond in the future. The average results may not in fact fit any one subject very well. It is argued, therefore, that if the experimental process is applied to one individual, one will at least get accurate information about that single individual which may be more useful than group averages, and it should still be possible to generalize to some extent to other similar individuals. Clearly, however, there will be objections similar to those of the use of repeated measures on the same sample with regard to sequence and carry-over effects. It is also arguable to what extent a sample of one individual can be representative of any group or population. Most research theory follows the argument that the larger the sample which can be assessed, the more representative it is likely to be and therefore the more widely the results can be generalized.

Typically, in a single-subject design, the subject will be studied first under baseline conditions, the conditions which prevailed before any experimental change was made. During this period, all the relevant variables will be measured, and in some ways, this phase can be compared to a no-treatment condition in group research. Following the baseline period, one new factor is then introduced, the independent variable, and the effect on the selected dependent variable

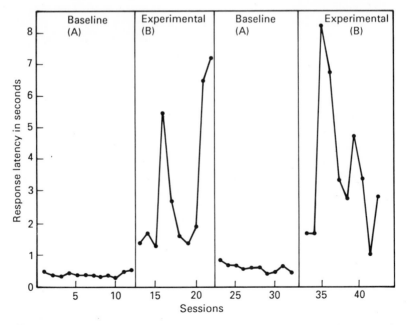

Fig. 16.3   The latency of the self-injurious behaviour plotted for each session of one trial for all conditions.

assessed. Provided the introduction of this factor is the only change, and that conditions are otherwise identical to the baseline, then it is argued that the change in the independent variable caused the change in the dependent variable.

An example of this design is shown in the experiment by Jones and Baker (1988) which is outlined in Fig. 16.3.

This experiment was designed to assess the effectiveness of a method of reducing self-injurious behaviour in a 9-year-old boy with a severe mental handicap. The problem behaviour in this case was the repeated striking of the side of his head with the palm of his hand at a rate in excess of 60 per minute. As a result, a restraining arm splint had to be used much of the time. In the baseline condition (A) the splint was removed. The dependent variable was the time from removal of the experimenter's restraining hand to the subject striking his head (response-latency). In the experimental condition (B), on removal of the splint, the boy was physically prompted to place a block in a box. This response was immediately rewarded and the hand again restrained by the experimenter. The experimenter's hand was then removed again and the response-latency recorded. Following this phase, a return-to-baseline (A) phase was carried out, followed by a further experimental phase. This repetition of the AB sequence helps to strengthen any overall conclusion from the experiment.

It can be clearly seen from Fig. 16.3, that in the experimental phase, the response-latency was much greater. That is, a considerably longer period elapsed before the boy started hitting his head. It was therefore concluded that the reinforced activity (placing the blocks) resulted in delaying the onset of subsequent self-injurious behaviour and thus in an overall reduction in the frequency of the behaviour. A causal connection was thus established between the independent variable (introduction of the reinforced activity) and the dependent variable (response-latency). It is not being claimed that this result applies to any other children with similar problems. This child was not selected as a sample of such children, but the experiment was carried out so that this one child's behaviour became predictable. However, it cannot be denied that this single-case experiment may give clues to what is more than likely to happen in similar circumstances with similar children.

The three basic experimental designs, comparison of independent groups, repeated measures (same subjects), and single-case, have been described. All have their advantages and disadvantages. Which type applies when any particular research question arises is not an easy matter and expert advice should always be sought before such a decision is made. Although the purpose of these basic experimental designs, and of many variations not mentioned here, is to allow clear-cut conclusions to be drawn, it must be said that the best-planned research will answer some questions, but will raise at least as many more that require further research. That is how science progresses.

REFERENCES

Campbell J. (1989) Dietary treatment of infant colic: a double-blind study. *Journal of the Royal College of General Practitioners*, **39**, 11–14.

Creason N.S., Grybowski J, Burgener S., Whippo C., Yeo S. & Richardson B. (1989) Prompted voiding therapy for urinary incontinence in aged female nursing-home residents. *Journal of Advanced Nursing* **14**, 120–6.

Dowding V.M. (1982) Distributions of birth-weights in seven Dublin Maternity Units. *British Medical Journal*, **284**, 1901–4.

Jones S. & Baker L. (1988) The differential reinforcement of incompatible responses in the reduction of self-injurious behaviour: a pilot study. *Behavioural Psychotherapy*, **16**, 323–8.

Rimer B., Levy M., Keintz M., Fox L., Engstrom P. & MacElwee N. (1987) Enhancing cancer pain control regimens through patient education. *Patient Education and Counselling*, **10**, 267–77.

Chapter 17
Action Research
Christine Webb

Action research is a relatively new approach in nursing but is rapidly attracting considerable interest because it is so highly suited to the kind of problem-solving and evaluation research which the profession needs. As well as being very similar in its methods to the stages of the nursing process, action research has parallels with other current trends within nursing. Nursing development units are being set up so that practitioners can implement and monitor research-based care and try to narrow the theory–practice gap. Action research also attempts to close the gap between the theory and practice of research, and to help participants to learn about doing research. The role of the researchers in action research is also to assist practitioners to take control of and change their own work. This parallels moves for nurses into patient/client advocate roles, empowering people to have more autonomy and control over their own health care.

This chapter will discuss these issues in greater detail, show what action research is, how the approach has come into being, and detail some action research projects in nursing.

WHAT IS ACTION RESEARCH?

Action research is a way of doing research and working on solving a problem at the same time. Researcher and participants work together to analyse the situation they wish to change: this may include doing some baseline measures using questionnaires, observation, or other research methods. After this assessment they can then plan the desired change, set their objectives, and decide how to bring about the change. While they are putting their plans into action, they continue to monitor progress, changing their plans if this is judged appropriate. At the completion of the change process, they will make a final assessment and draw conclusions, perhaps writing a report on the project for themselves and/or others.

Action research, in the view of Susman and Evered (1978), establishes the conditions for the development of others, and serves as a model of how to act in unpredictable situations. Through the use of interpersonal and problem-solving skills, action research becomes an 'enabling science' which focuses on the future and on planned outcomes.

According to Smith (1986), 'action research, as the name implies, is a process containing both investigation and the use of its findings'. She used an action research approach in a hospital for the care of elderly people to facilitate changes which would improve the quality of life for patients. Action research was chosen for this project because it places emphasis on the developmental aspects of research and can cope with the resistance which is often encountered when changes are introduced. Results are fed back into the change process while the

155

research is on-going, and the participating nurses are involved in the research alongside the research team. By being so closely involved in the study, the researchers are able to gain deep understanding of the setting and put forward realistic plans for change (Smith 1986).

Lauri (1982) introduced the nursing process in Finland using action research. She sees the role of the researcher as that of co-ordinator and consultant, and action research as an attempt to 'motivate the workers into developing the activity and into direct application of the results in practical work'. This is done mainly through consultation and work guidance, although education and group work may also be features.

Sandow (1979) used action research in an intervention study in which she acted as a resource-person to groups of parents of handicapped children and evaluated the outcomes. Sandow is not a nurse, but both her subject matter and methods were similar to those of Smith and Lauri. Sandow sees action research as offering 'a bridge between pure and applied research'. There are at least two participants – the practitioner/evaluator, and the recipient of the service, who is both 'subject' and 'client'.

Carr and Kemmis (1986) write about the use of action research in education but, if 'nursing' were to be substituted for 'education', what they write would be equally applicable to nursing. They state that professions have three distinctive features. Firstly, their work is based on theoretical knowledge and research. Secondly, they have 'an overriding commitment to the well-being of their clients'. Thirdly, members of a profession make independent judgements about how to act in particular situations.

Action research incorporates all three of these features: it provides a method for improving practice based on research organized by professionals, it takes a critical view of existing practice, and it provides a theoretical basis for professional decisions. In describing the role of the teacher-researcher in action research, Carr and Kemmis accurately portray the role of the nurse-researcher too.

Action research in facilitating change

What these definitions have in common is an emphasis on action research as a method of facilitating change through involving and motivating participants in a given project. Involvement is crucial for the researcher too, for it allows her to gain a much deeper understanding of the setting and the change processes than she would otherwise have. In other words, both sides in the research encounter stand to benefit. Participants are helped to implement the changes they desire and at the same time learn about how to do research, while the researcher also extends her knowledge and experience of the process of research and learns about the particular area being studied.

Contained within these definitions are clues about why the action research approach has been developed and what its origins are. These points will be dealt with in more detail in the following section because they lead on to a discussion of the particular methods used in action research projects, and to what makes action research distinct from previously established approaches.

WHY ACTION RESEARCH?

Action research has evolved in the social sciences in recent decades in response to criticism of the more traditional quantitative and qualitative approaches. These are discussed in detail in Chapters 15 and 13 respectively, but it is necessary to outline some of their features here in order to explain how the critical approach of action research has come about.

Quantitative research

Quantitative research – sometimes called positivism – was the original approach adopted by natural scientists studying physics, chemistry, astronomy, biology, and so on. This approach relied on the observation of phenomena and their behaviour, whether these were stars, chemicals, animals, or subsystems of these, such as the renal or cardiovascular systems. The fundamental aim was to control natural events by being able to predict what would happen and then to intervene to change things (Allen 1985). For example, if a law can be established which shows that bacterium X requires certain conditions to live and reproduce, then intervening to alter these conditions will result in the death of the strain and the treatment or prevention of infection.

Positivist researchers claim that their research methods are objective. The researcher studies a particular subject without having any preconceptions or preferences about the outcome of the study, and without interfering in the natural course of the events. In this sense, natural science claims to be value-free in that the personal values of the scientist are irrelevant to the scientific study.

However, this description is superficial and in some ways a caricature of what has come to be called 'the scientific method'. It is impossible for anyone to separate themselves as a scientist from themselves as a human being, and therefore a scientist's personal values and preferences inevitably creep into the research process. For example, someone who has a first degree in microbiology might choose to do research into the prevention of disease or, equally, into the development of germ warfare. The choice will depend very much on personal beliefs and values about the kind of research which is morally justifiable, a choice which can have very little to do with 'objectivity'.

It is equally possible to show that beliefs and values enter into all stages of the research process, from decisions about which methods to use (for example whether experiments on animals will be used), right through to what level of statistical significance to choose as accepting or rejecting the research hypothesis.

Furthermore, positivist scientists are increasingly realising that their research does have an intrusive effect on the subject matter they are studying. It seems obvious, for example, that experimental psychologists studying rats will influence the rats' behaviour by they way they handle them. Rough handling will induce stress and alter biochemical measures of anxiety which may well have an effect on the findings.

Qualitative research

In response to these and other criticisms of quantitative science, qualitative workers have developed different methods which they claim are more suited to the different subject matter which social scientists study, namely human beings. This second approach has also been called 'interpretive' science because its goal is understanding rather than control. Qualitative social scientists aim to understand or interpret people's behaviour by learning how they themselves make sense of the world in which they live. Communication is the means whereby interpretive scientists come to share the same understandings as their subjects and arrive at a consensus interpretation of the meaning of events.

The 'ideal' form of interpretive study is anthropology, where anthropologists spend an extended period of time living among a group of people in order to understand their way of life. Classically, anthropologists studied a society different from their own, and lived there, learning its language, joining in its kinship, work, leisure, and ceremonial activities. These anthropologists knew they had truly understood the society under study when they could live like a 'native' in that society quite naturally and spontaneously without having to think about how to behave. Today it is perhaps more common for this type of method to be used to study a group in one's own society but the methods are basically the same, as is the end point and aim, of being able to understand by empathy and consensus how and why the people being studied behave as they do.

Like quantitative approaches, qualitative approaches have their limitations. In both approaches, the researcher is the 'expert' who chooses what and how to study, who has the knowledge and expertise, and who does research 'on' the subjects – whether these are rats, bacteria, or humans. In other words, the research relationship is a hierarchical power relationship, and research subjects give up their time and energy to take part in the research but receive little or nothing in return. Both types of research can therefore be described as exploiting their subjects.

Inequality between the researcher and those studied in both quantitative and qualitative approaches is also evident in the degree of 'exposure' each receives. Research subjects make themselves vulnerable by disclosing their activities and meanings, and sometimes their deepest and most personal secrets to researchers. Researchers' personal lives, beliefs and feelings, however, are left out of the research. This can add to the false 'objectivity' of research because readers who do not know about the researchers' personal views cannot judge the extent to which these have influenced their interpretations of the data.

Related to these inequalities are the different rewards which researchers and researched obtain from participating in the study. Research subjects often gain nothing, other than perhaps the gratification of having a researcher show an interest in them and take what they are saying seriously. Once the researcher has collected that data, however, nothing changes for the subjects – they are left with their problems and concerns, and life goes on much the same as before. The researcher, on the other hand, stands to gain a great deal in terms of career advancement, financial rewards, and an enhanced reputation from publishing the research report.

Another frequent limitation of both quantitative and qualitative approaches is their reliance on a single research method; this will necessarily produce data of limited validity. For example, if nurses are asked in a questionnaire about their practice, different findings may be obtained than from an observation study in which what they do is seen directly. If the topic of the research were health teaching of patients, it is likely that in the questionnaires the nurses would over-estimate the amount of teaching they do; the observation study, however, would allow such a discrepancy to be identified. Using a single method, whether it is quantitative or qualitative, will show the researcher only one side of the topic.

Using a variety of different methods – or triangulation – will give a more full, rounded and valid picture.

A further criticism of interpretive research is that it gives a false impression about reality, but in a different way from that of quantitative research. Whilst not claiming objectivity, it does give the impression that the basis of all human relationships is communication. Therefore if something goes wrong in social life, we can put it right by improving communications. While there may be something in this, it is very often the case that features that lie beyond communications are at the heart of the problem and it is misleading to imply that people can change their own situations fairly easily by improving communications. For example, the nurse–doctor relationship is based on differences in power which can lead to doctors telling nurses to mislead or lie to patients about their diagnosis. Nurses are often afraid to 'disobey' doctors in this respect, and no amount of attempts to improve nurse–doctor communications may be able to persuade some doctors not to behave in this way. Nurses are not able to make fundamental changes in this aspect of their practice by improving communications because the underlying power structures which have been in place for centuries remain.

Critical science

In response to these and other criticisms and limitations of both quantitative and qualitative approaches (Allen 1985, Webb 1989), a third approach called critical science has emerged. Allen states that, 'the fundamental goal of critical science is to establish the conditions for open, unconstrained communication. This entails exposing hidden power imbalances'. He likens critical research to informed consent, in which all participants can act with autonomy and responsibility because obstacles which block or distort communication have been removed.

Critical science as an approach has therefore been developed to overcome problems and limitations with earlier quantitative approaches. Action research is one method of carrying out critical science, just as experiments are a quantitative method, and participant observation and unstructured interviews are qualitative methods. Having examined the origins of critical science and action research, it is now possible to look in more detail at how action research is carried out.

PERFORMING ACTION RESEARCH

Several writers have put forward schemes to illustrate the stages involved in carrying out action research, and it is easy to see how these mirror the problem-solving strategies which are also reflected in the nursing process. Towell and Harries (1979) describe a 'general model of the change process in project work', whose five major stages are illustrated in Fig. 17.1.

However, there are additional activities which run alongside and concurrently with these stages: these include seeking assistance, establishing a project committee, investigations to illuminate issues, choices by staff and working through their implications, and review of the changes introduced.

Whereas previous approaches to research have used a one-directional approach, moving from one stage to the next and so on to completion of the study, on-going monitoring, feedback to participants, and modifications to the innovation being introduced, are a crucial feature of action research.

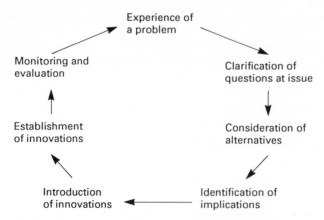

Fig. 17.1 The stages of action research.

Lauri (1982) emphasizes this constant reviewing and modification in her four-point list of the stages of action research:

(1) Preliminary diagnosis and the collection of baseline data;
(2) Processing the results with participants;
(3) Re-planning and re-implementation of the activity to be changed;
(4) Assessment of the changes and utilization of the results.

In summary, she writes that 'constant monitoring and evaluating of the activity is one of the leading principles of the action research.'

Hunt (1987) similarly drew attention to the cyclical nature of the action/evaluation process, feedback to participants as the study progresses, collaboration in setting and monitoring achievement of objectives, and use of group dynamics in carrying out the research.

Implicit in these descriptions of the action research process is that participants will be willing volunteers. They must want to examine their own practices and change them if deficiencies or better methods are identified. Otherwise, the action research will fail because collaboration will not be achieved between researcher and participants (Webb 1989). The starting point for action research is thus the recognition by workers of problems in their present working practices and a wish to change their activities (Lauri 1982).

Triangulation

A vital aspect of action research is its use of a variety of methods which give more valid data than a single method. This is called triangulation, as discussed earlier, and this is a term derived from surveying, where surveyors use a measuring instrument called a theodolite mounted on a tripod. However, triangulation does not mean the use of three methods together. What surveyors are doing when they take their readings is to measure a building or a road junction from a number of different angles in both the horizontal and vertical planes. These measurements then give them such a complete and detailed picture of the site that they can return to their drawing offices and construct scale diagrams and even models of it. This complete and full picture is what social researchers also aim for in using a triangulated approach. They might use several different methods to cross-check on data, for example, backing questionnaire data up with observations as already discussed. Or they might study more than one group of research subjects in different settings to compare their behaviour. Yet again, several different researchers might participate in the project, each bringing their own perspectives and skills to collecting and interpreting the data.

Methodological eclecticism

'Methodological eclecticism' is a technical term linked with triangulation by its rejection of the straitjacket of either quantitative or qualitative methods. Being eclectic means choosing freely from what is available according to one's preference. So a person with eclectic tastes in music might like Chopin, jazz, and 1960s music rather than sticking with one particular style. In action research, this free choice of different methods allows the advantages of some methods to offset the limitations of others, and enables one to 'have one's cake and eat it'!

Reflexivity

'Reflexivity' is another important concept within critical science and therefore also within action research. This term refers to the need for researchers to put themselves 'on the line' in their research reports in the same way that participants are made vulnerable by revealing their innermost thoughts and emotions. As well as making the research encounter a more equal one, and removing the exploitation which can be part of traditional approaches, researchers need to 'come clean' about themselves for other reasons. Readers of research reports can only make judgements about the quality of the research and the researcher's interpretations if they have access to all the data that went into the report. The beliefs and attitudes of researchers are part of this data and should be made available in the report.

Because action research is concerned with developing research methods as well as with introducing and evaluating changes in practice, researchers also need to write about the process of carrying out the project from their own point of view. Research methods textbooks can give the impression that doing research is like following a recipe, and that provided the instructions are followed, the product will turn out well. This is very misleading because in practice, research, just like cookery, seldom goes according to plan. The recipe may need to be varied because some of the ingredients may not be available. A cook can run out of margarine just as a researcher may not be able to obtain the sample originally planned. So changes and improvizations have to be made and these will affect the outcome of the cooking or the research. If research methods are to develop and people are to learn from others' successes and failures, researchers have a scientific obligation to 'tell it like it is'. They should be honest about how they did the research so that others may benefit and not feel inadequate if they have to deviate from their own research recipe for some reason.

A good tip when critically analysing a research report is to be suspicious if the report gives the impression that the study ran completely smoothly and no changes had to be made. Research is rarely so 'hygienic' and if the writer is hiding this, what else is also being kept from the reader?

If one were to search for one word to describe how action research is done, perhaps 'openness' would be the best one. Action research should be marked by an open attitude to the participants and the changes they wish to make in their work, to the research methods used, to making changes along the way, to investing the researcher's 'self' in the project, and to writing up the study in an honest and revealing manner.

ACTION RESEARCH IN PRACTICE

A look at three examples of nursing action research will illustrate how these underlying ideas are put into practice.

Putting research findings into practice

Hunt (1987) used action research in a project designed to assist a group of nurse-teachers to translate research findings into practice. Teachers and librarians from nine schools of nursing were invited to participate in the project, and in the first phase the librarians helped the teachers to carry out a literature search to identify research-based nursing practice literature. In phase two, evaluation and synthesis of the literature was carried out, using guidelines to standardize the critiques and develop the teachers' skills in this area. Subgroups of teachers worked on different topics, and in phase three groups (focusing on mouth care and on pre-operative fasting) attempted to translate their findings into practice.

The mouth care group prepared written summaries of their work and discussed these in workshops and study days with colleagues from both education and service areas. The procedure committee was also given a copy of the summary and teachers announced that this would form the basis of their teaching of learners after a certain date. Changing mouth care practice also involved liaising with the central sterile supplies department as well as the supplies department to curtail supplies of mouth care packs and substitute small toothbrushes.

The whole process took several years to run through, and even after this period of time some ward sisters did not use the guidelines although they had been involved in the workshops which discussed the changes. Hunt (1987) concludes that:

> 'this indicated the extent of the autonomy exercised by ward sisters in ignoring policy decisions and the lack of an effective management system to ensure that agreed practice changes were implemented and maintained.'

With regard to pre-operative fasting, the same process was gone through, albeit with slight variations. A similar lack of response on the part of some staff was felt by Hunt to reflect 'the traditional patient–professional relationship of passivity and control, in spite of the developing rhetoric' about patients' active participation in their own care.

Certain features of action research emerge clearly from Hunt's report, including the participation of teachers as research subjects in solving the practical problem of translating research findings into action. Evaluation was also continuous, in that reports on the three stages of the project are given. There is also a reflexive and critical discussion in the latter part of the article about the methods used, and the degree of success or failure they achieved. What seems to be missing is an account of the part played by the action researcher – presumably Hunt herself. It would have been fascinating and highly illuminating for later researchers to gain insight into the experiences of the researcher throughout the protracted process of trying to introduce change. What was the precise nature of her input to the project? How did she cope personally with the stress of her involvement over many years in a project that met with limited success? How did she attempt to overcome resistance?

Developing the nursing process

Lauri (1982) writes about her work as co-ordinator and consultant to a project in Finland whose goal was the development of the nursing process. She decided on an action research approach because 'its purpose is to solve practical problems and to be in direct contact with practical problem situations'. She identifies her role, as an outsider to the organization in which the work took place, as motivating the nurses into developing the nursing process and applying it directly in their practical work. Among the methods she used were educating nurses, work guidance, group work, literature reviews, consultation, and helping to develop nursing process documentation. She emphasizes the importance of agreement with participants on the objectives and content of the activities, and also on the responsibilities of the various participants. The investigator's task is seen as taking overall responsibility for the project if this is not done by someone from within the organization. Evaluation of her work was guided by the goal set at the outset, and a variety of questions were addressed, including:

(1) Has the action model based on the nursing process been achieved?
(2) Has it improved the nursing of the patient?
(3) Were any unexpected results achieved?
(4) Did any unexpected problems arise?

Lauri states the importance of collecting systematic information about developments in the various stages of the project, as well as about the reactions and attitudes of the nursing staff.

Unfortunately, she does not give the answers to these questions within her report and, like Hunt, does not discuss the details of her own role and experiences as researcher.

The action research project

Webb's report on her personal experiences of carrying out an action research project, on the other hand, does focus on these issues (Webb 1989). She spent three months working as a participant observer on her study ward, collecting baseline data using stress and ward learning environment questionnaires, measuring workload, and attempting some further measures. The aim in this initial period was to get to know the ward and its staff, to understand its methods and problems as an insider, and to build up credibility with staff in preparation for the subsequent action phase.

The conflicts of being closely involved in a ward where there were deep interpersonal conflicts are discussed. The strategies used – whether successful or not – to cope with ethical and practical dilemmas are described, and the writer's personal learning through the project are presented. Webb tells how difficult it can be not to take sides in a situation of conflict, and how this is made worse when, as a participant, a researcher becomes part of the conflict. Because she intended to act as a facilitator for the subsequent action phase of the project, Webb did not think it appropriate to take sides in a dispute because this could alienate participants. At the same time, she witnessed, and was on the receiving end of, difficult situations in which it was hard not to convey her feelings, and impossible not to be personally affected by the events.

To take one example, a discussion arose during ward report about a doctor having given confidential information to a patient's divorced wife when she had come to visit her ex-husband. The information concerned a diagnosis of cancer, which had not been given to the patient himself. Most nursing staff were angry about the doctor's action, felt that it was a breach of confidentiality, and that the doctor should not have behaved in this way. The ward sister, however, felt that it was up to the doctor to make his own decisions on the basis of his medical training, which she explained was longer and deeper than nursing training. Consequently she felt that it was not appropriate for nurses to challenge such a decision. Like most of the nurses present, Webb disagreed strongly with the ward sister's view, but felt that in the context of the project she (as a researcher) should be restrained in the way she expressed herself. It was more difficult when staff openly talked to the researcher about interpersonal problems on the ward. Webb tried to deal with these situations by using active listening techniques, and trying to get the nurses to explore how they could have acted differently to resolve the difficulties constructively.

Webb concludes that, despite the precarious nature of her negotiations through this phase of the project, action research is a powerful method for studying and implementing change in nursing research.

CONCLUSIONS

In summary, this chapter has attempted to show how action research is an approach which draws on the best of other approaches, and uses research to respond to the needs of those who are being studied as well as those of the researcher. This process brings out into the open many of the taken-for-granted assumptions of previous approaches. Issues of power, autonomy, ownership, and research purposes are placed on the agenda. However, action research cannot provide a ready answer to these dilemmas; as Light and Kleiber (1978) state, 'where each researcher draws her/his ethical and practical lines must be her/his own decision.' Nevertheless, they believe that action research leads to 'more human, more moral, and more perceptive field research.'

REFERENCES

Allen D.G. (1985) Nursing research and social control: alternative models of science that emphasize understanding and emancipation. *Image: The Journal of Nursing Scholarship* XVII (2), 58–64.

Carr W. & Kemmis S. (1986) *Becoming Critical* Falmer Press, London.

Hunt M. (1987) The process of translating research findings into nursing practice. *Journal of Advanced Nursing*, **12** 101–10.

Lauri S. (1982) Development of the nursing process through action research. *Journal of Advanced Nursing*, **7** 301–7.

Light L. & Kleiber N. (1978) Interactive research in a health care setting. *Social Science and Medicine*, **12**, 193–8.

Sandow S. (1979) Action research and evaluation: can research and practice be successfully combined? *Child: Care, Health and Development*, **5** 211–23.

Smith G. (1986) Resistance to change in geriatric care. *International Journal of Nursing Studies*, **23** 1, 61–70.

Susman G. & Evered R. (1978) An assessment of the scientific merits of action research. *Administrative Science Quarterly*, **23**, 582–603.

Towell D. & Harries C. (1979) *Innovations in Patient Care. An Action Research Study of Change in a Psychiatric Hospital.* Croom Helm, London.

Webb C. (1989) Action research: philosophy, methods and personal experiences. *Journal of Advanced Nursing*, **14**, 403–10.

Chapter 18
Historical Research
Anne Marie Rafferty

Much has been written about the purpose of history and the function of the historian although little of it in the field of nursing. The exceptions to this are the introductory chapters to the edited collections of Davies (1980) and Maggs (1983) and two methodological studies from America (Allemang 1987 and Matejski 1986). There is as yet no comprehensive review of research in either American or British nursing history although a useful guide to the American literature is provided by Dzuback (1983). Like 'nursing', 'history' may be defined by its subject matter, methods, or institutions. The study of history can be defined as 'the attempt to recreate the significant features of the past on the basis of imperfect and fragmentary evidence' (Barraclough 1955), or 'the continuous interaction between the historian and his facts, an unending dialogue between the present and the past' (Carr 1970). Historiography, with which I shall be more concerned here, addresses the methods used in the study and writing of history.

In nursing research, historians are a minority group and only rarely is their subject incorporated into the curricula of educational institutions. The reasons for this 'marginialization' are not clear, although, in a world dominated by science and technology, historians share in a sense of depressed importance experienced by those whose work is located in the humanities. There are exceptions to this 'rule', notably the Diploma in Nursing that is validated by the University of London and which has always contained a 'history' component. The number of programmes that contain a history strand may increase with the expansion of higher education programmes in nursing. The first part of the chapter is directed towards a more general discussion of the ways in which historical research differs from the conduct of other forms of research, notably 'scientific' models.

The aim of the second part of the chapter is not to explain how to undertake historical research, but rather to describe the many factors which come to bear upon the historical research process in nursing. Throughout the chapter, 'historian' denotes historical researcher.

HISTORICAL AND SCIENTIFIC RESEARCH

Why historical research?

The poor representation of history in nurse education programmes is no reflection of its importance nor of the contribution history has made and could further make to nursing research and knowledge. History may be pursued for its own sake, as an intellectual training, or as a contextual guide to decision-making. It may also have implications for the solving of problems in which an understanding of the past is a necessary precuror to subsequent investigation. Direct lessons from history are difficult to identify since the events of the past might be considered unique. Nonetheless, the study of the past has much to contribute to our understanding of contemporary problems, human behaviour, and the forces driving social change (Marwick 1970).

Research is concerned with describing and explaining the relationship between variables; historical research is concerned not only with the 'what' and the 'why' of variables of the past but specifically with the timing and definition of problems. Historical research may be differentiated from other forms of research by the chronological nature of the question(s) being asked. For example, in attempting to identify the 'causes' of wound healing, an historical survey of past treatments may cast light on the mechanisms underlying changes in the theory and practice of wound care. The Hippocratic and Galenic medical theory of the fifth century BC to the second century AD, for example, maintained that suppuration and the production of so-called 'laudable pus' was an essential part of wound healing (Cartwright 1977). This reasoning contrasts vividly with current theory of wound care, the object of which is to prevent infection. The observation of changes in 'nursing' theory and practice over time does not confer the right to ridicule the thinking and practice of the past. What the historian through research seeks to understand is how such theory was determined, in addition to the factors which promoted and sustained its existence. The historian's function is not to judge, praise or condemn the actors and actions of the past, but to understand how they came into being and the forces which shaped their existence. To take a recent example in this country, if studying the origins of Project 2000, one of the major questions the historian would ask is why has Project 2000 apparently succeeded as a reform strategy where others seem to have failed? What have been the factors which have promoted such change? The merits of the case? Demographic pressures? The social, political, and economic environment? Changes in the administration of the health and social services, and educational provision? All of these, and if so were all equally important? Immediately, we are confronted with the problems of historical evaluation. What in historical terms counts as 'success' or 'failure'? How can we measure historical change? Which outcome variables should we consider? Whose view(s) should we take into account? Which sources should we use? How should we order our enquiry?

Perhaps the value of historical research in nursing can best be illustrated by an example which has provided a corrective to the historical record. This 'revisionist' approach is admirably illustrated by Baly's study of Florence Nightingale and the politics of the Nightingale Fund (Baly 1986). Much of the difficulty of assessing the contribution of Florence Nightingale to nursing reform derives from the fact that much of the writing has been biographical rather than historical. Baly steers a balanced but mould-breaking path between the two extremes of the uncritical and heroic-centered work of Cook (1913) and the 'anti-hero' account of Smith (1982) in her account of the fate and fortunes of the nurse training experiments at St Thomas's. Much of Baly's research is devoted to the exposure of a number of myths concerning the Nightingale School and its training methods. Contrary to popular wisdom, St Thomas's was not originally considered by Miss Nightingale as an ideal institution for the Nightingale School on account of its insalubrious location, and its matron, Mrs Wardroper, whose competence to supervise nurse training was doubted by Miss Nightingale. Furthermore, far from providing a codified scheme of instruction and a model of training ready for export, the training provided was haphazard, the 'wastage' rate high, and only modest numbers of well-educated women came forward to be inculcated with the 'new' spirit of reformed nursing. Diaries, for example, which were kept by the probationers for inspection by Miss Nightingale, indicated that most of the probationers' time on the wards was unsupervised and that the intellectual content of lectures was pitched deliberately low and required supplementary interpretation and coaching from the Home Sister (Baly 1986, p. 174). Up until 1871, 188 nurses were accepted for training of whom 126 completed training. Of those remaining, three died, seven resigned, and 52 were dismissed, either for misconduct or ill-health. At least 36 of the 'survivors' left nursing within two years. Baly has calculated that it was unlikely there were more than 50 St Thomas's trained nurses at work in hospitals after ten years of the scheme (Baly 1986, pp 57–61). She concludes her study with the contention that the main contribution of the Nightingale Fund lay in secularizing nursing earlier than otherwise would have been the case (Baly 1986, p. 202). Although the Fund was doubtless important in marketing nursing as an acceptable form of employment for non-religious women, it should be seen more as a catalyst rather than a prime mover of change. Far from being in the vanguard of the professionalizing changes associated with nurses' registration, the St Thomas's faction was one of its staunchest opponents. The reputation of St Thomas's for 'progressive' change and reform requires definition and qualification. Baly's account demonstrates the value of the critical spirit for historical and nursing research. These and related points are elaborated elsewhere (Dingwall *et al.* 1988).

NURSING HISTORY AND THEORIES OF CHANGE

Historical research helps us to understand the process of change, be it in methods used to treat pressure sores, or the introduction of new ways of organizing care. One of the first evaluation studies of team nursing, for example, was published in the late 1950s by a Canadian nurse (Jenkinson (1953). Where did the idea and method originate? Was it significant that this innovation was promoted by a nurse from North America? What was it about the organizational climate at the hospital in question (St George's, London) which favoured the introduction of new ideas? Was the then Matron, Muriel Powell, a crucial influence in supporting the change? In relation to nursing research, historical research can help us to understand more fully the factors which transform a 'good idea' into standard practice why some research findings are implemented and not others.

Historical research provides one way of investigating the dynamics and direction of change. The historian's own views, opinions and preconceptions (not to mention funding policy) may be crucial determinants of the question selected for study and the mode of investigation adopted. Individuals may be attracted to different disciplines, topics, and techniques in research for a variety of reasons, some of which may be very personal. In qualitative research, the researcher's belief-system may be taken for granted as intrinsic to the research process and even formally integrated into the fabric of the account and analysis (Reason & Rowan 1981). In scientific research, where such store is set by objectivity, the accent is on eliminating the influence of the investigator, although studies in the history and sociology of science confirm that researchers' values, personal histories, belief systems, and ambitions can and do impinge upon scientific research (Barnes & Shapin 1979).

The 'progress' of historical research in nursing

It may be tempting to view the changes of the past as somehow inevitable and as the fulfilment of progress, and much history has been written from this point of view. This assumes that the past is governed by law-like mechanisms and ignores the conflict and complexities of rival forces competing for power. Much of the recent research in the history of nursing rejects this view as failing to account for the tensions between historical agencies and the intricacies of power differentials which favour one set of conditions rather than another. The past as representing 'progress', while psychologically gratifying, prejudges the past, and forces it into a mould which empirical research may contradict. For example, although increases in nurses' pay in the United Kingdom have occurred since the introduction of the National Health Service, the fluctuating pattern of relativities suggests that the story of nurses pay has not been one of onward and upward (Gray 1989).

Social and socializing history

So what have been the characteristic features of historical research in nursing? I have reviewed some of the major trends in the writing of nursing history elsewhere and argued that nursing history has been used to serve a number of professional or 'professionalizing' ends (Rafferty 1991). The extract below, taken from a recent textbook on nursing research (Stinson & Kerr 1986, p. 30) illustrates this approach:

'Historical knowledge in nursing is needed to provide knowledge and understanding of the achievements and of the contribution to the profession as well as to the larger society by individual nurses and groups of nurses and about significant forces than have shaped the character of the profession. The essence of nursing and the nature of professional identity will be more directly understood as a result of studies undertaken within such contexts. For those entering the profession, learning about the achievements of nurse leaders and the progress of the profession over time can provide a basis for professional socialization as well as encouraging new initiatives in desired directions, but the history of nursing is a factor which should enter into the perspective of every nurse, and at all career stages.'

The authors seem both unconscious and untroubled by the 'ideological' character of these prescriptions. Objectives such as these would not be acceptable to all historians of nursing, particularly those of a critical social history persuasion.

It is arguable, if we define research as concerned with the generation of new and verifiable knowledge, that historical 'research' in nursing has a rather recent history. Much of the early writing in nursing history was more concerned with synthesizing and reinterpreting existing knowledge rather than producing new knowledge through fresh investigation. The use of previously unexploited primary evidence and the development of novel interpretations is arguably the function of historical research. Both characteristics have been exemplified in studies of British nursing since the early 1960s, of which Abel-Smith's (1960) study of nursing professional politics is the earliest. Davies' (1980) innovative edited collection of social scientific aspects of historical nursing research provided a focus for feminist and labour history interpretations of nursing history. Maggs (1978) was one of the first nurses to treat nursing history as a case-study in social history. Social history has arguably exerted the greatest influence upon the conduct of historical research in nursing. Social historians are interested in the contextual and structural conditions which influence living and working patterns of groups, and individuals. It borrows methodological tools and insights from related disciplines such as politics and economics, feminism, labour history, psychology, and anthropology and thus represents an eclectic and multifactorial approach to the study of the past. The number of researchers in nursing history is nonetheless small and virtually no one earns their living full time from such work.

THE METHODS OF HISTORY AND SCIENCE

Sharp distinctions between the arts, social science, and science may be difficult to sustain empirically, especially when the boundaries themselves are historically determined. Soffer (1988) has described the development of disciplinary boundaries in university education with particular reference to history. At a common sense level, historical and scientific research are often regarded as being situated at opposite extremes of the research continuum; 'science' claims that its authority relies on the production of disinterested knowledge, whereas history is more generally associated with interpretation. These stereotyped distinctions, however, ignore the reality of research for both groups of workers, and the flow of cognitive resources between the two: scientists are not immune to drawing upon intuition in designing their experiments, and historians may test hypotheses against the evidence. Differences may be of degree rather than of kind.

Truth and objectivity

Where historical and scientific research seem to differ is in the potential to establish cause and effect relationships between variables, to control and manipulate variables, and to intervene and predict their behaviour. But even here, scientists have no monopoly: historians also talk of 'causes' although the meaning and application of the term may be different. Stone (1972) in his discussion of the causes of the English Civil War, divides the causal factors into three chronological groups: long-term preconditions, medium-term precipitants, and short-term triggers. The provision of conclusive proof is not a feature of historical research, which cannot easily rank the importance of different factors. 'Causes' may be more readily conceived of in terms of necessary and sufficient conditions. The lack of opportunity to generalize from unique events may be a further differentiating factor for historians. The cultural and economic success of science has, however, encouraged other forms of intellectual enterprise to emulate their methods. The move towards a more quantitative approach in history is characteristic of this trend. Quantiative methods in the history of medicine have been reviewed by Porter and Wear (1988) and more generally by Denley and Hoplain (1987). History, as science, approaches the past as objective, empirical, and recoverable reality; capable of reconstruction as it once was. Such an approach may be traced to nineteenth century confidence in positivism, a philosophical movement which presupposed that truth was represented by observable phenomena and verifiable facts. Positivism exerted a significant influence upon science, social science, and history itself, and close affinities developed between 'scientific' and 'historical' forms of research, in which history was seen as reducible to a set of universal laws (Burrow 1966).

The dominance of positivistic and reductionist approaches to research has been difficult to break. Historians such as Elton (1967), who study the philosophy of history, have tried to turn the 'superiority' of science argument on its head by arguing that history might be considered closer to objectivity since the material studied by the historian has had an existence independent of the observer. Scientists by contrast, through their experiments, create an artificially constructed reality (Elton 1967). It is arguable that participation in this form of debate only serves to legitimize the status of natural science as the yardstick by which all other forms of research should be judged. All disciplines have to contend with questions of validity and standards of practice. Insofar as judgments of both may involve high levels of 'expert' knowledge and opinion, both history and science may rely upon the agreed judgements by the scholarly community of what constitutes quality and acceptable standards of research practice. Both may therefore be vulnerable to nuances in judgement which impinge upon assessments of validity. Elton's position on the objectivity of history would be rejected by commentators who support the view that 'history' has no independent existence outside the historian who has brought it into being (Carr 1970).

Discovery is often perceived as the prerogative of the scientist, while recovery is the concern of the historian. Both imply uncovering something which exists but which has hitherto been invisible. Yet even the scientist's capacity to reveal material essence may rely purely on inferential and indirect evidence – as illustrated by the work of particle physicists: particles such as quarks or charms have not been visualized, but their existence is inferred from assumptions and physical measurements. Whilst historians may have difficulty in ascertaining the authenticity of the material, neither science nor history can exclude the exercise of imagination or speculation from their repertoire of methods. So far, I have argued for the comparability rather than the contrast between history and science. These are easier to sustain when considering the overall aims and objectives of researchers in each. These should not obscure major differences in subject-matter and method.

THE RESEARCH PROCESS IN NURSING HISTORY

Sources and sampling

It may at this point be worthwhile considering the range of resources upon which the historian of nursing might draw in order to construct an account. First I shall discuss access and availability. While both historians and scientists may have to negotiate access to the research site through gate-keepers such as ethical committees, health service administrators, and keepers of manuscripts, the historian may have his work predetermined by virtue of the preservation or destruction of records. The potential to generate data anew rests with the scientist. The historian traversing unknown territory may have little idea of what if anything her sources, once located, will reveal.

Historical sources are subject to a particular set of regulations concerning access and closure which may be crucial determinants of the research which can be undertaken. The 'thirty year rule' closes access to public records for thirty years after the date of the last item in the file. Public may be defined as those deriving from organizations which are accountable to public bodies such as Parliament. All records of National Health Service authorities fall into this category, and administrative records are only open 30 years after the date of the last item contained in the file. Medical records of patients in this country are only open after 100 years. In exceptional cases, organizations may decide to waive the rules normally governing access to material under their jurisdiction, and open files earlier than the statutory period to *bona fide* researchers, provided precautions to safeguard anonymity and the conditions of the Data Protection Act in publications, are adhered to. Public records may be stored at the Public Record Office (PRO), the Scottish equivalent (SRO), or a local repository such as the Greater London Record Office (GLRO) or (in Scotland) the Lothian Health Board Medical Archives Centre. Some hospitals store their own records, but the state of preservation varies enormously. Private organizations may also maintain their own records. The Royal College of Nursing (RCN) employs a full-time archivist for this purpose. Archives may be defined as 'a document which is produced by an individual or institution in the normal course of life and work and which provides a record or part of the history of that individual or institution' (Foster & Sheppard 1980, p. 200). While mainly referring to written manuscript materials and documents, the definition of archives has been broadened to include sound, pictorial, and photographic forms.

Primary and secondary source considerations

The scholarly merit of an historical work hinges upon the extent to which it is based upon primary sources. Primary sources are the raw unedited data (the minutes, papers, and correspondence of the General Nursing Council, for example) upon which historical interpretation is based. Secondary sources refer to the digested, interpreted, or reported data of primary historical material. Generally, the secondary literature is mastered before the primary data are mined to provide the necessary contextual material for the account, but this order may not be strictly adhered to as new lines of inquiry are generated and elaborated as the evidence is uncovered. Arguments will usually be suggested by the data, and are subject to change as different types of sources emerge and are explored and re-read at different stages in the research. Interpretation is a dynamic and interactive process.

The hierarchy and range of sources

In keeping with developments in other areas of historical research, notably that in the history of medicine, the scope of nursing history has broadened recently to encompass a wide range of sources (Webster 1983). There is no standard method for the organization of compiling of sources or evidence. These might include not only official and semi-official printed or written documents and private papers, but also literary accounts, biography, autobiography, and fiction, none of which should be overlooked. More recently, oral testimony has yielded useful data on the experiences of working nurses (Maggs 1983). Little account as yet has been taken of patients' views, but film, architecture, art, and photographic material have recently been incorporated within the inventory of sources and methods (Hudson-Jones 1988). All sources have their strengths and their weaknesses, and a comprehensive review of these is provided by the resource guide produced by Maggs and Newby (1984). One of the major advantages of using a range of tools and sources as data is the potential for verification of evidence and interpretation. Thus, official documents may be used in combination, if possible, with private diaries and oral testimony to check and confirm a line of enquiry. Different perceptions of the same situation or event are likely to emerge from different individuals with different agenda and interests. Whilst identification of areas of conflict and consensus may be important to the task of interpretation, it is not the responsibility of the historian to reconcile conflict or assign priority to one view rather than another. The uncovering of 'multiple realities' may be the very point of the investigative exercise and is especially important in tracking the pathways of decision-making in policy analysis. In many ways, historical research may be considered akin to qualitative research in its acknowledgement of multiple realities and triangulation of methods.

Voyage of discovery of journey without maps?

On a practical level, historical research can be both frustrating and rewarding. Hours spent searching for a particular source of evidence may yield little. Equally, it is possible to stumble upon a goldmine of information: a personal diary, an album of photographs, a clutch of newspaper cuttings. The records of the past were not written with the needs of the historian in mind, although public bodies do have preservation policies implemented by officials trained to evaluate the historical importance of documents. These policies may be regulated by resources and other factors not necessarily within the control of historians themselves. As nurses and historians, we should take an active role in trying to influence preservation policies to maximize their utility for future generations of historians, nurses, and researchers.

Although it is probably advisable to build a research project around a solid set of records, this assumes the archives have been used by, or are known to, the researcher already. This presupposes that the researcher has already undertaken sufficient work to have refined the research question in order to identify specific sources. Few may be able to afford the luxury of such in-depth preparatory or pilot work before submitting proposals for funding to vetting agencies. Nonetheless, it is possibly inadvisable to depend upon only one source of data, no matter how potentially rich.

The direction and outcome of the research will be dependent upon the use that can be made of the sources and, consequently, the questions asked may change dramatically in the course of investigation. The order of inquiry is negotiated and loose; there is no orderly progression of steps or stages to follow, and one is likely to come and go between primary and secondary material in response to the data. Practicalities such as the employment of an archivist may be crucial in determining the use of sources. The listing of holdings and cataloguing of material greatly enhances the efficiency of information retrieval. Much may also depend upon the experience and efficiency of the researcher, and few nurses, unless they have undertaken first degrees in history, are well-equipped for undertaking major research projects in history; much of what trained historians perhaps take for granted has to be learned along the way.

Generally speaking, however, the problem of historical research is not one of finding sufficient material, but of containing the huge volumes of paper generated by organizations. Documents, journals and personal papers should be systematically screened for relevant material and this can mean hours of laborious scrutiny and scanning. All research has its routine tasks but this is labour which may be crucial to how the account will be organized and presented. In determining the division of labour, it may be advisable to tackle the records of one organization at a time. If events are particularly current, it is desirable to interview the participants themselves.

Oral history requires special methodological considerations and has acquired the status of a sub-discipline within history itself (Thompson 1978; Seldon & Pappworth 1983). It may serve a variety of purposes: to fill gaps in the documentation, uncover details of decisions, generate evidence missing from the records, or allow the clarification of factual points. There are many pitfalls – as well as great potential – in the use of oral testimony, which reflects the personal relationships and histories of people in different positions within organizations. Oral history may be invaluable as an insight into an individual's thought processes, the discovery of new and important information, and, more generally, in enriching the quality of data.

In many ways, historical research may be compared to mining; extensive exploratory work may be necessary to refine an area for further investigation. Diligent excavation may reveal a wealth of resources. For this reason, and the fact that only in exceptional cases will records be susceptible to computer analysis, the process of extracting and analysing the data and formulating interpretations is time-consuming and labour intensive. One cannot readily feed the data into a computer and run a battery of tests or a statistical package to identify trends or characteristics. Much of the analysis has to be conducted without such aids to efficiency. This may be another reason why history has not featured as one of the more popular forms of research in nursing; it is expensive in time and resources, and there are no immediate spin-offs in terms of a product to justify research investment. It also tends to be an individualistic enterprise and frequently undertaken as part of a multidisciplinary project. One does not see much of the 'group' research activity of 'science' in history. There is no reason, however, why historical research should remain at the periphery of research activity in nursing. Not only can it be rewarding and intellectually challenging, but, as I have argued elsewhere, historical research may provide a valuable precursor to participation in policy making (Rafferty (1989). The vicious circle of an under-resourced discipline and its perceived low market value by potential researchers has to be broken if historical research is to attract committed and talented students of nursing.

CONCLUSION

The above discussion represents only the briefest outline of some signposts to historical research in nursing. Only the most tentative of conclusions can be offered at this point. One thing which does seem striking is that the occupational and academic history of the researcher seems the most important determinant of the content and analytic framework of accounts. Until the early 1960s, the writing of nursing history was dominated by nurses. Social scientists and historians arrived, relatively speaking, late in the day. Fuller details of the significance of the occupational backgrounds of historians for the writing of nursing history have been explored elsewhere (Rafferty & Dingwall 1989). The timing of the participation of different groups of workers is an obvious area for investigation but one beyond the scope of this chapter. The pre-eminence of the professionalization theme, which characterized the early writing in nursing history, was not broken by social scientists but was treated and evaluated in a different way. Subsequent interest in nursing by social historians (Maggs 1983; Summers 1988) has led to a new set of questions being asked about nurses as women workers, and the effect of class and gender and other socio-political and economic factors upon the working experience, and opportunities of nurses. Contact with social historians has arguable produced a more critical approach to evidence and sensitivity to contextualization. While this may be welcomed by some as an antidote to the congratulatory, individualistic, and progress-orientated accounts of the past, we should remember that all writing should be regarded in terms of the context in which it was generated. These points are also elaborated elsewhere (Rafferty 1990). If histories of nursing were written with certain commitments in mind, that does not necessarily mean they should be considered historiographically inferior. It is only where evidence has been deliberately distorted, to fit a social purpose or serve a legitimizing function, that history might then be considered ideological (Kragh 1987). Florence Nightingale's life as a 'heroine legend' is admirably illustrated by Whittaker and Olesen's study of the differential representation of her life by teachers in university- and hospital-based schools of nursing (Whittaker & Olesen 1964).

Access to historical research in nursing is mediated through normal academic channels but inquiries are welcomed by the History of Nursing Society based at the Royal College of Nursing in London. Help and advice can be offered by members of the Society and also through the Wellcome Units for the history of Medicine based in Glasgow, Manchester, Oxford, Cambridge, and the Wellcome Institute in London. The Society for the Social History of Medicine also welcomes nurses as members. A list of useful addresses are included in the publications of Maggs and Newby (1984) and Foster and Sheppard (1980). In America, a Center for Nursing History and Archives is affiliated to the University of Pennsylvania School of Nursing. The Mary Adelaide Nutting Collection at Teachers College, Columbia University, New York, contains important educational and clinical material and texts. Historical options are offered in Masters and Doctoral programmes at the University of California San Francisco jointly between School of Nursing and the Department of History of Health Sciences.

But what implications might history have for nursing research? In the haste to establish nursing as a research-based profession and generate new knowledge, there is the danger that the past may be discredited. Traditions, rituals and myths, as vestiges of the past, tend to be represented negatively and naively in the research literature as the 'enemies of scientific progress', the antithesis of rationality (Walsh & Ford 1980). But before we consign these symbols of the past to what E.P. Thompson, in quite a diffferent context referred to as the 'enormous condescension of posterity' (Thompson 1989, p. 12), we would do well to consider the functional as well as the alleged dysfunctional factors which have sustained their existence. An understanding of the context and culture which has brought past practice into being will enhance our understanding of innovation and inertia in nursing practice. Historical research has an important contribution to make to reflective practice and the management of change in nursing. We ignore it at our peril.

REFERENCES

Abel-Smith B. (1960) *A History of the Nursing Profession* Heinemann, London.
Allemang M.M. (1987) Oral Historiography. In *Research Methodology (Recent Advances in Nursing Series No. 17)* (Ed. by M. Cahoon), Churchill Livingstone, Edinburgh.
Baly M. (1986) *Florence Nightingale and the Nursing Legacy* Croom Helm, London.
Barnes B. & Shapin S. (1979) *Natural Order: Historical Studies of Scientific Culture* Sage, London.
Barraclough G. (1955) *History in a Changing World*, Blackwell, Oxford. 29–30.
Burrow J. (1966) *Evolution and Society: A Study in Victorian Social Theory.* Cambridge University Press.
Carr E.H. (1970) *What is History?* Macmillan, London, 24.
Cartwright F.F. (1977) *A Social History of Medicine* Longmans, London.
Cook Sir E. (1913) *The Life of Florence Nightingale*, **Vols 1 and 2**, Macmillan, London.
Davies C. (1980) The Contemporary Challenge in Nursing History, In *Rewriting Nursing History*, (Ed. by C. Davies), Croom Helm, London; 11–17.
Denley P. & Hoplain D. (Eds) (1987) *History and Computing*, Manchester University Press.
Dingwall R. Rafferty A.M. & Webster C. (1988) *An Introduction to the Social History of Nursing.* Routledge, London.
Dzuback M.A. (1983) Nursing Historiography, 1960–1980: An Annotated Bibliography. In *Nursing History: New Perspectives, New Possibilities* (Ed. by E.C. Lagemann), Teachers College Press, New York; 181–210.
Elton G.E. (1967) *The Practice of History* University of Sydney Press, 53.
Foster J. & Sheppard J. (1980) Archives and the History of Nursing. In *Rewriting Nursing History*, (Ed. by C. Davies), Croom Helm, London; 200–14.
Gray A.M. (1989) *The NHS and the History of Nurses' Pay.* Bulletin of the History of Nursing Group at the Royal College of Nursing: **2** (8): 15–29.
Hudson-Jones A. (Ed.) (1988) *Images of Nurses: Perspectives from History, Art and Literature*, University of Pennsylvania Press.
Jenkinson V. (1953) Case Assignment Method of Nursing. *Nursing Mirror*: **116**, December 18:i–iv.
Kragh H. (1987) *The Historiography of Science.* Cambridge University Press, Chapter 10; 108.
Maggs C.J. (1978) Towards a Social History of Nursing, part 1 and 2 *Nursing Times*, **74** Occasional Papers: 53–8.
Maggs G.J. (1983) *The Origins of General Nursing* Croom Helm, London.
Maggs C.J. & Newby M. (1984) *A Sourcebook in Nursing History.* King's Fund publications, London.
Marwick A. (1970) *The Nature of History.* Macmillan, London, p. 17.
Matajski M. (1986) Historical Research: The Method. In *Nursing Research: A Qualitative Perspective.* (Ed. by C.J. Oiler & P.L. Munhall), Appleton Century-Croft, New York.
Porter R. & Wear A. (1988) *Problems and Methods in the History of Medicine.* Croom Helm, London.
Rafferty A.M. (1991) Historical Knowledge in Nursing. In *Knowledge in Nursing.* (Ed. by K.M. Robinson & B. Vaughan), Heinemann, London.
Rafferty A.M. & Dingwall R. (1989) *The Sociology of the Professions: the Case of Nursing.* Paper presented to the Wellcome Unit for the History of Medicine, University of Oxford, seminar series on the professions.

Rafferty A.M. (1989) *Continuity and Change in Nursing Education: Project 2000 and the History of the Present*. Paper presented at National Conference on Continuing Nurse Education, Beyond project 2000, Birmingham Polytechnic.

Reason P. & Rowan J. (Eds.) *(1981) Human Inquiry: A Sourcebook of New Paradigm Research* John Wiley, Chichester.

Seldon A. & Pappworth J. (1983) *By Word of Mouth: Elite Oral History*. Methuen, London.

Smith F.B. (1982) *Florence Nightingale: Reputation and Power* Croom Helm, London.

Soffer R. (1988) The Development of Disciplines in the Modern English University. *The Historical Journal* **31**: 933–46.

Stinson S. & Kerr J. (Eds.) (1986) *International Issues in Nursing Research*. Croom Helm, London.

Stone L. (1972) *The Causes of the English Revolution* Routledge, Kegan Paul, London; 47–144.

Summers A. (1988) *Angels and Citizens: British Women as Military Nurses 1854–1914*. Routledge, London.

Thompson E.P. (1980), *The Making of the English Working Class*. Gollancz, London.

Thompson P. (1978) *The Voice of the Past*. Oxford University Press.

Walsh M. & Ford P. (1989) *Nursing Rituals: Research and Rational Practice*. Heinemann, London.

Webster C. (1983) Historiography of Medicine. In *Information Sources in the History of Science, and Medicine*. (Ed. by P. Weindling & P. Corsi), Butterworths, London; 29–43.

Whittaker E.W. & Olesen V.L. (1964) The Faces of Florence Nightingale: Functions of the Heroine Legend in an Occupational Subculture *Human Organisation* **23**: (2) 123–30.

Chapter 19
Descriptive Research
Diana E. Carter

INTRODUCTION

Descriptive research, which involves the systematic collection of information, aims to discover and describe new facts about a situation, people, activities, or events.

As with other types of research, descriptive research begins with the identification of a problem or problematic situation. The description and analysis of that situation may reveal relevant factors or relationships hitherto undetected. Descriptive research is an essential phase in the development of nursing knowledge, forming the basis for future research by serving as a mechanism for generating questions and hypotheses for further experimental study.

Many areas of nursing have been investigated in descriptive studies, including nurses themselves, characteristics of patients, and the content and methodology of nursing education. For example, Armstrong-Esther *et al.* (1989) described attitudes and behaviours of nurses towards the elderly in an acute care setting; McHaffie (1990) described the adjustment mechanisms of mothers of low birth weight babies, and Edel (1986) investigated and described the status of gerontological nursing curricula. The characteristics of nursing students, the environment in which nursing care is given, and the equipment used in the provision of that care, and specific nursing practices, are further examples of areas of nursing where descriptive research has been carried out.

THE NATURE OF DESCRIPTIVE RESEARCH

The focus of descriptive studies is on the situation as it is – conditions that exist, practices that prevail, beliefs and attitudes that are held, ongoing processes, and developing trends. The data obtained can be used to justify and assess current conditions and practice, or to make plans for improving them.

Descriptive studies vary enormously in their scope and complexity. For example, a large sample of subjects drawn from a defined population may be studied. This is sometimes referred to as *survey research*. At the other extreme, a *case-study* design involves the extensive study of a single unit (an individual, family, or group). In this instance, while the number of subjects is small, the number of variables examined tends to be large because there is a need to investigate all the variables that may have an effect on the situation being studied. Similarly, the information obtained in descriptive studies may be quite diverse, ranging from data on easily defined objective facts such as age, gender, income, and educational level, to subtle and personal realms of human experience such as feelings or attitudes. The methodology of descriptive studies varies widely;

methods of data collection include the use of questionnaires, interviews, and observation techniques.

Descriptive research frequently precedes experimental studies in that it often serves to generate hunches about the relationship among the various phenomena studied which can then be tested in an experimental study which may confirm or reject the hunches.

Descriptive studies are generally guided by research questions and/or research objectives rather than a research hypothesis *per se*. There is no attempt to introduce anything new or to modify or control the situation being studied. Because there is no manipulation of the variables under study, and as no attempt is being made to establish causality, the terms 'dependent' and 'independent' are not used when referring to variables. Whilst relationships between variables are identified in order to obtain an overall picture of the phenomena being examined, examination of the types and degrees of relationship is not the primary purpose of a descriptive study.

However, in common with all types of research, the descriptive researcher is trying to achieve a clear picture of the situation, and protection against bias is an important consideration. Measures taken to achieve this protection include definition of variables, sample selection, and the use of valid and reliable instruments and data collection procedures.

Definition of variables

Researchers refer to two types of definition – conceptual and operational.

A *conceptual definition* conveys the general meaning – in much the same way as does a dictionary definition (LoBiondo-Wood & Haber 1986) – but it does not help in relation to the measurement of a particular variable. It is necessary to go further than this and to describe *what* is to be measured and *how* this will be carried out. This is known as an *operational definition* (or operationalization), and involves specifying the tools or instruments required to make the observations or measurements (see Chapter 8). Such a procedure makes it possible for others to replicate the study and it also renders the findings of the study more reliable.

Sampling

Samples vary considerably in the extent to which they represent the population, but the researcher who pays particular attention to the representativeness of the sample increases the possibility of generalizing the findings to a larger group.

Many descriptive studies include a large number of subjects obtained through random sampling, which, it is hoped, will increase the generalizability of the findings to a wider population. However, some studies use non-random sampling techniques, and while they may produce important relevant findings, such findings cannot automatically be extrapolated to similar situations. More details of sampling techniques can be found in Chapter 21.

Reliability and validity

Instruments to be used for the collection of data must first of all be tested for reliability and validity. Reliability refers to the degree of constancy or accuracy with which the instrument measures an attribute, while validity is the degree to which it measures what it is supposed to be measuring. There are many methods of assessing aspects of an instrument's reliability, and also a variety of approaches in relation to validity which are referred to elsewhere in this text.

Perhaps an important point to note here is that even though an instrument has been previously tested in another study, it is advisable to re-test it as it has been shown that neither reliability nor validity is constant – both can change over time.

Methods of data collection

As mentioned above, data collection in descriptive studies may involve the use of interviews, questionnaires, and observation techniques.

Interviews and questionnaires

Interviews and questionnaires both involve direct questioning of subjects. Qualitative descriptive research frequently employs unstructured interviews, while quantitative descriptive studies – which call for instruments that will facilitate the collection of numerical (quantifiable) data – often use questionnaires and structured interviews. Both interviews and questionnaires are useful for obtaining data about the subjects of a study. The data may pertain to:

(a) *personal background information* such as age, marital status, educational level, and professional qualifications;
(b) *behavioural information*, including what the subjects did in the past, do at present, or intend to do in the future – for example, previous smoking habits, dietary intake, intended career moves;
(c) *level of knowledge or information* on a particular topic, such as pre-operative patients' knowledge of post-operative care;
(d) *opinions, attitudes and values* or how the subjects feel, or what they believe.

Observation

Observation techniques are also frequently used in descriptive nursing research studies. The focus of observation may be the behaviours and characteristics of individuals, including physical appearance, verbal and non-verbal communication behaviours, and actions. Environmental characteristics may also be observed as an individual's surroundings can have a considerable effect on behaviour.

Where a particular situation is being observed, the researcher's participation in that situation can range from one of non-participation, where the emphasis is solely on the observation and recording of events, to one of active participation, where you are actually a part of the situation as well as an observer and recorder of events.

If you are using interviews, questionnaires, or observation as means of collecting data, you need to give some consideration to the validity of each of these methods. For example, subjects' verbal or written responses to interview questions or questionnaire items about how they carry out a particular task, may bear little or no resemblance to how they actually perform it. Similarly, there is no guarantee that the behaviour you observe is a true reflection of how subjects behave when there is no observer present. Interviews, questionnaires, and observation are dealt with in more detail in Chapters 22, 23, and 24. The remainder of this chapter will look at the different types of designs that can be used when conducting descriptive research.

DESCRIPTIVE DESIGNS

Opinions differ as to which non-experimental research approaches should be classified as 'descriptive', and some research texts do not include exploratory designs in this category. One of the reasons for this is that, in descriptive studies, the research question presupposes a prior knowledge of the problem and you must be able to define what and who are to be measured and the techniques of doing so. However, it is worth briefly considering what I will call 'exploratory descriptive designs'.

Exploratory descriptive designs

As the name suggests, this type of design is appropriate for areas about which nursing has little theoretical or factual knowledge. The researcher is exploring a particular area to discover what is there, the meanings attached to the discoveries, and how these can be organized. This type of study calls for intuition and insight on the part of the researcher. It also calls for a degree of flexibility so that you can follow through a new lead and move the study into new areas as you proceed and as your knowledge of what is being studied increases.

The approach in such studies is frequently qualitative (see Chapter 13), integrating a variety of data collecting methods such as participant observation and unstructured interviews. This type of approach does not rely on pre-coded instruments and the possibilities of discovery and of understanding unknown phenomena are enhanced. Van Maanen's (1988) study of perceptions of health among elderly Britains and Americans adopted such an approach. Because of the exploratory nature of the study, few if any of the variables are under the researcher's control – they are simply discovered and observed as the researcher comes across them.

Simple descriptive design

In this type of design, the variables of interest have been previously studied – either independently (as in an exploratory study) or with other variables. The variables are partly controlled by the situation (as in exploratory designs) but they are also partly controlled by the researcher, who chooses the sample for the study. This

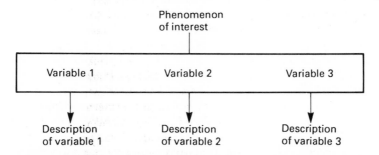

Fig. 19.1   Simple descriptive design.

design is used when the researcher wishes to examine the characteristics of a single sample – as shown in Fig. 19.1.

After determining the phenomenon of interest, you identify and define the variables within this and then proceed to use the appropriate data collecting techniques in order to obtain data which describe the variables. The number of variables to be examined and described will be determined in part by the complexity of the phenomenon being studied and also by the overall aim of the study. For example, Armstrong-Esther *et al.* (1989) identified professional education, age, marital status, frequency of contact with elderly people, age of parents, preferred area of clinical work, and relevant nursing courses, as variables to be described in their investigation of the attitudes of health care workers toward elderly patients in acute care settings; they then proceeded to gather data pertaining to these through the use of a questionnaire.

Comparative descriptive design

The comparative descriptive design is appropriate if you wish to examine and describe particular variables in two or more groups. Figure 19.2 shows an example of the comparative descriptive design.

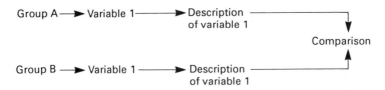

Fig. 19.2   A comparative descriptive design.

This type of design can be seen in the study, carried out by Ronayne *et al.* (1989) of the beliefs about smoking and attitudes towards amputation held by patients who decided either to stop or to continue smoking following a diagnosis of chronic peripheral vascular disease. By subjecting the collected data to inferential statistical techniques such as *t*-test and chi-square (see Chapter 28), the researchers were able to determine statistically significant differences between the groups' beliefs and attitudes.

Time dimensional designs

Time dimensional study designs developed within the discipline of epidemiology (which is concerned with the occurrence and distribution of disease among populations). The designs were developed to help determine the risk and causal factors of illness states. Examples of this approach are longitudinal and cross-sectional designs.

Longitudinal designs

A longitudinal design would be used if you wanted to examine changes in a group of subjects over a period of time (Fig. 19.3). For example, your study may be concerned with the development of manual dexterity among student nurses. Using a longitudinal design, you could measure the students' manual dexterity at various stages during their training programme.

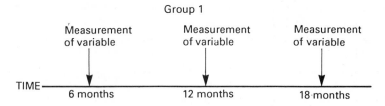

Fig. 19.3 Longitudinal design.

A descriptive study by Jackson (1990) of the use made of community services by elderly people discharged from hospital used a longitudinal design, the subjects being interviewed at six-week intervals over a three-month period.

As can be readily appreciated, the use of a longitudinal design tends to be expensive and also calls for long-term researcher and subject commitment in many instances. On the other hand, it is generally recognized that research problems which involve trends, changes, or development over time, are best addressed through longitudinal designs.

Cross-sectional designs

This type of design involves the collection of data at one point in time. It is a design that would be appropriate for examining groups of subjects in various stages of development simultaneously (Fig. 19.4).

Group	Stage of development	At same point in time
1	End of year 3	Measurement of variable
2	End of year 2	Measurement of variable
3	End of year 1	Measurement of variable
4	Start of year 1	Measurement of variable

Fig. 19.4 Cross-sectional design.

To refer back to my earlier example of a study concerned with the development of manual dexterity in student nurses, by employing a cross-sectional design, you would be able to describe groups of students at different stages of their training programme at the one time. Hence the collection of data can be 'telescoped' into one period, the duration of which is determined only by the length of time it takes to collect the data. While this type of design may be more economical in terms of time and money than the longitudinal design, it does make the assumption that the stages of development are part of a process which will progress across time. A comparison of longitudinal and cross-sectional designs is shown in Fig. 19.5.

Retrospective study designs

Retrospective studies are sometimes referred to as 'ex post facto' studies and they attempt to link the present situation with what happened in the past. In other words, both the proposed cause and the proposed effect have already happened, and you attempt to identify the factor(s) which resulted in the effect. However, it is recognized that your knowledge of the proposed cause and the proposed effect can sometimes bias the investigation. Additionally, there is the problem that if you

Longitudinal	Cross-sectional
Costly in terms of time, effort and money.	Less time-consuming, less expensive, more manageable.
Confounding variables could affect the interpretation of the results.	The confounding variables of maturation resulting from elapsing time is not present.
Depth of response can be obtained.	Less ability to establish an in-depth developmental assessment of the inter-relationship of the phenomenon being studied.
Early trends in the data can be investigated.	
Subjects may respond in a socially desirable way that they believe is congruent with the researcher's expectations.	

Fig. 19.5   Comparison of longitudinal and cross-sectional designs.

are interested in something which happened a long time ago and which has resulted in the effect, then the subjects' ability to accurately recall the information may be suspect.

Prospective study designs

Prospective studies are very like longitudinal studies in that they start in the present and end in the future. Looking to the future, the researcher is interested in describing the effect(s) of a cause (or causes) which may already have occurred. However, such studies are less common than retrospective studies in that it can take a long time for the phenomenon of interest to become evident. It is acknowledged that prospective studies are stronger than retrospective ones because of the degree of control that can be imposed on extraneous variables that might confound the data. A prospective design was used by McHaffie (1990) in her study of adjustments made by mothers following the delivery of low birth weight babies.

CONCLUSION

Many variables in nursing are not amenable to experimental manipulation, and this is one reason why descriptive studies can be of great value. The descriptive researcher – in search of meaning – is concerned with observing, describing, and documenting aspects of events, phenomena, or situations, as they occur naturally, and the information obtained can often form the foundation for the development of nursing theories.

This chapter has introduced some of the aspects related to descriptive research and has briefly considered a number of types of descriptive design which are frequently employed by researchers conducting this type of research.

REFERENCES

Armstrong-Esther C.A., Sandilands M.L. & Miller D. (1989) Attitudes and behaviours of nurses towards the elderly in an acute care setting. *Journal of Advanced Nursing*, **14**, 34–41.

Edel M. (1986) Recognizing gerontological content. *Journal of Geriatric Nursing*, **12** (10), 28–32.

Jackson M.F. (1990) Use of community support services by elderly patients discharged from general medical and geriatric medical wards. *Journal of Advanced Nursing*, **15**, 167–75.

LoBiondo-Wood G. & Haber J. (1986) *Nursing Research – Critical Appraisal and Utilization*. C.V. Mosby, St Louis.

McHaffie H.E. (1990) Mothers of very low birth-weight babies: how do they adjust? *Journal of Advanced Nursing*, **15**, 6–11.

Ronayne R., O'Connor A. & Scobie T.K. (1989) Smoking: a decision-making dilemma for the vascular patient. *Journal of Advanced Nursing*, **14**, 647–52.

Van Maanen H.M. Th. (1988) Being old does not always mean being sick: perspectives on conditions of health as perceived by British and American elderly. *Journal of Advanced Nursing*, **13**, 701–9.

Chapter 20
Evaluation Research
Senga Bond

What sets evaluation research apart from other forms of research is its prime intention to contribute to policy making – be it at the level of an individual work unit like a school of nursing or a hospital ward or, at the other end of the continuum, at the highest level of government. That the then Secretary of State for Health recently spurned the collective proposals of the Royal Colleges that there should be evaluations of the proposed changes to the structure of the Health Service as outlined in the White Paper 'Working for Patients', points to the political context in which evaluations may or may not take place.

Well-conceived, well-designed and conducted, and thoughtfully analysed evaluations have the potential to provide insights into how services or projects are operating, the extent to which they are meeting intended goals or needs of recipients, their strengths and weaknesses, and their cost effectiveness, and so to potentially provide fruitful directions for the future. Evaluations should provide relevant information for decision makers and so contribute to setting priorities, guiding the allocation of resources, and guiding the modification and refinement of project structures and processes. With such a broad range of possible functions, it is not surprising that evaluation conforms to a number of different models, differentially appropriate to a range of circumstances and interests, and having particular strengths and weaknesses in different contexts.

THE PURPOSES OF EVALUATION

Table 20.1 points to some different evaluation models and the particular characteristics they emphasize. This list should immediately alert the potential evaluator to the wide range of activities and meanings involved in the idea of 'an evaluation' and the range of investigative activites that could be involved. Usually, however, there are three main categories of purpose which guide the request for, or the decision to undertake, an evaluation. These are needs assessment, formative evaluation, and summative evaluation.

Needs assessment

The first is not evaluation of an existing project at all but a means of seeking an assessment of needs, problems or conditions which should be taken into account and addressed in future planning. In this kind of situation, there is generally a need for information, or a feeling that things are not as they should be, and there is a need to clarify goals, assess the extent to which they are shared, identify whether clients perceive problems, and decide whether there needs to be new forms of action. Examples of this kind of inquiry would be, 'What is the overall magnitude

Table 20.1   Some models of evaluation.

Model	Emphasis
Goal-orientated evaluation	Evaluation should assess the extent to which the specified goals of an innovation are achieved, i.e. the effectiveness of an innovation.
Decision-orientated evaluation	Evaluation should facilitate intelligent judgements by decision makers.
Responsive evaluation	Evaluation should describe the processes involved in a scheme or innovation and relate this to the value perspectives of key people.
Evaluation research	Evaluations should focus on explaining the effects of innovations and generating generalizations about their effectiveness.
Goal-free evaluation	Evaluation should assess the effects of innovations over and above their own specified goals and focus on the extent to which client needs are met as well as unintended consequences.
Advocacy-adversary evaluation	Evaluation should derive from the argumentation of contrasting points of view.
Utilization-orientated evaluation	Evaluation should be structured to maximize the utilization of its findings by specific stakeholders and users.

(based on Herman, Morris & Fitz-Gibbon, 1987)

of the population requiring a service?' 'What is the nature or range of facilities likely to be required?' 'How will a new service be monitored?' 'What do consumers feel about services offered?'

Formative evaluation

This kind of evaluation has as its main thrust the provision of information which will improve the running or development of an ongoing service in relation to its value. It will involve monitoring the implementation of an innovation, the functioning of an existing service, and the processes of achieving goals. The thrust is to understand how well a service or project is moving towards its objectives so that remedial action may be taken when things seem to be going amiss and modifications are required, or to recognize when things are going well. Parlett and Hamilton's (1972) influential paper deals with conducting formative evaluations.

This time-consuming activity involves detailed assessments of the many processes involved in an innovation and in feedback activities to the participants so that they can act on the insights gained. In some respects, formative evaluation embodies components of action research (see Chapter 17) since its thrust is to make changes for improvements. These changes may involve personnel, their activities, organization, or technologies in use. An example of formative evaluation is work undertaken to study management practices in a new residential unit, staffed by nurses, for the care of long-term psychiatric patients (Garety & Morris 1984). This study relies on already developed scales to assess staff orientation and attitudes as well as direct observation of the ways that staff interact with patients in order to decide whether care practices are related to styles of interacting with patients.

Summative evaluation

The main goal of summative evaluation is to present information about the effectiveness and value of an innovation. It may relate to the decision to continue or discontinue an innovation and whether or how to expand or reduce it.

Carrying out this kind of evaluation may involve comparison, either between different innovations within a programme, or with a control group which is not receiving any intervention. An example of summative evaluation is the work carried out on NHS Nursing Homes set up in three experimental sites and compared with hospital accommodation (Bond *et al.* 1989a).

COMPARING EVALUATION AND RESEARCH

It should now be clear that there are many purposes to evaluation and many different ways of going about it. Thus different people involved in evaluations will not only see different purposes in it, but will hold conflicting expectations of it. It is fundamental to carrying out an evaluation that these purposes and expectations are clarified at the outset.

Evaluation applies the methods of social research; the principles and methods which apply to the other kinds of research described throughout this text therefore apply here too. What distinguishes evaluation research is not method or even subject matter, but intent – the purpose for which it is done.

Table 20.2 describes some of the characteristics which apply to evaluation and to research. The focus in evaluation relates to the underlying purposes and, while evaluations are intended to inform decisions – and hence action – there is nothing inherently action-oriented about research *per se* (with the exception of action research). While nursing research tends to have an applied focus, it need not have, since the prime purpose is to seek new understandings and add to our store of knowledge. Thus evaluation research straddles the twin ideals of knowledge generation and informing decisions, and has to adapt to fulfilling both purposes.

Most evaluations are local, although they may have more general implications. Research has a main characteristic the generalizability of its findings. Thus evaluation research must be set at this wider level and make clear the parameters which limit the extent of its generalizability. If we take the NHS Nursing Home research as an example, there are some findings which may have relevance for the private nursing home sector. However, because the study was wholly based in the NHS, and we know that clients in NHS nursing homes are more psychologically dependent than are those in private establishments (Bond *et al.* 1989b), there would be danger in extrapolating findings for this reason apart from any others.

Table 20.2 Characteristics of research and evaluation.

Characteristic	Evaluation	Research
(1) Focus	Decisions – evaluation seeks understanding to facilitate decisions	Conclusions – research seeks understanding as its primary goal
(2) Generalizability	Low – results are often applicable only to the setting studied	High – results should be applicable to comparable settings
(3) Valuing in inquiry	Worthwhileness	Truth
(4) Measurement principles	Important	Important
(5) Scientific principles	Important	Essential
(6) Sampling techniques	Desirable	Crucial
(7) Random selection of subjects	May be feasible	Important if possible
(8) Descriptive and inferential statistics	Utilized	Utilized
(9) Audience	Identified and important	May or may not be identified
(10) Politics	Recognized and accommodated	Usually considered improper
(11) Replicability	Usually not possible	Very important
(12) Setting	Very significant	Minimally important
(13) Reporting	Internal and political	External, public and open
(14) Theory building	Not usually	Central and important

Those who seek evaluations are interested in the worthwhileness of findings in terms of their value for decision making. This tends to be the major criterion in considering whether the evaluator has done a good job. For research, the essence lies in the truth of the findings – can the research be believed – irrespective of any other value it may hold. Evaluation research, then, has to conform to the canons of science and the principles of measurement to arrive at information which is valid. While evaluators also use methods which conform to measurement principles, adhering to good science is usually less important than empiricism. Often, evaluations are the art of the possible – and often it is not possible to adhere absolutely to good science because the practical context in which evaluations are done just does not permit this. It is not always possible, for example to adequately sample those who are exposed to new developments – for practical or political reasons – so the evaluation exercise is carried out in such a way that the findings are restricted and interpretation not straightforward. Thus, while the statistical and measurement aspects of evaluations may be similar to those carried out in research, the underlying design and/or sample selection is often, of necessity, less rigorous. This is one of the reasons that the findings in evaluations are more constrained than are those of research.

Evaluations tend to be sought, or are carried out, in-house; alternatively, an external consultant may be employed. The customer and audience for the evaluation therefore is well identified in advance and should have had a major say in how the evaluation has proceeded. The relevance of the findings, however, may prove to be of value to a wider audience, but this is not necessarily the case. In research, the audience is not targeted in advance, unless the research has specific practical relevance in commerce, industry, or public service. Indeed research, especially fundamental research, should in many respects be impartial to particular applications, and focus exclusively on a search for truth. Marie Curie had no application in mind in her life work to isolate a new chemical element. The search was to increase our knowledge. In research *per se* then, the political context of research is played down while in evaluations and evaluation in research, the political context is both recognized and taken into account while the researcher, rather than the focus of the study, attempts to remain impartial. Thus, in doing evaluation research, there has to be a balance between disinterest and the political context in which the results are to be produced and used.

In the NHS nursing home study, where care was nurse, rather than medically managed, there were obvious vested interests, and the evaluation research had to take these on board while designing a study which had high scientific rigour. This scientific approach to evaluation research meant that the study was long and time-consuming and the products, in the form of scientific publications, were made available to a wide audience of different stakeholders in the provision of care, not only to the customers who commissioned the study. Evaluations tend to be wanted rather more quickly than is possible in carrying out rigorous research, and the findings are generally of more local interest, with publication limited to local reports. The characteristics of evaluation mean that often there is little to add to a general body of knowledge or to theory-building while at the same time contributions to theory are of central importance to research. Thus evaluation research should inform theory as well as provide information which has relevance in its own right. Evaluations on the other hand, which only approximate the requirements of research, will be unlikely to contribute to theory.

The above discussion indicates why there is a distinction between many evaluations and research. However, it is possible to do evaluations which are themselves research, so long as the study can accommodate both the rigour of research and the political and practical requirements of evaluation. Evaluation research describes an endeavour which is partly social, partly political, and only partly technical.

DETERMINING THE EVALUATION APPROACH

While a clear specification of the reasons for undertaking an evaluation should be established at the outset, it is equally important to ascertain what evaluation customers will accept as credible information. This is where the professional standards of researchers are challenged in finding ways to carry out credible work within the constraints laid down both by customers and the situation in which they are being asked to work. Nevertheless, since the 1960s, evaluation research has itself developed the range of methods it uses to provide information.

Like most of social science, early evaluation looked to logical positivism to justify its method choices. Congruent with this approach was the preference for using goals articulated in advance as a basis for formulating causal hypotheses which could then be tested experimentally. This kind of thinking relies on assumptions that the implementation of a programme or policy is homogeneous across sites and unvarying over time, that goals are explicit and shared, and that there are effects which are amenable to valid measurement using experimental designs. This approach to evaluation was epitomized in the classic texts of Suchman (1967) and Campbell (1969) which advocated methods approximating experiments. However, field experiments are only feasible where:

(1) The programme under trial is a simple one with clearly defined aims;
(2) There is a need to establish its effectiveness;
(3) Inputs are specific and measurable;
(4) People can agree on how outcomes can be measured;
(5) Randomization is both politically feasible and administratively possible;
(6) Clinical objectives do not intrude;
(7) Non-co-operation or attention can be kept within acceptable bounds;
(8) Results are likely to be useful and timely (Booth 1988).

Few innovatory programmes and evaluation studies meet such guidelines.

The assumptions of the value of experiments have come under attack not only in evaluation research but also in science as a whole. A basic difficulty lies in the nature of experiments themselves which, while probing connections between 'independent' and 'dependent' variables, cannot assign causality nor explain why a treatment is or is not effective. Quasi-experimental methods (Cook & Campbell 1979) have also been criticized in recent years because of difficulties in interpreting treatment-related selection. Full explanation of why an innovation achieves its effects is extremely useful in specifying the factors which have to be present if an innovation is to be successful when transferred elsewhere (Cronbach 1982). Together with a recognition of the need for explanatory knowledge, came the recognition that it is important to let evaluation issues emerge from intensive on-site knowledge, rather than formulating them prior to data collection at the outset. Innovations change in unanticipated ways; they are not stationary targets, and they are conceptualized by actors with different viewpoints, realities, and meanings. Thus evaluators who came to recognize this used ethnographic methods based on a phenomenological viewpoint. In so doing, they are prepared to use methods which take on board such different perspectives, and which are inductive in their logic. This approach involves constructing and testing explanations of what is observed from the data, and seeking data to enable explanations to be constructed rather than setting out hypotheses in advance and pre-determining the data to be collected. More recently, case-study research (Yin 1989) has gained prominence as an evaluation strategy. Case studies include the collection of multiple dependent variables to assess whether there is a pattern of results.

These developments in different philosophical and methodological approaches to evaluation underscore the values of a pluralistic approach to evaluative research. There are merits in the different approaches, and each add in different ways to the carrying out of successful evaluations. While quantitative methods, particularly pragmatic randomized controlled trials (Schwartz & Lellouch 1967), are designed and interpreted in such a way that they enable a decision to be taken about the more favourable of two treatments, such methods, despite their scientific rigour, cannot begin to uncover the sequences of intention, action, interaction and reaction which constitute the day-to-day implementation of a service or policy. Trials are limited to deciding whether there is a difference between treatments; they cannot explain *why* such a difference is found. It is for this reason that qualitative methods of research have become attractive.

Using qualitative approaches, Smith and Cantley's (1985) evaluation of a psychogeriatric service enabled the elucidation of the unanticipated occurences and developments that took place as a new service was implemented. There is a needed respect for a diversity of approaches. Because of the desirability of contributing data about structures, processes and outcomes of the NHS nursing homes, the approach taken in that research was to use a range of methods within a single complex research study. This kind of research is expensive and time-consuming, but its comprehensiveness enables not only decisions to be taken about the most appropriate policy to adopt, but also contributes to understanding the means whereby the policy may be successfully disseminated to new sites. However, strategies which cannot be adaptive are 'doomed to reflect only that which stood still long enough to be measured' (Rist 1984).

EVALUATION RESEARCH: AN EXAMPLE

An example may help elucidate some of these points. Let us say we are going to evaluate the impact of a seminar programme for new staff nurses. The idea behind the programme is to offer continuing education about topics which new staff nurses have themselves identified as of interest and importance to them in their new roles. These topics were obtained by a needs assessment survey of new staff nurses in the unit, carried out at a single point in time.

Since releasing staff for educational purposes involves opportunity costs – the staff or the staff replacing them could be occupied in some other activity – there is a need from managers to know whether they are worthwhile, but without necessarily proceeding to a cost-effectiveness study. Nevertheless, it may be worth costing the exercise in terms of hours of time of staff nurses, lecturers, and seminar leaders, as well as the administrative costs of the programme.

The approach to be taken is both formative evaluation and summative evaluation – the series will be evaluated while in progress and adjustments made on the basis of what is discovered, as well as on the basis of an assessment of perceived benefits at the end of the series. The task has been given to a member of staff in the continuing education department in the health authority. How should she go about it?

The seminars have been set up during the afternoon 'overlap' – the time when it is assumed that staff are most available. A number of lecture sessions have been arranged around an apparently sensible sequence of topics interspersed with discussion seminars. A number of targets for evaluation are immediately apparent and methods of collecting data suggest themselves. These might include some of the activities listed in Table 20.3.

By using formative methods, it may very quickly become apparent that while the

Table 20.3 Some steps in an evaluation.

Evaluation question	Data to illuminate the questions	Method of collection
Is the timing of seminar/ discussion seminars appropriate?	Proportion of target staff attending	Staff sign attendance sheet and calculate %
	Attention given by staff to lecturer/degree of participation in seminar groups	Observe behaviour, note and count questions asked, assess quality of debate
Is the content of the seminars appropriate?	"	Number of staff attending different topics
		Observation of behaviour, count questions, number dozing, rate extent of interest expressed by seminar participants
Is the method of presentation appropriate	"	Number of staff attending different kinds of seminar
		Observation of behaviour, count questions, number dozing, rate extent of interest expressed by seminar participants
Is the sequence appropriate, i.e. lecture followed by discussion seminar		Observe points brought forward from lecture to seminar
Are there important topics missing or inadequately addressed	Opinion behaviour on ward	Questionnaire or structured interview with staff nurses who attended
Has the seminar programme influenced the staff nurses' performance?	Behaviour on ward	Questionnaire or structured interview with staff nurses *and* ward sister regarding staff nurses' performance

early afternoon seems an appropriate time, low attendance permits a rapid search for the reasons. It may be that staff are not available or that they feel reluctant to take time out for educational purposes or feel too tired to absorb information. It may be found that other times are more appropriate and more convenient or that there may be more to be gained by seeking a block of time in whole days or over a few days. New formats may also be tried for the programme.

Moving to the end point – do the seminars influence the staff nurses' performance? A means of obtaining some behavioural assessment rather than only self-opinion would be helpful; in this kind of small study it is unlikely that direct before/after behavioural comparisons or comparison with a 'control' group would be possible, but an indication may be obtained by asking the staff nurses' immediate manager to assess changes. Of course, there will be effects of time-in-post and maturation into the new staff nurse role which confound the efforts of the programme, but there is nothing that can be done about this except for comparison with a group which does not have the opportunity to attend the seminar programme. To begin to do this kind of comparison, and to develop behavioural measures of educational effectiveness, would extend the evaluation into a much more rigorous design, endowing it with research credibility. Knowledge would be gained not only about the effectiveness of the seminar programme – or what may replace it as a result of the changes brought about by the formative work – but also about the development of staff nurse behaviour over time.

Of course, some readers who are already knowledgeable about pedagogic processes may have set up their educational initiative in a very different way at the outset, basing it on different educational theories. Nevertheless, the sound evaluation of innovations, whatever their nature, is crucial in deciding their worth – the more bold and radical the innovation, the more critical the need to evaluate it.

CONCLUSION

Services are difficult things to do research on. They are multidimensional, complicated, elusive, and always 'on the move'. Research methods employed must also be subtle, sophisticated, and valid; they must be sufficiently dynamic to adapt to both the changing characteristics of clients and the changing perceptions of their needs. They must also be responsive to changing social, political, and economic climates – as anyone doing health service research in the 1990s will be only too aware. Nevertheless, attempting to provide as scientific a base as possible for service development is an infinitely interesting – and challenging – occupation. So long as policy makers are willing to take account of the findings produced through evaluation research, it is potentially also a very useful and rewarding activity.

To carry out evaluation research demands the application of research principles to the evaluation process. This is an activity of an entirely different order to other approaches to evaluation which lack scientific rigour, and may amount to no more than a group of professionals sitting around a table and passing opinions. For this reason it is important to understand the distinctions between evaluations and evaluation research, and to consider the substance of their findings for policy decisions. Unfortunately, all to often decisions are taken before evaluations are reported or without due attention to their findings. It is worth stressing again the importance of involving policy-makers in the evaluation process to gain their commitment to the implications of the findings.

REFERENCES

Bond J., Bond S., Donaldson C., Gregson B. & Atkinson A. (1989a) Evaluation of an innovation in the continuing care of very frail elderly people. *Ageing and Society*, **9**, 347-81.

Bond J., Atkinson A., Gregson B., Hughes P. & Jeffries L. (1989b) The 1984 and 1987 surveys of continuing care institutions in six health authorities. **Vol. 4**, *Evaluation of Continuing-Care Accommodating for Elderly People*. Health Care Research Unit, University of Newcastle upon Tyne.

Booth T. (1988) *Developing Policy Research*. Gower, Aldershot.

Campbell D.T. (1969) Reforms as experiments. *American Psychologist*, **24**, 409–28.

Cook T.D. & Campbell D.T. (1979) *Quasi-experimentation Design and Analysis Issues for Field Settings*. Houghton Mifflin, Boston.

Cronbach L.J. (1982) *Designing Evaluations of Educational and Social Programs*. Jossey Bass, San Francisco.

Garety P.A. & Morris I. (1984) A new unit for long-stay psychiatric patients: organisation, attitudes and quality of care. *Psychological Medicine*, **14**, 183–92.

Herman J.L., Morris L.L. & Fitz-Gibbon, C.T. (1987) *Evaluation Handbook*. Sage Publications, New York and London.

Parlett M. & Hamilton D. (1972) *Evaluation as Illumination: A New Approach to the Study of Innovatory Programs*. Occasional paper, Centre for Research in the Educational Sciences, University of Edinburgh.

Rist R. (1984) On the application of qualitative research to the policy process: and emergent linkage. In *Social Crises and Educational Research*, (Eds. L. Barton & S. Walker). Croom Helm, London.

Schwartz D. & Lellouch J. (1967) Explanatory and pragmatic attitudes in therapeutic trials. *Journal of Chronic Diseases*, **20**, 637–48.

Smith G. & Cantley C. (1985) *Assessing Health Care: A Study in Organisational Evaluation*. Open University Press, Milton Keynes.

Suchman E. (1967) *Evaluative Research*. Sage Publications, New York and London.

Yin R.K. (1989) *Case Study Research. Design and Methods*. Sage Publications, New York and London.

Chapter 21
Survey Design and Sampling
F. Ian Atkinson

The intention of this chapter is to introduce the general principles of survey research design and methods of random sampling. Broadly, survey research can be seen as either descriptive or analytical in purpose. Descriptive surveys aim to make descriptive statements about a study population. The intention of analytical surveys is to explore associations between the different variables under study. While it is useful to distinguish these two main purposes, in practice, much survey work is carried out for both descriptive and analytical reasons.

A major feature of a survey is that information is obtained from a sample of subjects who are selected from a study population and then, on the basis of this information, the whole study population can be described. In other words, population parameters can be estimated on the basis of sample statistics. Already this has introduced terms which now need to be defined.

The term 'population' refers to all those people about which a researcher wishes to make statements. In research, it is up to the investigator to define the population of interest. For example, if you wanted to make statements about the prevalence of smoking among ward sisters in a single Health Board or Health Authority area, then the population would be all ward sisters employed in that Health Board or Authority. Populations for surveys are not always people, they may be items. If hospital officials wanted to make a statement about the quality of a consignment of disposable syringes delivered to a hospital, then every syringe in that consignment would constitute the population of interest. A 'sample' refers to the group of people that a researcher selects from a defined population and these are the individuals about whom information will be collected. This information can be summarized as 'sample statistics' (for example, the average age of a sample). A population 'parameter' refers to a measurable characteristic of a study population which is not known but which is estimated on the basis of a sample statistic in descriptive surveys.

By their very nature, descriptive survey findings do not allow statements of 'fact' to be made about a population parameter. Indeed, any statement about a population, based on sample findings, can only be a probability statement, meaning that there is a chance that it could be wrong. The challenge is to reduce the chance of this final statement being wrong to an acceptable and calculable level. This can only be achieved by giving attention to the design of surveys and the principles which need to be applied here are outlined below.

At this point, it might be reasonable to ask, 'If there is a chance that the final statements about a population will be wrong then why bother doing surveys at all? Why not get information from everyone, for example, all the ward sisters, then statements of fact could be made about how many smoked and no one could question the findings.

To collect information from everyone in a population involves carrying out a census and, although the idea may hold some attractions, a consideration of the nature of a census as compared to a survey shows that things are not so simple. First, it is very difficult to get information from everybody in a defined population; there are always some who either can't be contacted or decline to help with an investigation. Even in the national census, where people are compelled by law to complete and return a form, there are still those who refuse. As a consequence, the researcher may still be unable to make factual statements about the population. Second, a census can be very expensive to carry out. Third, in some instances, it might be entirely impractical to get complete information from a population. In the example of a consignment of disposable syringes, if each was to be tested for contamination then none would be left for the hospital to use. In addition, some populations change so that they can not be counted in any event; they may also be so large or inaccessible that counting them becomes impossible.

For practical reasons, survey designs and methods may have to be used in order to study populations. In Britain, much of what is known about the nation's health, social conditions, standards of living, work, education, social attitudes, and behaviour, is based upon survey findings (see, for example, Office of Population Censuses & Surveys (OPCS) 1987 and Government Statistical Service 1990).

SOURCES OF ERROR

One of the major objectives of any survey research is to achieve the highest possible degree of accuracy in the findings. Generally there are seen to be three main sources of inaccuracy, or error, in survey work. These are known as sampling error, non-response error, and response error.

Sampling error

The avoidance of sampling errors is central to the design of surveys and by giving attention to the sampling procedures employed they can, to a large extent, be avoided. The problem for the researcher is how to select a sample which will represent the population under study. A system of selection is needed to ensure that the researcher, and factors extraneous to the research, have no influence whatsoever on the selection procedure. If there is a possibility that individuals with particular characteristics might stand a higher chance of being included in a sample than do others in the population, then the final sample could represent a population different from the one intended for study. Consequently, the research findings could be inappropriately applied to what is essentially a different study population. This problem is referred to as sampling error or bias.

As an example, imagine you needed to assess the numbers of nurses with a positive or negative view towards proposed changes in salaries and conditions of service. In order to estimate the feeling of the profession in a particular hospital, it is decided to sample nurses and ask them how they will vote on the agreement. The population here would be all nurses, both qualified and in training, at the hospital. A sample might be taken by a convenient procedure involving the researcher sitting in a hospital corridor and asking the views of all who came by. Unfortunately, and unbeknown to the researcher, this corridor leads to an area stocked with journals and daily newspapers, all of which contain detailed comment on the issue. The outcome of this might be that a high proportion of nurses who answered the questions were aware of the full implications of the proposed agreement and would not support it. Had the sample been obtained by other means, or in another part of the hospital, then an entirely different picture could have emerged in the findings because a less well informed group of nurses would have been selected. As it was, the sample selected was biased and did not represent the whole population of nurses in the hospital.

How then can a sample that might represent a defined population be selected? In order to obtain such a sample, a method is needed that will remove all biases in selection. The only way this can be achieved is by incorporating a system of randomness into the selection procedure. The term 'random' does not mean haphazard or careless but refers to a precise method of selection where all individuals in a defined population stand an equal chance of being selected for inclusion in the study sample.

Simple random sample

There are many types of sample design which incorporate the principles of random selection. Here, only the 'simple random sample' is outlined and used to introduce the basic principles of random sampling. An easily understood and full exposition of variations in the design of random samples is provided by Moser and Kalton (1971).

The procedures involved in selecting a simple random sample are illustrated using a practical example of sampling people from a population of 100 patients who attended an out-patient clinic, the purpose being to estimate the average age of the population. The procedures involved in this exercise are identical to those which would have to be followed in real sample selection.

After defining the study population, the first stage of sample selection is to obtain a list of all individuals in that population. This list is known as the 'sampling frame' and from it the sample is chosen. It is essential that the sampling frame gives a complete coverage of the population otherwise it will not be adequate for its purpose. Clearly, if some members of the population are not included in the list, they stand no chance of being selected and the resulting sample might be biased. Obtaining an adequate sampling frame often poses problems for research which involves human populations.

Once the sampling frame is obtained, individuals are numbered consecutively starting at 0. For the purposes of this practical exercise, the population is represented by all the people included in Fig. 21.1. The members of this population have already been given consecutive numbers starting at 0 and finishing at 99. The two-digit number underneath each person represents their number in the sampling frame. The number above each person represents their age.

Imagine that a sample of 15 people is required; all that is needed is a list of 15 two-digit random numbers and the people on the list with those corresponding numbers are taken for the sample. Random numbers can be obtained in several different ways but the example of the tombola drum method gives the clearest understanding of the nature of randomness. To generate random numbers using a tombola involves marking ten discs with a single digit from 0 to 9. The discs are placed in the drum which is then spun and a single disc picked out. The number is written down, the disc is put back in the drum and the process is repeated until

The Population

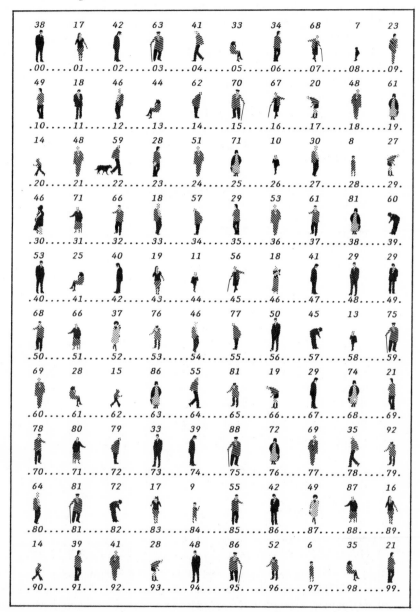

Fig. 21.1 The population. One hundred patients who attended an out-patient clinic.

sufficient numbers have been obtained to select the sample. This process ensures that all numbers have an equal chance of being selected which in itself is the property of randomness. If a tombola drum was used to select a sample of 15 people from a population of 100, then the procedure would have to be repeated a total of 30 times. This would provide 15 two-digit numbers between zero ('00') and

(99), thereby covering every numbered individual in the population. Such a procedure could become rather tedious if a large sample was required so random numbers are published in sets of statistical tables (Lindley & Scott 1984); they can also be easily generated by a computer. Figure 21.2 shows a table of such random numbers generated by a computer.

28	98	16	42	02	52	11	94	58	65
07	48	17	11	90	06	44	16	83	92
44	96	27	13	38	71	70	45	61	13
96	18	84	58	25	95	37	11	12	77
75	**87**	41	62	61	85	62	35	84	02
69	**81**	00	90	65	10	96	03	27	96
40	**96**	08	06	39	39	51	43	13	59
45	**21**	62	59	92	62	57	03	02	74
14	**74**	29	57	32	57	52	12	39	44
82	**25**	38	03	30	96	74	70	86	13
59	**80**	06	78	09	29	10	43	09	68
76	**34**	36	58	48	33	86	09	31	34
37	**04**	38	11	74	28	03	79	12	52
68	**89**	13	93	80	58	75	32	40	47
74	**45**	59	62	02	15	87	95	63	44
31	**20**	12	19	74	31	71	10	51	30
53	**51**	86	80	74	48	56	06	15	30
52	**28**	71	45	61	22	01	03	47	89
57	**41**	82	32	86	09	02	01	98	12
47	43	77	34	65	32	83	34	20	36

Note: The 15 highlighted numbers indicate those selected for the example given in the text.

Fig. 21.2   Random numbers.

For our sample, 15 two-digit numbers between 0 and 99 have to be found and they are chosen in the following way. First select a point in any row and any column of Fig. 21.2. Imagine that the third column along and the fifth row down is chosen; that is, number 8. A two-digit number is required so two columns have to be used. The first number then is 87 and the person who has number 87 in the sampling frame (Fig. 21.1) is selected for the sample. The second number is then selected by going down the column so the next person to be included in the sample is number 81. This process is repeated until a list of 15 random numbers have been obtained. If by chance the same number is encountered twice, then that person is not included in the sample twice. Rather, selection continues until a set of unique numbers (15 for this sample) have been obtained. The sample selected in this example is shown in Fig. 21.3.

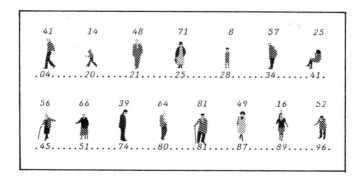

Fig. 21.3   The sample selected.

In some sample designs, a particular subject might be included in the sample more than once and this is called sampling with replacement. In social surveys, this is not generally done and is termed sampling without replacement.

When this procedure has been completed a simple random sample consisting of 15 individuals has been selected. A sample has no particular property which could be tested to see if it is representative of our population. All that is known about it is that it was just as likely to be chosen as any other sample. Any 'test' of randomness can only be applied to the process by which the sample was selected.

In order to introduce the idea of how survey findings can be generalized to a whole population – in other words, how population parameters can be estimated on the basis of sample statistics – a sample average (mean) is used to illustrate the general principles. Estimation from other types of sample statistics, for example proportions, variance, and differences, are in principle similar to procedures applied to the mean and are considered by Armitage and Berry (1987).

The reason for selecting this sample was to calculate the mean sample age in order to estimate the mean age of the population. As already noted, the number above each person in Fig. 21.1 represents their age, in years, so the mean age of the sample can be calculated as 45.8 years. In real research, the value of a population parameter is not known, but in this case the true population mean can be calculated and it is 46.09 years. Notably, these two numbers are not the same, and if more samples were taken it is likely that they too would have mean values which were different from the true population mean. This raises the question, 'If sample means vary, then how can the true population mean be estimated with any confidence on the basis of one sample?'

The answer to this question lies in the fact that although the mean values obtained are determined randomly, if a large number of different samples are selected, the mean values obtained begin to vary in an astonishingly predictable way. If a very large number of samples were taken from the population and the mean age of each was plotted on graph paper, eventually a symmetrical bell shaped curve, approximating the profile of a 'normal' distribution, would be produced (readers not familiar with the normal distribution curve should consult Chapters 27 and 28). The curve produced by this graph is known as the sampling distribution of the mean and is very important in establishing levels of confidence in survey findings. If an infinite number of samples were taken, and the average of all the sample means calculated, the result would be exactly equal to the true population mean. In terms of the sampling distribution curve, this implies that the value at its centre equals the true population mean. Further, the larger the sample size used to make these calculations, then the more compact this curve would become. These phenomena can only be guaranteed to occur when the samples are selected using random methods.

The actual calculations required to estimate the levels of confidence in the estimated population parameter, is outwith the scope of this chapter. However, an understanding of the use of the normal distribution indicates that it is many times more likely that a sample is picked with a mean near to the centre of the sampling distribution than one with a mean at the 'tails' of the curve. Areas enclosed by the standard normal distribution represent the probability of observing a value, in this case a sample mean, from a normally distributed variable such as the sampling distribution of the mean. Using this knowledge, the chances of a sample mean falling different distances from the true population mean can be calculated. It is by using these tools for analysis that levels of confidence in survey finding are estimated. Readers who wish to follow up the subject of making population estimates and calculating confidence limits are referred to Chapter 28 of this book and to Armitage and Berry (1987).

In research practice, obtaining truly random samples is extremely difficult and often impossible. The main difficulty lies in obtaining sampling frames which are adequate for their purpose. As an example, consider where complete lists of stroke sufferers, physically disabled people, low birth weight babies, and practising registered nurses, might be obtained from. Each of these populations have been the subjects of survey type nursing research but any sampling frames that have been applied must be extremely dubious in terms of the statistical model upon which descriptive surveys are based. Obtaining an adequate sampling frame of practising registered nurses might appear to be simple, but in fact proved to be difficult in a study recently carried out in Edinburgh (Macmillan *et al.* 1989). The sample for that study was selected from names and addresses appearing in Health Board or Health Authority pay-rolls. By the time the sample was selected and questionnaires posted, a considerable number of staff had left their posts and could not be contacted.

This is not to say that survey research becomes invalid because of this difficulty, rather it just becomes difficult to extrapolate the findings to wider populations. Often it is the insights attained through the analysis of associations between different variables affecting a sample which prove to be the most valuable part of survey findings.

Sample size
There are no simple answers to the question of how large a sample should be recruited for survey work. There are formulae in the literature (Armitage & Berry 1987; Moser & Kalton 1971) which can be applied to the problem but they alone still can not provide definitive answers. These formulae take into account factors, including the levels of confidence, which need to be attained in the findings: the size of the population, and the variability of our measures when they are applied to the study population.

Accuracy in survey work is determined by careful design and execution of the research and large samples alone do not in any way guarantee the accuracy of findings. To illustrate this point, many research textbooks describe an American survey which aimed to predict the results of a presidential election and used a sample size of ten million people. Because of the ways in which the sample was selected, incorrect conclusions were drawn about the forthcoming election result.

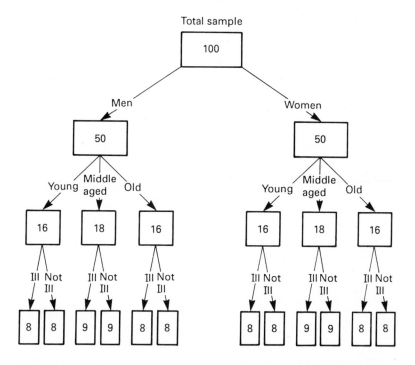

Fig. 21.4   Sizes of sample sub-groups following division by three variables.

In practice, sample size is to a large extent determined by the ways in which the data are to be analysed. If it is intended that the information should be tabulated, this means that respondents will have to be divided into different categories, for example, male and female; young, middle aged, and old; those who are ill or not ill (Fig. 21.4). Figure 21.4 illustrates the rapid reduction in the sizes of sub-groups for analysis after dividing a sample of 100 people by only three variables (sex, age band, and illness). In this example, it would be impractical, because of the small numbers after the third division, to control for the influence of both age and sex when examining the effects of another factor on the health of the sample. In Fig. 21.4, the splitting into sub-groups occurs equally at each division. In research practice, this equality rarely occurs and after three divisions it may be found that some sub-groups contain no respondents at all.

The process of dividing and sub-dividing can only be continued so long as there remain workable numbers of respondents in the sub-groups and, even with a large initial sample, only a few divisions can leave such small numbers that conclusions could not be drawn from them. It is important therefore to clarify which sub-division of the sample will be the final one, and what would be the smallest desirable number of respondents to have within it for the purposes of analysis.

This procedure can, of course, lead an investigator into estimating that enormous samples are required but here an unavoidable constraint thwarts these intentions – the limitations of time and resources. The process of collecting data from respondents can be costly and time consuming so, inevitably, considerations arising from the organization and funding of research impinge upon the nature and size of research endeavours.

Non-response error

The second of the three main sources of error, noted at the beginning of the chapter, was non-response error. As an essential part of sampling, precisely who is to be included in the sample is determined. Then it has to be ensured that information is obtained from everyone included. If some of the sample either refuse to help with the survey or for some reason can not be contacted, then there is a risk of introducing error into the findings through non-response.

To illustrate the mechanics of this type of error, imagine that for the previous example of the survey of the numbers of ward sisters who smoked, a simple random sample was taken, but only one half of the sisters agreed to help with the research. Their decisions to help or not might have been influenced by their own smoking behaviour. Imagine that those who did smoke felt threatened by the thought of having to answer questions on the subject while the non-smokers felt no inhibitions. As a result, a high proportion of non-smokers and a low proportion of smokers would provide data for the research. The consequences for the survey findings would therefore be to under-estimate the numbers of ward sisters who smoked.

In dealing with respondents, every effort must be made to encourage them to provide the information required. A careful choice of research topic, clear explanations as to the purpose and importance of the study, well constructed questionnaires and interview schedules, all contribute towards motivating respondents to co-operate.

When faced with a non-response problem, the question which has to be addressed by the researcher is, 'Do those people who have responded differ from those who have not responded in ways relevant to the aims of the research?' Finding an answer to this question may not be easy but it could be crucial for the validity of the research project.

Response error

The final source of inaccuracy is termed response error and takes two forms, random error, and systematic error.

Random error

Random error broadly refers to making mistakes in measurement and/or in the recording of data. This type of error always occurs in any endeavour which involves measurement of any kind and there is a well developed 'law of errors'. Because mistakes in this type of error behave in a random way, in the long run, they even each other out and will not unduly affect the findings of research involving groups of respondents. This can be illustrated using the example of estimating the average age of a sample. An interviewer might inaccurately record a respondent's age because of fatigue or a lapse of concentration, but the recording made is just as likely to be above as below the respondent's true age. If it is truly random error, then an equal number of over-estimates as under-estimates will be made in the course of collecting data from the whole sample. When the average age is calculated, the numbers will balance each other out and a correct mean age will be produced. In other words, random error tends to control itself statistically.

Systematic error

Systematic error is rather different in its mode of operation and arises from problems in the way in which phenomena are measured. Using the example of age, imagine that the phrasing of the question predisposed respondents to say they were younger than they really were. The outcome of this would be to systematically under-estimate the age of the whole sample. Because the researcher might be unaware of the bias in the question, these errors would not be accounted for in the presentation of research findings. Even if the loading in the question was eventually discovered, it would be impossible to make corrections to the data obtained. Consequently, systematic error has to be guarded against from the outset of the research. This will involve the careful testing of questions used in interviews or questionnaires, and precise calibration of all measuring instruments being used for the research.

This chapter has attempted to acquaint the reader with the basic principles upon which survey research is based. The main sources of error in survey findings, how they operate, and how they might be controlled, has been discussed. This short consideration can only offer an intending researcher an introduction to survey design and sampling but it is hoped that it will provide an initial grounding for further study in the area. Survey research can be applied in many fields of inquiry and its principles will continue to provide an indispensable tool for planners, policy makers, and all those who, for whatever reason, need to describe and analyse the characteristics of populations.

REFERENCES

Armitage P. & Berry G. (1987) *Statistical Methods In Medical Research* 2nd edn., Blackwell Scientific Publications, Oxford.

Office Of Population Censuses & Surveys (1987), *The General Household Survey*, HMSO, London.

Government Statistical Service (1990), *Social Trends*, No. 20, HMSO, London.

Lindley D.V. & Scott W.F. (1984), *New Cambridge Elementary Statistical Tables*; 78, Cambridge University Press.

Macmillan M., Atkinson F.I., Prophit P. & Clark M. (1989) *A Delphi Survey Of Priorities For Nursing Research In Scotland*, Nursing Research Unit Report, Dept. Of Nursing Studies, University of Edinburgh.

Moser C.A. & Kalton G. (1971), *Survey Methods In Social Investigation* 2nd edn., Heinemann Educational, London.

Other recommended reading

Marsh C. (1982) *The Survey Method: The Contribution Of Surveys To Sociological Explanation*, Contemporary Social Research Series No 6, George Allen & Unwin, London.

C: Data Collection

The selection of a data collection instrument offers considerable scope and choice. This section is not intended to present a comprehensive range of data collection methods, but to introduce a small variety of techniques.

Each of the data collection methods selected for inclusion has been well tested, and has been more or less widely used in nursing research.

The material presented in relation to interview, questionnaire, observation, and the critical incident technique, provides a *basis* for understanding each of these methods and, for potential researchers, an overview of a number of data collection methods for consideration and further study using the references given at the end of each chapter.

Chapter 22
Interview
Philip J. Barker

The interview is the most ubiquitous means of data collection at our disposal. Nurses interview patients and their carers routinely, as part of everyday practice. The 'ordinary' status of the interview may suggest simplicity. In this chapter, the factors which 'everyday interviewing' and the 'research interview' share, will be discussed, and this discussion will be supported by some illustrations of the key distinctions between them.

The research interview can have three possible uses:

(1) to explore a subject area, as a preliminary form of inquiry. In the exploratory interview you identify situations, events, and their relationships to one another, which form the basis of hypotheses.
(2) to collect data as part of the formal care of the study. The data collection interview measures a specific variable, or set of variables, usually by means of a carefully constructed set of questions, or schedule.
(3) to supplement other methods of inquiry.

You may wish to collect additional information, following some unexpected results, or wish to validate responses obtained by other means (e.g. mail questionnaire); you may also wish to probe more deeply into the subject's responses to the original question set.

The objective of the interview (data collection) will be considered at more length in Chapter 23. Here, consideration is given to the interpersonal context of the interview: what needs to take place between interviewer/interviewee; how the interview should be structured; and potential problems involved in interviewing different groups across different subject areas.

GENERAL PRINCIPLES

The quality of the information generated from the interview is dependent to a great extent on the behaviour of the interviewer. Even in a structured interview, where the interviewer is guided, wholly or in part, by a set of questions, certain characteristics of the interview can influence the outcome.

General interpersonal style

The interviewer needs to be able to engage the interviewee in a relationship involving more than a simple question and answer session. You need to be able to show attentiveness; listening actively to what is being said; sitting an appropriate distance from the person; adopting a posture which suggests that you are relaxed and open to the responses of the interviewee. Throughout, you should maintain steady eye contact, appropriate to what amounts to a deep conversation. These considerations illustrate the 'helping' status of the interviewer, whose behaviour acts as facilitator for the interviewee's responses, helping the person feel comfortable and relaxed (Keenan 1976).

Introduction and rationale

The first requirement of the interviewer is to 'set the agenda' for the interview. An explanation must be given of the aims and objectives of the interview, how it is to be conducted, why the respondent was chosen, and for whom the data are being collected. A clear statement should also be made concerning the anonymity of the person and/or the confidential nature of any information collected. It is also advantageous to invite any questions regarding the nature and objectives of the interview, before beginning.

This kind of 'openness' is essential for dealing with three major obstacles. Firstly, the respondent may mistake you for some other form of 'official': this might prejudice the responses given. Second, the respondent may censor his responses if an unambiguous guarantee of confidentiality is not offered. Finally, you may be seen as someone who is testing, or checking up on, the respondent: this may generate levels of anxiety which preclude appropriate responses.

Establishing rapport with the respondent requires the exercise of traditional pleasantries, and the interpersonal style already noted. These features support

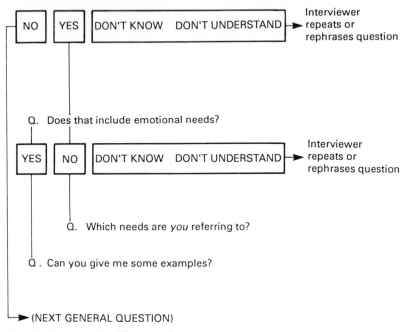

Fig. 22.1 Example of filter question.

the 'declaration of intent' offered by you; both are designed to reduce anxiety and facilitate comfort.

Questioning

You require a plan for the interview: this will address the main subject areas for enquiry, and a procedure for pursuing clarification of responses to the main questions. This plan – in the form of an interview schedule – is discussed briefly in Chapter 23. The interview schedule serves to standardize the interview: each respondent is asked the same questions, in the same sequence, in a similar manner. Questions are worded in such a way that they are understandable to all respondents. Where the respondent fails to understand the question, this is repeated first, before you try to explain the question further. In this sense you treat the interview schedule as a scientific instrument: offering the same cues to a wide ranging population of respondents.

Where the questionnaire involves 'filter questions' (if 'Yes', move to question 26, for example), respondents can become confused over which item to answer next. The problem does not arise where well-trained interviewers can move quickly from one optional question to the next, apparently asking the respondent only one series of questions. Where respondents do not understand the question, you can repeat or clarify the question as shown in Fig. 22.1.

Amplifying responses

In a few situations, the interview may focus upon yes/no answers; alternatively, the respondent may be invited to select a response from a range of alternatives. Such a schedule might be better framed as a self-report questionnaire, since here the facilitative presence of the interviewer seems to be redundant.

Collecting data by formal interviewing involves a three-stage process:

(1) First of all, you ask the respondent the questions;
(2) You then invite the respondent to either add further information *or* clarify his/her initial response;
(3) Finally, you reflect back the core of the response, seeking confirmation that your understanding is correct.

Example

INTERVIEWER: 'How do you feel about working with people with AIDS?'

RESPONDENT: 'I'm not sure. I guess I feel a bit wary. There is so little we know.'

INTERVIEWER: 'Can you tell me a bit more about that: what you are wary about?'

RESPONDENT: 'Well, the virus, I mean. They say that we are not at risk providing we take the right precautions, but there are reports of people catching the virus. Without having full contact: you know blood, body fluids and that.'

INTERVIEWER: 'You feel that your own welfare might be under some kind of threat?'

RESPONDENT: 'That's right. I think we focus too much attention on the patient's welfare.'

The interviewer here tries to 'probe' in a non-directive manner (Graesser &

Black 1985), helping the respondent to identify a response, to consider it further, and finally to confirm or revise the response. In some interviews, the respondent is asked more direct questions, where responses are not considered in this manner. Reed's (1986) study of chemically dependent nurses employed a structured interview schedule covering personal history, family history, educational background, health history, drug history, attempts to cope, consequences of addiction, and relapse history. All but one of the 42 questions asked required Yes/No answers, or a response chosen from identified options. In some of the questions, the respondent was invited to supply additional information (Have you ever been arrested? Yes/No. If yes, please list charges). This format was essentially fact-based: most of the data collected were unambiguous and focused upon recall of actual events. Davis's (1984; 1986) descriptions of the experiences of student nurses, employed a less structured schedule. Given that the respondents in these reports were trying to clarify what they felt about past experiences, the semi-structured approach was the more appropriate.

The structure of the interview and the form of the questions relate strongly to the aims of the study. Where the researcher has a clearly defined objective, involving the collection of discrete, factual information, the need for amplification of responses will be limited. Where the interview is used as an exploratory tool, to build hypotheses, or to canvas attitudes, beliefs, or other less clear-cut forms of data, careful amplification of responses will be vital.

TRAINING INTERVIEWERS

Selection

The use of an interviewer to collect information from subjects allows for a greater degree of flexibility than would prevail through the use of a self-report questionnaire. The interviewer is able to clarify and modify questions to elicit a response and can also modify her presentation or approach to enhance the respondent's motivation. Interviewers often change the tone of their voice or speech rate to establish rapport with the subject. Such adjustments may keep respondents interested and responsive throughout the interview. Such flexibility, however, may be gained at the expense of a standardized interview. The researcher may be left wondering whether or not differences among respondents reflects their individual differences or those of different interviewers. Researchers are generally advised to recruit interviewers with relatively similar characteristics; after which all are trained in the use of a standardized procedure.

Personal characteristics

Personal factors such as age, sex and race of interviewers can have a major effect on the interview data. You need to pay special attention to the recruitment of interviewers with characteristics likely to facilitate the positive relationships necessary for exploratory questioning to occur. It is generally advisable to employ interviewers of the same sex as the subjects where possible, and to use interviewers who are close to the age-group of the subjects. Young people may respond to much older interviewers by either being subservient or rebellious; older subjects may feel offended by very young interviewers who might be seen as inexperienced. The ideal age range is between 25–45: very young people often lack tact and the necessary interpersonal skills; much older people are often unwilling to follow instructions carefully (Topf 1988).

The interviewer's general appearance can also be important. Traditional rules about 'plainly attired interviewers' being most successful (Brown 1937), or 'prosperous looking' or 'too glamorous' interviewers being a disadvantage (Parten 1950), are probably no longer valid. However, despite the major cultural changes of the past two decades, it would be inappropriate to consider that 'anything goes' when recruiting interviewers. Individuals presenting with any 'extreme' characteristic, whether of accent or dress style, are perhaps best avoided. Similarly, individuals who are extremely enthusiastic or pessimistic about the study, expressing strong political affiliations, with past negative experiences of interviewing (or a related area such as sales), or possible contaminating views about the therapeutic potential of interviewing, are probably at risk of prejudicing the outcome.

Training in the standard interview

Prospective interviewers need to be aware from the outset of the importance of adhering to the interview rules. Interviewers should be discouraged from introducing new questions: all additional questions aimed at exploring or amplifying prior responses should be programmed as part of the schedule. The interviewer needs also to be aware that changing the emphasis on specific words can change the context of the question. Oppenheim (1968) noted that changing the emphasis of the following question:

'Who do you say *that*? . . . to . . . Why do *you* say that?'

represents a significant change from a 'challenge' to a more 'personal inquiry'.
Preparation of interviewers should comprise the following:

(1) Interview rehearsal under role-play conditions, followed by feedback. Ideally, these rehearsals should be audio- or video-taped;
(2) The interviewer should learn to code the role-play subjects' responses from the recordings, comparing these codings with those of more experienced interviewers;
(3) Once the basic format is established, emphasis should be given to the dangers of adapting wording or emphasis, or to omitting questions or part-questions;
(4) Brainstorming sessions, where the interviewers anticipate problems which might occur 'in vivo' are helpful for establishing a 'resolution menu'.

It is important that interviewers are 'valued' by the researcher. The preparation should be sensitively staged, and should enhance the interviewer's motivation to use the standardized guidelines positively, rather than serve to provoke unnecessary anxiety or irritation.

Motivation of the interviewer

Perhaps because of the apparent simplicity of interviewing, research assistants who are employed to collect such data require careful preparation. Interviewers need to be made acutely aware that there is more to interviewing than asking people questions and getting information from them. The interviewer needs to have an overview of the research process, identifying the interviewer's part in the overall plan; information about the drawing of the sample; and how the data are to be analysed. The information should also provide an understanding of why she has been trained in certain interview techniques.

The interviewer also needs to be motivated by the researcher. It is inadequate to assume that the interviewer will bring enthusiasm to the job: this feeling should be instilled in the interviewer. Emphasis needs to be placed upon why the study is important, and why it is necessary to pursue a particular line of questioning. Finally, emphasis must be given to the craft of the interviewer, emphasizing the importance of the interviewer's skills.

Monitoring

Attention also needs to be paid to maintaining the effectiveness of the interviewer across time: especially where the project has a long duration, or interviews are widely spaced. The gradual loss of efficiency is known as 'interviewer drift'. Possible causes are:

(1) *Loss of the original frame of reference.* Once the interviewer has ended the preparatory training, she no longer has others to compare with and may lose the objective criteria necessary to maintain appropriate standards;
(2) *Loss of reinforcement.* Under training conditions, the researcher provides the observer with encouragement to stay 'on target'. In the field, practical problems, or, in the respondents, recurring incompatible views, may lead him/her to embrace different standards.

To avoid such problems, the interviewers require regular supervision to allow detection of any significant drift (Collins 1988). Group sessions, reviewing the interview procedure, inviting the identification of problems associated with 'drift', can all be effective. Alternatively, tape recording a proportion of the interviews and checking these for irregularities, may serve as a 'quality control' procedure.

SPECIAL CONSIDERATIONS

As noted above, some interview situations require careful consideration in the selection of an appropriate interviewer. People with major emotional problems, mental illness, or mental handicaps, may demand the selection as specially trained interviewers, using interview schedules which acknowledge the cognitive or emotional disabilities of the subject (Flynn 1986). Where highly 'taboo' topics are examined, as in sexual abuse, the characteristics of the interviewer and the schedule are crucial (Quinn 1989). In this context it is worth noting that expectations of difficulty are often confounded. Rodgers' (1987) study of older people, for example, found that the subjects' recall of information was not significantly less 'faulty' than that of other age groups. The assumption that all older people are likely to encounter difficulty with interviews may be no more than an assumption.

ADVANTAGES OF THE INTERVIEW

Collecting information through direct, face-to-face contact with the subject, has some advantages, as is outlined below, over self-report questionnaires completed independently.

(1) People are more likely to discard questionnaires or leave sections blank; faced with an interview, the likelihood of a fuller response to all questions is more likely;

(2) Some subjects will be unable to complete self-report questionnaires through blindness, illiteracy, poor education, or limited comprehension or reasoning. Very young, older, or anxious people may also be put off by the demands of the self-report questionnaire;

(3) Areas of uncertainty or ambiguity can be clarified, avoiding the misinterpretations and possible awareness of conclusions which might arise from the questionnaire;

(4) Some forms of interview allow the subject to expand on their response: this is rarely possible or likely in a self-report questionnaire. The subject may talk expansively where he/she would not write detailed or lengthy responses;

(5) The interviewer can control the context of the response by her presence: it is not unknown for respondents to questionnaires to to seek assistance from friends or colleagues, thereby contaminating results;

(6) Additional data on the performance, attitude, and degree of understanding of the subject, can be collected by the interviewer. The supplementary observations may be used to qualify final conclusions, or as preparation for the design of other interview schedules and research hypotheses.

CONCLUSION

Interviews are a costly method of data collection, but offer significantly better returns: both in terms of the overall quality and the quantity of responses. Interviews are a more appropriate method of data collection for a wider range of populations and the interviewer always has an opportunity to 'rescue' a respondent from confusion or fatigue: options which are not possible under self-report conditions. In addition to the general standardized 'exploratory' interview discussed briefly in this chapter, interviews can employ any one of the vast range of structured measures noted in Chapter 23. These range from the use of 'general' semantic differentials (White 1986) to highly 'specific' pain questionnaires (Wilkie 1990). Interviews can be unstructured, aiming to explore through use of a 'topic guide' the subjects' experience (Skidmore 1986). At the other extreme, interviews can be conducted by telephone, allowing the participation of a wider range of geographically distant subjects.

REFERENCES

Brown L. (1937) *Market Research and Analysis*. Ronald Press, New York.
Collins C. (1988) Interviewer training and supervision. *Nursing Research*, **37** (2), 122–4.
Davis B.D. (1984) Interviews with student nurses about their training. *Nurse Education Today*, **4** (6), 136–40.

Davis B.D. (1986) The strain of training: being a student psychiatric nurse. In *Psychiatric Nursing Research* (Ed. by J. Brooking). John Wiley, Chichester.

Flynn M.C. (1986) Adults who are mentally handicapped as consumers: issues and guidelines for interviewing *Journal of Mental Deficiency Research*, **30** (4), 369–77.

Graesser A. & Black J. (Eds.) (1985) *The Psychology of Questions* Erlbaum Associates, Hillsdale, N.J.

Keenan A. (1976) Effects of non-verbal behaviour of interviewers on candidates' performance *Journal of Occupational Psychology* **49**, 171–6.

Quinn K.M. (1989) Influences of an interviewer's behaviours in child sexual abuse investigations. *Bulletin of the American Academy of Psychiatry and Law* **17** (1), 45–52.

Oppenheim A.N. (1968) *Questionnaire Design and Attitude Measurement* Heinemann, London.

Parten M.B. (1950) *Surveys, Polls and Samples* Harper, New York.

Reed M.T. (1986) Descriptive study of chemically dependent nurses. In *Psychiatric Nursing Research* (Ed. by J. Brooking) John Wiley, Chichester.

Rodgers W.L. (1987) Interviewing older adults: the accuracy of factual information. *Journal of Gerontology* **42** (4), 387–94.

Skidmore D. (1986) The effectiveness of community psychiatric nursing teams and base locations. In *Psychiatric Nursing Research* (Ed. by J. Brooking). John Wiley, Chichester.

Topf M. (1988) Verbal interpersonal effectiveness *Journal Psychosocial and Mental Health Nursing* **26** (7), 8–11; 15–16.

White T. (1986) Factors influencing general practitioners to refer patients to community psychiatric nurses. In *Psychiatric Nursing Research*, (Chapter 12) (Ed. by J. Brooking) John Wiley, Chichester.

Wilkie D.J. (1990) Use of the McGill Pain Questionnaire to measure pain: a meta-analysis *Nursing Research* **39** (1), 36–41.

Chapter 23
Questionnaire
Philip J. Barker

INTRODUCTION

The word 'questionnaire' is an umbrella term for a variety of instruments, some involving straightforward questioning, with 'closed' (Yes/No) answers; others inviting more 'open' responses, by use of checklists, ratings, or open-ended comments. Some questionnaires involve combinations of two or more different approaches. Where the questionnaire is employed within an interview, it may be described as an *interview schedule* (see Chapter 22). Where subjects provide attitudinal data, using some scaling technique, it may be described as a *rating scale*. It is appropriate to view these technical differences as representative only of the diversity of questionnaire design and application.

Emphasis is given in this chapter to the methodology of questionnaire construction: this is relevant both to self-report surveys (the mail questionnaire), and the use of questionnaires in direct interviewing, as described in the previous chapter. The general principles of questionnaire design are assumed to be similar in both situations.

THE FUNCTION OF THE QUESTIONNAIRE

The first requirement of the questionnaire is that it be suitable to collect data which can be used to test the hypothesis(es) of the study. Consider a study which asks the following question:

'what is the effect of "peer support" on the "mood levels" of clinicians working in terminal care?'

You need to be able to express, first of all, a relationship between the two variables: how are 'peer support' and 'mood levels' related? The resultant *hypothesis* is a conjectural statement about the possible relationship between two or more variables. In the *null* form (see Chapter 16), the hypothesis might state that '"peer support" has *no effect* upon "mood levels" of terminal care clinicians'. 'Peer support' might involve behaviours which are defined *by others* as 'supportive' (in the study setting they would be *perceived* by the clinicians to be present or absent); and 'mood levels' might represent *internal*, self-reported experiences. A questionnaire, completed either independently (self-report) or within an interview (interview schedule), might be the most appropriate mechanism for collecting information on the clinicians' 'perceptions of others' and related 'emotional experience'.

The questionnaire, in this example, would aim to study the terminal care situation, highlighting the *actual*, rather than the *hypothetical*, relationship between the experimental variables. For this reason, the questionnaire must ask questions which have a direct bearing upon the variables under study: 'peer support' and 'mood levels'. Each of these terms must be defined in operational terms, to ensure that the respondent is in no doubt as to which perceived behaviours and personal experiences are under study. In this sense, the first requirement of the questionnaire is to be *valid*: it must measure what it claims to measure.

The questionnaire should collect this information with the minimum distortion: the questions should elicit, as closely as possible, the true response of the individual. Questions should not 'lead' the respondent into making responses; and should be open to analysis which does not require corruption of the actual answers (see Chapters 27–29). These general aims are pursued by giving consideration to the *overall* design and *administration* of the questionnaire. Design issues relate to language, frame of reference, information level, nature, sequence, and form of questions. Administration will be discussed briefly in the case of self-report (survey) questionnaires: Chapter 22 (The Interview) discusses administration in some more detail.

GENERAL PRINCIPLES

The primary aim in designing the questionnaire is to *communicate* with the respondent. The respondent needs to understand the questions, and needs an appropriate structure to facilitate his response. To achieve this aim you must acknowledge the central role of *language*, and the general context in which the questions are set (the *frame of reference*), and the nature of the responses expected (the *information level*).

Language

The first priority is to choose language which allows the optimum exchange of ideas. Key words should be within the comprehension of the respondent: colloquialisms or clichés should be clarified or avoided. It seems self-evident that an interview schedule designed to elicit the respective attitudes of medical staff and patients towards 'quality of care', might differ both in terms of the questions asked, and the language used to define the questions. Consideration is given to the possible levels of literacy, ethnic and cultural background, as well as age and understanding of respondents. Technical language may be unintelligible to some; direct reference to taboo subject matter, such as sexuality or sexual abuse, may be anxiety provoking. The form of language chosen will facilitate communication, avoid patronizing people (by being too simplistic), or confusing, embarrassing or upsetting them by use of inappropriate terminology or expressions.

Frame of reference

The questionnaire needs also to introduce topics in a form which links in to the respondent's idea of what is or is not relevant to the study. As noted in the previous chapter, the respondent is given an 'agenda' for the interview: this prepares him for the line of questioning involved. Care is taken to ensure that the questions develop in a manner which fulfils the respondent's notions about reasonableness and logic.

For example:

Q. 1: 'Have you had a distressing emotional experience at work within the last month?'
Q. 2: (If yes) 'What effect did this have upon you, personally?'
Q. 3: 'Did that experience have any effect upon your work?'
Q. 4: (If yes) 'In what way?'

Information level

The questionnaire should also take care not to assume that a specific level of information is possessed by the respondent. The respondent may feel embarrassed or resentful if a question cannot be answered: this may prejudice the rest of the interview. Alternatively, the person may pretend to knowledge which he does not possess in order to avoid embarrassment.

DESIGN OF THE QUESTIONNAIRE

Nature

The questionnaire should investigate the *minimal* amount of the person's experience necessary to inform you about the research question. Many questionnaires begin by collecting details about the respondent: such as personal characteristics, history, and social context. The questionnaire should collect only as much information as is necessary to fulfil the specific aims of the study. For this reason, 'general life histories', used as a preamble to different studies, may be time wasting by being over-inclusive, or may fail to focus on the relevant biographical or demographic data.

The questionnaire can be used to collect basic information: identifying whether or not certain events have occurred; whether people agree or disagree with specific views or attitudes; whether or not they would like to see certain events occurring in the future. These 'black-and-white' questionnaires are relatively simple to administer or complete, but need to be carefully designed to ensure that the questions represent the most comprehensive response to the research question.

Alternatively, you may wish the respondents to *quantify* some experience, using a scaling technique as an adjunct to the Yes/No question, or selecting from a range of responses to provide a measure of frequency or severity. The respondents might also provide a 'qualitative' measure of some experience or attitude, using a rating scale or drawing from a list of adjectives, in an effort to explain more specifically how they feel or what they believe. The basic *nature* of the questionnaire is, however, determined by the research question: what do you want to *know*?

Question form

The form of the question involves the nature of the response expected. Two forms are possible: 'open' questions are structured to allow the respondents to answer in their own words, briefly or at length; 'closed' questions invite the respondent to select from pre-assigned categories of response.

Open questions

Here the respondents are asked to supply *any* kind of information they consider appropriate. Examples of open questions are:

(1) How do you feel about men in nursing?
(2) What aspects of your training did you find most rewarding?
(3) How can we integrate research findings into clinical practice?

Such open-ended questions *assume* that the respondent has feelings, recollections, or views on the topics addressed. The manner in which the question is asked allows the respondents 'space' to consider their responses: these can be developed and clarified by 'funnelling', as described in the *sequence* section below. The main advantage of open questions is that the respondents are allowed to define their own frame of reference. Although the three examples above specify a general target area (*feelings* about men; rewarding *aspects of training*; *integration* of research), the respondents have a range of options open when 'framing' their reply. The open question also allows you to evaluate both *attitudes* and *information* level: the respondents may be unaware of the position of men in nursing, or of specific research examples pertinent to their area of work. The open-ended question allows you to assess what the person thinks or feels, and also what the respondent 'knows' about the subject. However, if the respondent is asked to give an estimate of the number of men in nursing, or to discuss a specific research example, a perceived 'information deficit' might generate anxiety, obstructing an appropriate response, perhaps even prejudicing the response to the rest of the questionnaire. The open nature of the question also allows an opportunity to collect information or to identify areas of interest not anticipated in advance.

A number of drawbacks are involved in the use of open questions. Respondents may answer at great length, making data analysis difficult. Where respondents answer in great detail in the early stages, fatigue may present a problem in the later stages. Comparison of responses to the same questionnaire across time may also be difficult, especially where respondents phrase their answers differently on different occasions.

Open questions are most appropriate where the subjects are being invited to assess a personal experience, or as part of an exploratory study, aimed at developing appropriate closed questions.

Closed questions

These invite the respondent to choose from a range of possibilities. The simplest questions involve 'strict alternatives' or 'dichotomous' questions. Examples of closed questions are:

(1) Are you employed at present: Yes/No?
(2) Nursing is a genuine profession: Agree/Disagree.

Where more freedom is required to answer other questions 'alternative statements' are appropriate. For example:

How often did you meet with your supervisor?
(   ) more than once a day

(   ) daily
(   ) once every two days
(   ) every two to three days
(   ) every three to seven days
(   ) less than every seven days

Alternatively, a 'checklist' or *matrix question* can be used, as shown in Fig. 23.1.

How important are the following people to your care and treatment?

	Not important	Some importance	Very important	Of great importance
General practitioner				
Health visitor				
District nurse				
Consultant psychiatrist				
Social worker				
Clinical psychologist				
Community psychiatric nurse				

Fig. 23.1   Example of a checklist or matrix question.

Respondents can also be asked to select from a 'menu' of responses which are *factual*:

Are you: – 'single, married, divorced, separated';
         – 'unemployed, employed, self-employed, retired'. (Underline)
or *attitudinal*:

Which of the following statements *most* reflects your present opinion:
– Benzodiazepines should never be prescribed to patients with anxiety
– benzodiazepines are useful only in low dosages, over a short term
– benzodizepines are effective in short- to medium-term treatment of anxiety
– the disadvantages of long-term usage of benzodiazepines are exaggerated

Finally, respondents may be asked to *rank order* their responses along some continuum: such as 'importance', 'preference' or 'danger'.
How important are the following 'personality' characteristics in teaching staff?

Rank order the characteristics indicating 1 for the 'most important' through to 5 for 'least important':

    (   ) humorous
    (   ) creative
    (   ) analytical
    (   ) warm
    (   ) challenging

The longer the questionnaire, the more appropriate are 'dichotomous' questions, which speed up the answer rate, thereby reducing the risk of respondent fatigue. The major drawback to this form of question is the 'forced' nature of the response: people need to commit themselves strongly to one answer or the other. This may lead to information loss or may prove off-putting to the respondent.

Any of the 'multiple-choice' options can help the respondent recall or clarify events, beliefs, or feelings. There is some danger, however, that the set of optional responses might 'suggest' that such experiences have occurred or that such views have been or are held.

Length and wording

As noted earlier, the language used in the questionnaire is of central importance. Questions should be phrased with the lowest, rather than the average educational level of the target population in mind. Analysis of the comprehension level of the questionnaire is possible through use of standardized methods such as the FOG index (Gunning 1952) or Reading Difficulty Formula (Flesch 1949). (For a wide-ranging discussion of issues and methods related to communicating with patients see Ley (1988).)

Questions should be as short as possible. Oppenheim (1968) maintains that the maximum length of any question should be 20 words. It could be argued, however, that it is not the number of *words* which is important so much as the number of *ideas* contained within the question. The following two examples are of similar length: the former, however, involves two questions, whereas the latter has only one:

'Have you ever worked with people who abuse alcohol either in hospital or in the community?'

'Can you tell me if you have any experience of working with people who have abused alcohol?'

Special attention should be paid to vague or ambiguous terms or phrases which can mislead or confuse the respondent. Terms such as 'occasionally' or 'often' should be defined in terms of some specific time scale or frequency; technical terms should be paraphrased in the appropriate vernacular. All questions should be worded positively: 'Does this ever happen? . . . rather than negatively . . . This doesn't ever happen, does it?' If the respondent answered yes (or no) to the latter, it would not be clear whether this meant 'yes . . . this doesn't happen . . . or yes it does'. Questions which focus upon sensitive areas, such as sexual behaviour or the abuse of drugs, require careful wording. Kinsey *et al.* (1953) acknowledged that respondents might be embarrassed by questions about their sexual behaviour. Their solution, which has been widely copied, involved *assuming* that low-valued, or unusual forms of behaviour were possessed by the respondents, thereby relieving them of the burden of denial. Respondents are more likely to give details about some negative or low-valued behaviour if the question, 'When did you first begin to feel stressed at work?' is asked. The alternative version 'Did you ever feel that you couldn't cope with work?' is more likely to be answered negatively. In this context, it should be remembered that all questionnaires and interview schedules represent an intrusion into the private life of the individual. Care needs to be taken to spare embarrassment and to promote honest responses. Where highly taboo topics form the basis of the measure, self-report questionnaires may be more appropriate than use of the interview schedule.

Question sequence

A well-designed questionnaire should involve progressing easily from one question to the next, in a sequence which appears logical to the respondent. Indeed, the respondent should be able to anticipate the next question. This 'logical' sequence might differ significantly from the 'order' which is most pleasing to the researcher. The sequence can be determined by 'funnelling' questions: asking the most general, unrestrictive questions first as a preamble to successively more specific questions:

Example:
QUESTION 1: 'What do you think of the present state of nursing education?'
QUESTION 2: 'What are your thoughts about the proposals to develop wider post-basic training opportunities?'
QUESTION 3: 'What aspects of clinical nursing would benefit most from further training input?'
QUESTION 4: 'What sort of things should we be doing differently there?'
QUESTION 5: 'Some would say that we just can't afford such developments at present, what do you think?'

The *funnel technique* provides a means of access to the person's true views or opinions, avoiding distorting the answer by the contaminating proximity to answers which might be conflicting in nature. In the example above, the respondent is given a great deal of freedom on the first question, then is asked to discuss the topic more specifically. Questions 3 and 4 allow the respondent to clarify his own views about the topic, before being asked the crucial final question. If question 5 was asked alone, or even after question 2, a different response might be forthcoming.

In self-report questionnaires *filter questions* may be employed to guide the respondent through different groups of questions. The respondent who answers 'No' to one question may be asked to 'proceed to question 6'. This procedure can cause confusion. An alternative format, where the 'route' is illustrated graphically, is shown below:

'Does the community team have an office base in the community?'
NO   YES
'If "yes", what proportion of the team work from this base? ____

Does the community team comprise only one grade of nurse?'
YES   NO
'If "no", indicate the number of different grades of staff' ____

Other considerations

Take every precaution against influencing the response, whether by design or default. Leading questions or the use of loaded words, as noted above, can cause considerable influence. Equally, failing to cite the range of alternatives may represent a form of *bias* (Oppenheim 1968): For example:

'*Do you prefer working with patients of your own sex?*'

is less appropriate than:

'*Do you have any preferences for working with men or women patients, or doesn't it matter?*'

Care also needs to be taken in ordering the sequence of questions requiring yes/no answers. Cronbach (1950) described the phenomenom of *response set* where the same response is given repeatedly despite the question. One possible solution is to employ multiple choice questions rather than strict alternatives. Another option is to vary the positioning of the responses. For example:

Q. 1 . . . . Yes/No/Don't know
Q. 2 . . . . Don't know/No/Yes

Similarly, the *layout* of the self-report questionnaire can affect the responses. These should be clearly worded and attractively presented. The immediate visual impact will either arouse the respondent's interest, or discourage completion. All self-report measures should carry (on a separate page) a clearly written introduction, providing a general explanation of the purpose of the questionnaire. Instructions for completion should include a completed example: this should be similar in form, but should not include one of the actual items from the questionnaire.

The layout should also employ emphasis, using different type sizes, bold type or underlining, to help guide the respondent. If questionnaires are to be returned by post, the page size should allow easy folding into a stamped addressed envelope. Some studies even suggest that light-coloured paper is more attractive, in the case of postal returns, yellow, closely followed by pink, having better return-rates over other colours (Eastwood 1940).

Finally, all questionnaires should be submitted to a *pre-test*: this is a trial run designed to evaluate the adequacy of the tool in measuring the research variables, isolating any bias, vagueness, and otherwise inadequate questions. This test should be conducted with a small sample of subjects drawn from the study population.

SCALING METHODS

Scales involve a set of symbols or numbers so constructed that they can be assigned by rule to subjects, or their behaviours, indicating the subject's 'possession' of whatever the scale claims to measure. Typically, scales measure *attributes* or constructs: warmth, hostility, anger, or dependency, for example. Subjects can rate themselves, or may be judged, by independent raters. A variety of scaling methods are possible:

Agreement–disagreement scales: three variants of this scale are in common use. In the first variant, subjects are asked to 'agree or disagree' or indicate yes or no. In the second variant, subjects are asked to choose from three or more responses: 'yes – don't know – no'; or 'strongly agree, agree, no opinion, disagree, strongly disagree'.

Visual analogue: here, subjects are invited to indicate, with a cross or tick, where on a continuum between one attribute and another they believe they (or others) lie. These scales are *bipolar*, inviting the respondent to provide a judgment somewhere between one end of the continuum and the other.

Example:
In general, how would you define the patients in your ward?

Independent   ——————————————————————   Very dependent

(indicate by placing a X on the line)

Alternatively, the continuum can incorporate the points used to measure the respondent's score. The most common scale used is 7 points:

Independent   ——————————————————————   Very dependent

| 1 | 2 | 3 | 4 | 5 | 6 | 7 |

Likert scales: Attitudes can be measured more specifically using 'degrees' of agreement or disagreement. The Likert scale involves statements which are considered to be approximately equal. Typically, the Likert scale employs 10–20 statements which are considered to be approximately equal. The respondent ticks the item which most approximates their attitude or opinion. Respondents to Barker's (1988) Depression Locus of Control Scale, were asked to indicate their responses to statements such as:

'Good mental health is largely a matter of good fortune.'

using the scale:

agree strongly	–1
agree a lot	–2
tend to agree	–3
tend to disagree	–4
disagree a lot	–5
disagree strongly	–6

The Likert scale uses equal numbers of positive and negative statements, avoiding a 'don't know' response. The *orientation* of the statement can be either positive or negative: the statement above could be re-phrased:

'Good mental health has nothing to do with luck or good fortune?'

Semantic differential: here, the respondent is asked to rate a specific concept, across a number of characteristics, using seven-point bipolar ratings. The semantic differential uses bipolar adjectives, such as happy–sad; good–bad. In the example below, the respondents are asked to give their views of community psychiatric nurses:

Community psychiatric nurses (CPN's) are:

Responsible ——————————————————————— Irresponsible

7	6	5	4	3	2	1

Ineffective   ——————————————————————— Effective

1	2	3	4	5	6	7

(The above scores are entered by way of illustration only. The boxes would be left blank, to avoid 'leading' the respondent. As the example shows, characteristics should be reversed, in terms of their positive-negative values, to avoid the fixed response set discussed earlier.)

Typically, the respondents' attitude towards each concept is evaluated across a number of dimensions: *evaluative* – judging how valuable, good, fair (etc.) is the concept; *potency* – how strong, large, effective; and *activity* – how active, fast, efficient. In a study of general practitioners' attitudes towards the service provided by CPN's compared with six other occupational groups, White (1986) used a 14-scale semantic differential.

USE OF QUESTIONNAIRES

The survey questionnaire

Researchers have consistently employed *mail questionnaires* as a relatively economic and expedient method for collecting data from either large population samples (see chapter 21) or from subjects who are geographically inaccessible. Studies might aim, for example, to follow-up subjects discharged from experimental nursing projects, or to study graduates from basic or post-basic educational programmes. In either case, direct interviewing might either be costly in terms of interviewer time, or impossible, in terms of travel restrictions.

Self-report format: The survey questionnaire can take a number of forms. Biographical (demographic) data is a common constituent, serving to identify key characteristics of the population surveyed. The rest of the questionnaire can employ either yes/no, or either/or questions; multiple choice questions: ratings, or open-ended comments.

Examples:

(1) During your stay in hospital were you given information about your condition? YES/NO

(2) All long-stay residents should be transferred to alternative facilities in the community. Agree/Disagree

(3) When you were admitted to hospital, were you given information about:
    - your condition   Y/N
    - your nursing care   Y/N
    - visiting arrangements   Y/N   Please circle yes (Y) or no (N)
    - your medical treatment   Y/N
    - other hospital services   Y/N

(4) How do you think your training affected *your* subsequent professional practice, or attitudes? The 1–5 scale indicates 1 = very negative effect; 3 = no effect; 5 = very positive effect.

Clinical practice	1	2	3	4	5
Management skills	1	2	3	4	5
Development of your service	1	2	3	4	5
Patient/client involvement	1	2	3	4	5
Staff support	1	2	3	4	5

(5) What aspects of the programme did you find unsatisfactory? Describe briefly.

The design of the mail questionnaire is also important. Shorter formats produce better response rates over longer questionnaires. As noted earlier, care needs to be taken over the presentation of the questionnaire: typing, lay-out, language. A clear, concise, and friendly accompanying letter, supported by a stamped self-addressed envelope, can also enhance response rates. As will be noted later, care needs to be taken over the wording of items, to avoid leading the respondent, or confusing through use of vague or ambiguous terms. Some studies provide small financial incentives contingent upon completion. Even where funding would allow, the researcher needs to carefully consider ethical issues and the risk of offending some respondents.

Despite their practical advantages, where mail questionnaires are employed alone, a number of drawbacks have consistently been cited: poor response rates; inability to check accuracy of responses; and difficulty in making valid generalizations from the resultant unrepresentative sample (see Campbell & Katona 1953; Parten 1950; Warwick & Linninger 1975; Williams 1987). Robinson (1989) noted that methods of improving response rates, and reducing sampling bias, remain elusive. Most authorities suggest that the selective nature of the responses call any conclusions into question (Parten 1950). In White's (1986) study of the attitudes of general practitioners employing the semantic differential (noted above), despite the brevity of the questionnaire, a response rate of only 72% was achieved. In Kerlinger's (1986) view returns of at least 80–90% should be sought. Failing this, non-respondents should be studied to learn something of their characteristics.

SUMMARY

The various questionnaire formats described in this chapter are designed to collect information from the subject. The information can be *facilitated* by an interviewer (the interview schedule) in a face-to-face or telephone interaction. More often the information is elicited through self-report, where the questionnaires are either mailed to the respondent, or delivered and collected at a later date by the researcher. The former is more appropriate for larger samples, distributed widely; the latter for smaller, local samples. As with all methods of data collection, it is necessary to evaluate the potential usefulness of any instrument or method prior to its use within the formal study. As with other methods, estimates of validity and reliability (see Chapters 27, 28 and 29) will indicate the extent to which the instrument will usefully measure the research construct.

In designing any of the questionnaire formats described in this chapter, much emphasis should be given to the importance of rigorously testing the formats (Oppenheim 1968). You must establish that the tool reduces to a minimum errors of comprehension, or completion; whether committed by interviewers or respondents.

The advantages of the use of questionnaires, within an interview schedule format, were described in the previous chapter. Researchers who elect to employ self-report questionnaire methods are likely to be influenced by the following factors:

Self-report questionnaires are:
(1) Less costly than interviews, in terms of time and energy;
(2) Able to gain access to larger samples;
(3) Appropriate for subjects geographically distant from the researcher;
(4) More anonymous than direct interviews;
(5) Less threatening, especially where 'taboo' material is under review;
(6) Less prone to bias, evident in the interviewer interpretation.

These advantages need to be balanced, however, against numerous disadvantages associated with such formats. The key difficulty involves the often blunt refusal of respondents to complete, and/or return, the questionnaires. In a related vein, some subjects may ask friends or relatives to assist, or even complete the questionnaire independently, thus prejudicing the sample. Similarly, people with handicaps may be restrained from completing self-report measures, while other subjects may fail to comprehend the meaning of specific questions: this potential problem demands significant rigour in the construction and pre-testing of the format. Finally, questionnaires can often only address the research themes superficially. It is clear, however, that the constraints of time, money, and availability of support workers, will make self-report measures an attractive proposition to many researchers.

REFERENCES

Barker P. (1988) Chapter 11 in *An Evaluation of Specific Nursing Interventions in the Management of Patients Suffering From Manic Depressive Psychosis* PhD thesis, Dundee Institute of Technology.

Campbell A. & Katona G. (1953) The Sample Survey: A Technique for Social Science Research In *Research Methods in the Behavioural Sciences* (Ed. by L. Festinger & D. Katz). Holt, Rinehart and Winston, New York.

Cronbach L.J. (1950) Further evidence on response sets and test design *Educ. Psych. Meas.* **10**, 3.

Eastwood R.P. (1940) *Sales Control by Quantitative Methods,* Columbia University Press, New York.

Flesch R. (1949) *The art of readable writing,* Harper, New York.

Gunning R. (1952) *The technique of clear writing,* McGraw-Hill, New York.

Kerlinger F.N. (1986) *Foundations of Behavioural Research* 3rd edn. N.Y.: CBS Publishing Japan.

Kinsey A.C., Pomeroy W.B. & Martin C.E. (1953) *Sexual Behaviour in the Human Male* W.B. Saunders, Philadelphia.

Ley P. (1988) *Communicating with patients: Improving communication, satisfaction and compliance* Croom Helm, London.

Oppenheim A.N. (1968) *Questionnaire Design and Attitude Measurement* Heinemann, London.

Parten M.B. (1950) *Surveys, Polls and Samples,* Harper, New York.

Robinson D. (1989) Response rates in questionnaires *Senior Nurse,* **9** (10) 25-6.

Warwick D & Linninger C. (1975) *The Sample Survey: Theory and Practice,* McGraw-Hill, New York.

White E. (1986) Factors influencing G.P.'s to refer patients to community psychiatric nurses. Chapter 12 in *Psychiatric Nursing Research* (Ed. by J. Brooking) John Wiley, Chichester.

Williams C.A. (1987) Research by mail and other distractions *Journal of Professional Nursing,* **3** (6), 327; 376.

Recommended Reading

Bircumshaw D. (1989) A survey of the attitudes of senior nurses towards graduates *Journal of Advanced Nursing* **14** (1), 68-72.

Fenton M.V. (1987) Development of the Scale of Humanistic Nursing Behaviours *Nursing Research,* **36** (2), 82-7.

Flagler S. (1989) Semantic differentials and the process of developing one to measure maternal role competence *Journal of Advanced Nursing* **14** (3), 190-7.

Gulick E.E. (1987) Parsimony and model confirmation of the ADL Self-care Scale for multiple sclerosis persons. *Nursing Research,* **36** (5), 278-83.

Holmes S. (1989) Use of a modified symptom distress scale in the assessment of the cancer patient. *International Journal of Nursing Studies,* **26** (1), 69-80.

Humphris G.M. & Turner A. (1989) Job satisfaction and attitudes of nursing staff on a unit for the elderly severely infirm, with change of location. *Journal of Advanced Nursing,* **14** (4), 298-307.

Chapter 24

Observation

Philip J. Barker

INTRODUCTION

All data collection methods involve extensions or consolidations of the researcher's everyday behaviour. This is most true of observation: everyone uses their senses to collect information about 'their world', interpreting such 'data' to 'make sense' of their experience of their world. Observation could be defined as a 'heightened' form of such everyday sensation: the *systematic* use of the researcher's sensory mechanism, within a *rigorous* framework. In everyday 'observation' we *trust* the evidence collected by our senses. In the research setting, observation is characterised by *doubt*: you take nothing on trust, constantly seeking to define, clarify, redefine, and measure *objectively* the events which occur.

Why be objective?

The use of observational methods can be arduous. The researcher who selects an observational framework will have considered alternatives and found them wanting. Interviewing people (Chapter 22), or inviting them to complete self-report rating scales or questionnaires (Chapter 23), gives the following information: What the subjects' *think* they do, or how they *feel* about their own, or others' actions. The attitudes people have towards themselves or others, or their experience of their own lives, is a laudable object of study. Such personal 'subjective' experience, however, tells us little about what *actually* happened. The researcher who selects an observational framwork wants to know what *really* did take place, between whom, and to what end. In some cases you may also be interested to extend this 'awareness' through direct measurement: how often did this take place, or for how long; in effect, what was the magnitude of the event? In all cases, however, a similar aim is expressed, to *describe*, if not also to *explain* events in the research setting (Sackett 1978).

What to observe?

Observational methods can be used to collect data from across a wide spectrum. The following represents the most commonly selected 'target areas':

(1) *Individual characteristics*
Information which defines either the constant characteristics of the study population, such as apparently enduring or, alternatively, more temporary patterns of behaviour, physical states, or physiological reactions, are a key feature of many observational studies. In nursing research, data which defines the health

or illness characteristics of the individual, and gross or subtle fluctuations in their presentation, will have a major bearing upon the definition of nursing 'needs' and measures of nursing 'outcomes'. Similarly, the defining characteristics of nurses may provide the most important form of data for educational or managerial studies, investigating anything from the experience of training, to sickness and absenteeism. For example:

(2) *Non-verbal communication*
Facial expression, gestures, body postures, interpersonal distance, are important elements in the communication process, and represent an important area for nursing researchers. Some theorists would argue that these behaviours often define the meaning of the communication more clearly than verbal behaviour, which can be deceptive and misleading. *How* nurses interact with patients, other staff or one another, may be of as much significance, as *what* they say to one another (Wolfgang 1979).

(3) *Verbal behaviour*
The content and structure of communication is an accessible, if difficult, area for observers. The *manner* in which nurses interact with patients, relatives, other professional groups, or each other, are important areas of research. How such verbal interactions take place under specific conditions, such as in emergencies, where violence, hostility or other emotional conditions, such as death, provides a sharper focus to the research goals.

(4) *Everyday living skills*
The activities which patients perform as part of their everyday routine provides another important research target. Patients' engagement in self-care, social, and recreational activities, tells the researcher much about their needs, progress, or deterioration, if not also about the effects of the nurses' intervention (Smith, Hogan & Rohrer 1987).

(5) *Nursing skills*
This group represents a parallel set of observations, focused more specifically upon technical aspects of the nurse-patient relationship: how nurses admit patients to hospital, complete specific assessments, conduct tests or other procedures, or prepare and complete care plans, are typical examples of observational subject matter.

(6) *Environmental characteristics*
Information concerning the *stimulus* conditions under which all of the above behaviours take place, provides the definition of the 'scenario' in which nursing care takes place (Owens & Ashcroft 1982).

DIRECT (NON-PARTICIPANT) AND INDIRECT (PARTICIPANT) OBSERVATION

Observation can be employed in two ways: *direct* observation, which is characterized by objectivity, a systematic framework, and the use of formal recording technologies; and *participant* observation, where the observation collects information from 'within' the research setting. In the former, the observer tries to remain apart from the study situation, aiming to collect objective data uncontaminated either by the observer's presence or her value system. In the latter, the researcher aims to become a member (albeit temporarily) of the group under study. In such *participant observation* the researcher becomes involved with the object of study, such as a group of nurses or patients, and collects data through *logs* or *field notes* (Patton 1987; Samarel 1989). All observation is dependent upon the quality of the data recorded. In participant observation, overt recording materials may represent an obvious intrusion. In participant observation, formal recording methods are often dispensed with: instead, mental notes are translated afterwards into log or field note form. Proponents of participant observation argue that more unstructured methods allow a deeper insight into the 'workings' of the research setting, and often eschew more structured methods on the grounds that they are mechanistic, offering only a superficial, if not artificial, account of the research setting. Alternatively, critics of participant observation are concerned about the extent to which such a method may be prone to observer bias or 'observer effect': how does the observer retain objectivity if she is part of the study situation; and how can the study group fail to be affected by an observer living in their midst?

Participant observation is representative of the *qualitative* approach discussed in Chapter 13. Given the methodological conflict between indirect and direct methods, the former is not featured formally in this chapter, although many of the general principles governing the 'why's' of observation remain similar for both approaches. Instead, emphasis is given to *direct observation*, which involves establishing a *quantitative* picture of the research setting by collecting more objective data from 'outwith' the setting under study.

The observer

The ideal observer of any social situation would be a machine programmed to recognize and monitor those aspects of social behaviour of interest to the researcher. Human observers may be expected to follow the research protocol, but may end up being led by their own instincts or prejudices. Kerlinger (1979) has observed that scientific objectivity has little to do with the presumed objectivity of scientists themselves: it is a quality of the methodology. This view is important for the selection and training of observers: few are likely to be 'naturally objective'; but all must be prepared specifically to use the research methodology which has been confirmed as an objective procedure.

THE WORLD OF OBJECTIVE OBSERVATION

What is objective observation?

All methods of observation have *some* objectivity. The extent to which any *method* of observation can be called objective, depends on the degree of agreement between two observers using the observational method. The methods discussed in this chapter do not possess any monopoly on objectivity. The only difference between the methods here and, for example, participant observation procedures, lies in the extent to which any two observers using the procedure might agree on what is taking place. Objective observation, like other forms of observation, involves *inference*: judgements and decisions concerning 'what' to observe, and 'what' different variables might 'represent'. These involve assumptions about the meaning of behaviour if not about the whole world. All methods of observation end up classifying and categorizing variables: they all involve assumptions about the meaning of the events which have been observed (Jones & Nisbett 1987). Direct observation can be defined as *more objective*, but *no less inferential*, than other methods to the extent that different observers will end up with a similar 'picture' of the observed setting, providing that they employ the same observational procedure (Weick 1985).

Naturalistic observation

Studies which elect to use an observational method tend to focus upon the 'natural' environment: for example, caring behaviours actually performed in a specific clinical setting. Naturalistic observation draws heavily upon the principles and methodology of ethology: naturalistic observation can be defined as the practice of noting and recording facts and events in accordance with, or in imitation of what has been called, 'the essential character of the thing' (Jones, Reid & Patterson 1974).

Before you can record this 'essential character', a clear definition of the 'thing' must be developed: this should allow all observers to recognize 'it' when they see 'it'. Although direct observation involves a specific focus upon events occurring under specific conditions, this does not obviate the need for clear definition of the events and conditions. At some stage in the research process, you will make *inferences* about the relationship between the actual behaviour of the subjects and related environmental events. Such inferences depend upon empirical evidence: evidence which must be *as free of ambiguity* (and inference) *as possible*. The defining features of naturalistic observation, therefore, are:

(1) Recording of behavioural events *where* they occur;
(2) Emphasis upon *operational definitions* of the observed behaviour *and* related environmental events;
(3) Recording of events *when* they occur;
(4) Recordings conducted by impartial, *reliable* observers (Boice 1983).

OBSERVATIONAL TARGETS

Observational units: large or small?

Observational targets are commonly divided into *molar* or *molecular* targets. Molar behaviour involves large units of activity, such as 'co-operativeness', 'interaction', 'aggression', 'helping'. Molecular behaviours involve small, often highly specific, units of behaviour: 'nodded head (in agreement)', 'made eye contact', 'hit other', 'supported patient's arm'. Researchers are often divided ideologically between the value of either of these approaches: proponents of the study of molar behaviour suggesting that this represents a 'real' event, which becomes lost in the minutiae of molecular examples, which are often not valid representations of the area of inquiry. Molecular advocates suggest that molar studies often fail to attain adequate levels of reliability, as observers cannot agree as to whether or not these ill-defined events have occurred. You need to carefully consider the balance between both approaches. A highly reliable observational method can be developed if you define all the components of the target behaviour operationally. 'Helping' could be defined as:

'Holding patient's arm; supporting cup; giving instructions; making encouraging statements; pointing; opening doors; holding part of patient's clothing' . . . and so on.

Observers using such molecular definitions might attain a high degree of agreement on their occurrence. In the process, it could be argued that the pursuit of reliability has led to the loss of validity of the observational procedure. Were all the occurrences of these behaviours representative of 'helping'? It is possible that on some occasions some of these molecular actions had other functions?

Molar definitions, which involve broader 'natural' definitions, may appear more valid. 'Helping' might alternatively be defined as:

'giving physical support; listening attentively; interacting harmoniously to assist the attainment of the patient's own goals.'

Such definitions allow the observer to capture something of the 'flavour' of the event. Because of their inherent ambiguity, these definitions might lead to interpretation, probably resulting in a lowering of reliability.

The item pool

The so-called item pool may be determined in advance or may require a preliminary descriptive study of the research environment. Typically, a 'running narrative' might be employed to describe in some detail the activities of the subjects in relation to a variety of environmental effects. The researcher may decide to devote a period of time to *continuous direct observation*, recording as much of the general activity in the research setting as possible, afterwards abstracting behaviours and setting events which appear congruent with the research aims.

Operational definitions

The study which elects an observational methodology is likely to be concerned with the *discrete*, or actual relationship, between sets of variables: such a relationship is often assumed to be *causal*. It should not be forgotten, however, that although it is helpful to *think* causally, causal laws cannot be demonstrated empirically (Blalock 1961). It is sufficient to demonstrate the strength of a *relationship* between two sets of variables: this does not demonstrate, however, that p causes q.

The researcher has a large universe of actions, events and situations available which might *define* the subject area. From this universe, specific patterns of behaviour, and specific setting conditions, need to be identified, to narrow the focus of the study and to make observation viable. Once identified, these must be defined operationally, to provide the researcher, and more importantly the observers, with a 'working definition' of each behavioural response or setting event which might comprise the observational target. As noted above, the *item pool* is defined first, either by pre-selection, or by a preliminary 'journalistic' description of the study setting. In some studies, the item pool may be almost 'self-selective'; a study of the nursing care of people suffering from incontinence might elect to observe the frequency of *micturition* in different situations. Given that micturition involves voiding urine, the researcher may define some forms of micturition as 'continence' (when the subject urinates in a toilet facility); others as 'incontinence' (urinating in bed). These behaviours are defined *not* in terms of what the subject does, but in terms of the *stimulus conditions* under which the behaviour occurs. If you wish to *explain* some aspect of the study environment which is presently unclear, every effort should be made to define both the social behaviour of the subjects and the environmental stimuli under which these behaviours might appear.

Stimulus conditions

Bijou and Baer (1961) define three stimulus sources:

(1) *The physical environment:* any aspect of the physical world of the subjects. The details required in an operational definition of this class would involve size, colour, texture, weight, etc. of objects within, or of, the environment itself. Other sensory stimuli which might be incorporated within this environment, such as sounds (music, bells, birds), or light (flickering neon, bright sunshine) should also be included.

(2) *The social environment:* this would include details of the number, status and geographical relationship to the subject of others, and will provide basic data. Additional stimulus classification would involve defining the behaviour of significant others towards the subject: this might involve single class stimuli (nurse prompts subject to drink from cup), or multiple stimulus classes (nurse talks to subject; guides subject's arm; nurse holds plate on table).

(3) *The internal environment of the subject:* in field studies undertaken in the natural environment, it is probably impossible to monitor this class of stimuli: examples including, hunger, thirst, pain, visceral activity. In a seminal study, Bijou, Peterson and Ault (1968) suggested that contemporary research methods were inappropriate for measuring such 'biologically anchored variables'. It is clear that in many settings, nurse researchers must work towards incorporation of such variables in an effort to provide a more satisfactory explanation of the interactions between nurses and patients. In some nursing research studies, contemporaneous monitoring of some internal variables may be possible through use of physiological and biophysical measures.

Subject behaviour

Operational definitions of behaviour should contain sufficient information to measure the occurence of the event reliably. The definition should not be overly complex: 'cry' might be defined as:

'repeated, usually low-pitched, vocalizations, "waah, aaah-hah"'.

The definition serves *only* to help the observer classify the occurence, and to distinguish, where possible, one behaviour which might be confused with a similar pattern. Clearly, subjects might be 'crying' with frustration . . . in despair . . . or with joy. The 'meaning' of the behaviour may emerge by identification of complementary behaviours (such as gestures or body posture) or by recording the environmental context (stimulus conditions).

Observer effect

Many researchers who are unused to direct observation, fear that the presence of the observer will be a major, and continuing, disruptive influence. Although the entry of an independent observer to the research setting can have an initial disturbing effect, providing that certain considerations are applied, this disruption will be short-lived (Heyns & Lippet 1954). Subjects could be observed discretely from a distance, by audio or video recording or through viewing screens. These methods involve no disruption of the natural behaviour of the study group but do represent a major intrusion of a highly unethical nature and should be rejected from consideration. The observer needs to have a clear view of the research territory, while remaining unobtrusive. Direct observational data is often collected by research assistants who initially explain in full the purpose of their presence in the setting, and ask for the consent of the group to be observed.

OBSERVATIONAL METHODS

The two main classes of observational method are *automated* and *pencil and paper*.

Automated methods allow the observer to monitor single or multiple responses in real-time (event recorders). However, the advantage of sensitive, real-time, recording may be outweighed by considerations of cost and the level of sophistication and training required of observers in their use. Less complex automated devices, such as tally counters, hand-held or worn or the wrist, pedometers, and stopwatches, are used as an adjunct to pen–paper methods. In some situations audio or audio-visual recording may be appropriate: these recordings allowing more discrete analysis by pen-paper methods later. Situations which might justify the use of such observations are:

(1) When the action is so rapid that other methods of observation are inadequate;
(2) When the action is complex;
(3) When distinctions between one behaviour (or behaviour of one subject) and another is difficult.

In any of these situations, replay, pause, and slowing of the recorded action allows more detailed analysis. Unless such automated devices are used unobtrusively, however, they are also likely to represent a major source of 'observer effect'. The disruptive influence of such devices with children has long been reported (Hutt & Hutt 1970). This may be the case with other 'sensitive' populations: such as hospital patients, and the nurses caring for them.

Pencil and paper methods embrace a wealth of possibilities. In principle, all forms of 'observing and recording' would be included under this heading. For the sake of simplicity, only *formal* forms of observing and recording will be addressed here: those with a high degree of objectivity.

Observational rating scales

Observers can measure the subject by use of rating scales which are similar to the self-report measures described in Chapter 23. The most commonly used methods are:

- *The category rating scale:*   here the observer is asked to quantify the presence of specified behaviours. The observer is asked to select a category, from a menu, which best characterizes the behaviour or characteristics of the subject. The observer then rates the degree of the category present. The category item 'empathic' might be:

> *How empathic is the nurse?*   (tick one only)
> Very empathic   ( )
> Empathic   ( )
> Not empathic   ( )
> Not at all empathic ( )

Alternatively, the item could be defined further:

> *How empathic is the nurse?* (tick one)
> Always very empathic; can predict the patient's emotional state   ( )
> Mostly empathic; shows understanding of patient's feeling   ( )
> Rarely empathic; often fails to acknowledge patient's feelings   ( )
> Mostly unempathic; ignores patient's feelings   ( )

- *The numerical rating scale:* this format is similar to the Likert scales described in Chapter 23. Here the observer gives a numerical rating, or score, according to the perceived presence of some attribute, characteristic, or pattern or behaviour (Downing & Brockington 1978). The observer might be asked to rate a range of characteristics or behaviours 'using the following scale':

> 0 – absent; not performed
> 1 – minimal; performed infrequently or to limited degree
> 2 – moderate; performed intermittently or to some extent
> 3 – considerable; performed consistently or to great extent

- *The graphic rating scale:* similar to the linear analogue scale (Chapter 23); this scale employs a line or bar, with accompanying descriptive statements:

> *Describe the subject's presentation between 8 am and 12 md:*

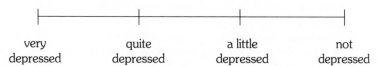

| very | quite | a little | not |
| depressed | depressed | depressed | depressed |

These scales can be presented in several ways: continuous lines, unmarked lines with two extreme definitions, identified intervals (as above), or segmented lines. Their key feature is that they fix a continuum in the observer's mind, suggesting intervals or degrees of the characteristic or behaviour. In Guilford's (1954) view, their virtues are many and their faults are few.

Observational rating scales can be used to measure virtually any variable which can be defined operationally by the researcher. In addition to behaviours, or behavioural characteristics, such scales might measure, for example:

(1) The quality of nursing assessments;
(2) Nurses' handwriting in care plans;
(3) Student nurses' use of theoretical concepts in written assignments;
(4) Nurses' emotional state under interview conditions.

Despite their potential, or perhaps because of their apparent widespread 'usefulness', a word of caution is appropriate. Even where scales are well-designed, they are prone to bias. One form of bias is the famous *halo effect*. Rugg (1921) defined this as a 'general mental attitude' towards the personality of other people which dominates our attitude towards their particular qualities. In research terms, this means that the observers' measure of some specific quality, behaviour, or other attribute of the person, may be dominated by their overall view of the person.

A further problem with ratings is the tendency of observers to err on the side of severity or leniency – observers may be too critical and tough – or they may 'feel sorry' for the subjects. Another dimension of this problem is the *error of central tendency*, where (usually) novice observers avoid all extreme judgments and consistently give the subjects an intermediate rating. All such problems indicate the need for rigorous preparation and monitoring of observers.

Direct observational methods

Actions which are short-lived and have a discrete beginning and end can be counted, using a frequency record. This is known as a frequency count. Any event which can be expressed *appropriately* as a number can be measured in this way. How often, for example (within a stated time frame) subjects:

(1) Are reported absent;
(2) Speak to patients;
(3) Are called out of meetings; or
(4) Request analgesic medication

can all be expressed as numerical frequencies. The major criterion for selection of this method is that the observer can identify the beginning and end of each event *precisely*.

The frequency count is most useful when the events occur at a moderate rate: neither too often nor too infrequently. Where high rates of occurrence exist, hand-held tally counters or more sophisticated automatic recording devices can be used as an adjunct. The major failing of this method is that, except where automated devices are used, the resultant measure gives no indication of distribution across time. Measures of the frequency of some event, per hour, day, week, and so on, is possible but, without the use of automated devices, or an alternative recording format, fluctuations in rate across time are lost.

Duration

The duration record measures the elapsed time of a given behaviour during a specific observation period. This is appropriate for behaviours of variable duration: talking, watching television, changing a catheter, for example. The observer needs to be able to identify the beginning and end of the behaviour, and must acknowledge all temporary cessations in the performance. The major drawback is that it is almost always confined to single-subject observation. It can, however, be incorporated easily with other methods into a multi-method observational format.

Latency

How long subjects *take* to respond to a given stimulus provides an alternative temporal dimension. For example, how long nurses take to:

(1) Respond to a patient's call for assistance;
(2) Locate emergency resuscitation equipment;
(3) Reach agreement on a specific issue of ward policy.

In some cases, the measure involves the time taken to begin the behaviour: in others, the time taken, from the cue, to complete the action.

Sampling behaviour

Two major methods of sampling behaviour are possible. These give an estimate of the frequency of some specified behaviour across time. This approach is used when the straightforward frequency count is found wanting.

The interval record

This method determines whether or not the behaviour has occurred within a specific time interval. Three variants are possible.

(1) In the first, an arbitrary time interval is selected, such as one minute. Any occurrence of the behaviour within the interval is recorded. A checklist of behaviours is commonly incorporated, and the serial occurrence of the different behaviours is recorded using serial numbers. This provides a total frequency for each behaviour, and an illustration of the temporal relationship of one behaviour to another. It provides only a crude estimate, however, of the time spent engaged in each behaviour.

(2) Alternatively, the time interval selected may be short enough to accommodate *only one* occurrence of the behaviour. If the observer determines that the behaviour to be observed lasts, on average, 20 seconds, this time interval is used to monitor its frequency. The common rule is that the behaviour is recorded as having occurred only if it occurs during *most* of the time interval. This method allows an estimate of the frequency of the behaviour, its rate across time, and the approximate amount of time spent engaging in the behaviour.

(3) Where the observer tries to measure more complex patterns of behaviour, including their relationship to the environment, the interval recording method requires further modification. In Figure 24.1 below (Barker 1977), the observer is collecting data on the behaviour of a young child in a playroom. Given the number of categories of behaviour and location included, a 10-second time interval is used:

	1	2	3	4	5	6
Location W: Wall D: Door F: Floor C: Chair T: Table	F	F	F	C	F	T
No object ST: Standing SI: Sitting W: Walking C: Crawling SP: Spinning	SI	SI	ST	SI	W	ST
With self B: Blowing V: Vocalizing R: Rocking H: Hitting WA: Waving arms WL: Waving legs RH: Rubbing hands RF: Rubbing face	R	R	WA	RH	V	H

Fig. 24.1 Example of data collection sheet: observation.

5 seconds to *observe*, and 5 seconds to *record*. The observer enters only the *code* for the location or behaviour in each time cell.

The time sample

This method involves brief observations, usually momentary, designed to identify whether or not a specific behaviour was occurring *at that particular time*. This can be used for single behaviours with single subjects, or with multiple behaviours across groups. This format allows a rough estimate of the frequency of patterns of behaviours across time, requiring no special equipment, and limited training of observers (Weick 1985).

GENERAL CONSIDERATIONS

Narrow or broad focus?

The major difference between recording methods, apart from those already noted, lie in their specificity or generality.

Specific observational systems measure either single or multiple classes of behaviour:

(1) Single response classes: focus upon one behaviour to the exclusion of all others:
(2) Multiple class responses: focus upon several behaviours. Typically, these are divided into mutually exclusive categories (behaviours which cannot occur at

the same time as others in that class); and concomitant behaviours (behaviours which can be contemporaneous with others).

General observational systems involve recording not only the subjects' responses but also the setting stimuli; the behaviour of other people in the environment, and other events which might be related to the subjects' actions. This form of observation is most valuable since it allows an opportunity to infer connections between the relative frequency of responses and their temporal relationship to other stimuli.

Training observers

A well-developed observational method is only as good as the skill of the observer. Observers require the following preparation:

(1) *Orientation to the study:* observers need to know how the observation format has been developed and why specific behaviours and/or settings have been selected. These boundary considerations are important if the observer is to develop an unusual perception of perhaps familiar patterns of behaviour.

(2) *Unstructured observation period:* observers should be offered an opportunity to study the research setting *without* the aid of the observational schedule. This exercise should provide the observers with an awareness of their need for clear definitions and a formal observational structure.

(3) *Formal introduction:* Even the simplest recording tool is likely to appear daunting at first glance. For this reason the observers should be guided patiently through the observational method, and should be provided with clear instructions as to the researcher's expectations.

(4) *Role-play:* Initial training should be conducted under role-play conditions, perhaps using a video recording, or group of actors, the action being stopped at strategic intervals to allow questions and clarification.

(5) *Pilot observation period:* the observers should spend a period of time completing the measures under full research conditions. Data from this pilot are discarded following critical analysis of the experience of the observers and the establishment of inter-observer reliability. This period can also be used to 'acclimatize' the subjects to the observer's presence, thereby reducing the potency of observer effect when formal data collection begins.

Reliability and validity

The use of formal means of direct measurement and clear operational definitions is not always sufficient to guarantee reliable data collection. Agreement between observers is essential if the measures are to be described as objective. Disagreements between observers can occur for the following reasons:

(1) The operational definitions may be inadequate;
(2) The observational code may be inadequate;
(3) The observers may be inadequately trained;
(4) The procedure for calculating reliability may be faulty.

The pilot observation phase is used to investigate these first three possibilities. At least two observers should study the same situation independently: their data is subsequently analysed to assess the degree of agreement. The most commonly used statistical methods for computing reliability is the correlation coefficient (see Chapters 27 & 28). The *acceptable* degree of agreement between observers is a moot point. Commonly, however, a reliability coefficient of less than 0.8 is deemed to be unacceptable.

The validity of observational methods has largely been neglected in the social science research literature due in part to the absence of external criteria to validate the kind of variables studied. Reliability and validity are closely connected. Clearly, an observational method which is not reliable cannot be valid. However, it can be reliable without necessarily being valid. Validity is concerned with the extent to which the observational method measures what it claims to measure. Does the interval measure illustrated in this chapter actually measure 'free play', or is it measuring something similar, but not identical. (For further discussion see Boice 1983; Brink & Wood 1989; Polit & Hungler 1985.)

SUMMARY

Observational methods are highly appropriate for nursing research studies, given that nurses spend much of their professional lives observing patients. Many nursing research questions may best be studied by collecting data from 'outwith' the research setting rather than by interviews or use of self-report measures. This applies equally to descriptive and experimental studies of nursing care, as well as to studies of the organizational context of nursing and the function of nurse education environments. Observational methods have a special appeal since they offer an opportunity to collect data 'at first hand', studying what actually takes place in any given setting.

Despite this appeal, observation is fraught with many ethical and practical problems. It was noted in the introduction that unless subjects agreed to being 'studied', any observational system, no matter how innocuous, would be unethical. It is clear that many people, patients, and nurses themselves, find observation too intrusive. Weick (1985) observed that people have strong needs not to examine their lives: observers threaten this avoidance. Even if consent is gained, the emotional state of the observer can bias the resultant data. Although steps can be taken to prepare and monitor observers, it seems unlikely that many observers will adopt a 'camera-like' persona. Despite these reservations, it is clear that many aspects of nursing will only be understood further by use of observational methods. Researchers are required to develop the necessary rigour central to the design of valid instruments and the accompanying discipline needed to ensure their reliability.

REFERENCES

Barker P. (1977) The ABC of ABA: Observational method in applied behaviour analysis. In *Observational Methods in Nursing Research* (Ed. by R. Dingwall & M. Colledge), Department of Health and Social Security, London.

Bijou S.W. & Baer D.M. (1961) *Child Development: A systematic and empirical theory* Appleton-Century-Crofts, New York.

Bijou S.W. *et al.* (1968) A method to integrate descriptive and empirical field studies at the level of data and empirical concepts. *Journal of Applied Behaviour Analysis* **1** (2), 175–91.

Blalock H. (1961) *Causal inferences in nonexperimental research*, University of North Carolina Press, Chapel Hill, NC.

Boice R. (1983) Observational skills. *Psychological Bulletin* **93** (1), 3–29.

Brink P.J. & Wood M.J. (Eds). (1989) *Advanced Design in Nursing Research* Sage Publications, London.

Downing A.R. & Brockington I.F. (1978) Nurse rating of psychotic behaviour *Journal of Advanced Nursing* **3**, 551–61.

Guilford J. (1954) *Psychometric Methods* (2nd edn.) McGraw-Hill, New York.

Heyns R. & Lippit R. (1954) Systematic observational techniques In *Handbook of Social Psychology*, (Ed. by G. Lindsey) Addison-Wesley, Baltimore, MA.

Hutt S.J. & Hutt C. (1970) *Direct Observation and Measurement of Behaviour* C.C. Thomas, Springfield, Illinois.

Jones E.E. & Nisbett R.E. (1987) The actor and the observer: Divergent perceptions of the cause of behaviour. In *Attribution: Perceiving the causes of behaviour.* (Ed. by E.E. Jones), Lawrence Erlbaum, Hillsdale, NJ.

Jones R.R., Reid J.B. & Patterson G.R. (1974) Naturalistic Observation: in *Clinical Assessment* (Ed. by P. McReynolds), **Vol. 3**, Jossey-Bass, San Francisco.

Kerlinger F. (1979) *Behavioural Research: A conceptual approach* Holt, Rinehart & Winston, New York.

Ownes G. & Ashcroft J.B. (1982) Functional analysis in applied psychology *British Journal of Clinical Psychology* **21**, 181–9.

Patton M.Q. (1987) *How to use qualitative methods in evaluation* Sage, California.

Polit D.F. & Hungler B.P. (1985) *Essentials of Nursing Research: Methods and Applications* Lippincott, Philadelphia.

Rugg H.O. (1921) Is the rating of human character practicable? *Journal of Educational Psychology*, **12**, 425.

Sackett G.P. (1978) (Ed.) *Observing Behaviour* (**Vol 2**) University Park Press, Baltimore, MA.

Samarel N. (1989) Caring for the living and dying: a study of role transition. *International Journal of Nursing Studies*, **26** (4), 313–26.

Smith D.W., Hogan A.J. & Rohrer J.E. (1987) Activities of daily living as qualitative indicators of nursing effort. *Medical Care*, **25** (2), 120–30.

Weick K.E. (1985) Systematic observation methods. In *Handbook of Social Psychiatry* (Ed. by G. Lindsey & E. Aronson), (**Vol 1**) Random House, New York.

Wolfgang A. (Ed.) (1979) *Nonverbal Behaviour: Applications and cultural implications* Academic Press, New York.

Chapter 25
The Critical Incident Technique
Desmond F.S. Cormack

The critical incident technique is a set of procedures for collecting direct observations of human behaviour in such a way as to facilitate potential usefulness in solving practical problems. An incident relates to any observable human activity that is sufficiently complete in itself to permit inferences to be made. This data collection technique was popularized by Flanagan (1954), an American psychologist, who wrote one of the earliest comprehensive descriptions of it.

The use of this technique by war-time researchers demonstrates how it was applied during the early stage of its development. Although the situation and problems described below are clearly not related to nursing, the same principles apply irrespective of the situation being researched. The problems facing the researchers towards the end of the 1939–45 war related to establishing those factors (incidents) which enabled United States Army Air Force crews to achieve success during their combat flying missions. Following each mission, crew members were asked to report incidents observed by them which were effective or ineffective in terms of achieving a successful flying mission. The questions put to the crew members related specifically to the activities of the officer leading the mission: they were asked, 'Describe the officer's action', and 'What did he do?' Analysis of several thousand responses (critical incidents) from crew members enabled the researcher to describe what the officer leading such a mission would have to do to achieve success and what he should not do to avoid failure.

It is not difficult to see how such a technique might be used in nursing to establish the factors that relate to, for example, giving a good nursing report. In this example, respondents such as nurses, who receive nursing reports, may be asked to describe activities (critical incidents) which result in an effective report being given by the nurse in charge of the ward. Examples of what nurses might say in response to that question are, 'The ward sister gave *all* nurses a report', or 'She gave us a report on *all* patients', or 'The report was very clear and specific'. A question relating to ineffective reporting might get replies such as, 'Sister is very vague when she tells us about the patients', or 'She occasionally forgets to tell us really important things', or 'Only the staff nurse gets the report'. Analysis of respondents' responses will enable the researcher to compile a description of effective and ineffective report-giving.

The use to which the researcher puts the information collected using the critical incident technique, depends on the purpose of the research. For example, the analysed critical incidents may be used when teaching nurses how to give nursing reports, or they may be used when assessing the ward sister's ability to give a report. The teacher or assessor is able, as a result of having effective/ineffective report-giving analysed in this way, to have specific and critical elements of the report-giving process in mind when teaching or assessing. In short, they will no

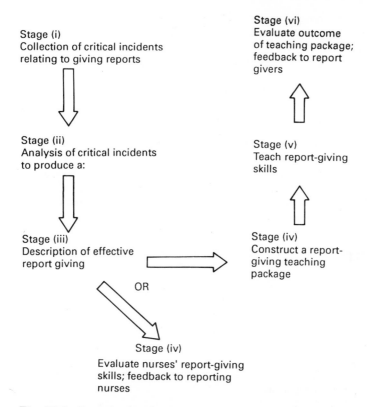

Stage (i)
Collection of critical incidents
relating to giving reports

Stage (ii)
Analysis of critical incidents
to produce a:

Stage (iii)
Description of effective
report giving

OR

Stage (iv)
Evaluate nurses' report-giving
skills; feedback to reporting
nurses

Stage (vi)
Evaluate outcome
of teaching package;
feedback to report
givers

Stage (v)
Teach report-giving
skills

Stage (iv)
Construct a report-
giving teaching
package

Fig. 25.1 Example of application of critical incident technique.

longer teach and assess in terms of what they *think* is important from a highly
personal and often biased viewpoint. Rather, they will teach and assess in terms of
specific criteria arrived at as a result of having applied this technique. Figure 25.1
shows how the critical incident technique may be used to improve the quality of
report-giving.

A major advantage of the critical incident technique is that it depends on
descriptions of *actual* effective events, rather than on descriptions of things as they
should be. Thus the technique is more concerned with the real, rather than the
imagined world, and is able to take account of the constraints and limitations under
which we all live and work. Critical incidents have been described as '. . . snapshot
views of the daily work of the nurse . . . the advantages of this technique are that
they provide a sharply focussed description in which opinions, generalizations and
personal judgments are reduced to a minimum.' (Clamp 1980.)

THE USE OF THE CRITICAL INCIDENT TECHNIQUE IN NURSING

The critical incident technique, as a means of collecting nursing research data, has
been widely used in the United States for more than twenty years. It has been
used, for example, to identify the role of the private duty nurse, to identify criteria
for the evaluation of student nurses, and to develop an evaluation procedure for
assessing staff nurses. Two important reference works on the use of the technique

in the US are those by Fivars and Gonsell (1966) who used it to identify problems in nursing, and the major work by Jacobs *et al.* (1973), who undertook a nationwide study of the work of the psychiatric nurse.

Nurse researchers in the United Kingdom are increasingly using the critical incident technique, see Long (1976), Clamp (1980), and Cormack (1983), who used it to describe the work of the psychiatric nurse in a sample of 11 Scottish hospitals.

The versatility of the critical incident technique is undoubtedly considerable, and it is particularly effective in obtaining data relating to actual nursing activities which are considered to reflect effective or ineffective nursing practice. One disadvantage of this technique is that it relies on the memories of respondents, their ability to distinguish between effective and ineffective nursing, and their ability to recollect specific and concrete examples of nursing. However, the advantages of this technique considerably outweigh the disadvantages.

APPLICATION OF THE CRITICAL INCIDENT TECHNIQUE

Having decided that this particular data collection technique is most suited to your needs, you can then proceed through a series of six phases (as shown in Fig. 25.2).

(1) Decide who should provide critical incidents
(2) Consider the number of critical incidents required
(3) Design a data collection form
(4) Decide where to collect critical incidents
(5) Decide how to collect critical incidents
(6) Analyse critical incidents

Fig. 25.2 Application of the critical incident technique.

These phases are in addition to those described in other chapters that relate to the research process in general. To illustrate the application of this technique, it will be assumed that you are seeking to obtain incidents which will enable you to describe the work of staff nurses in a particular hospital.

Decide who should provide critical incidents

You will first have to identify the group, or groups, of people who will be able to give an informed description of effective/ineffective nursing. It is often useful to include a range of respondent groups who are close to the work of the nurse. Bearing in mind that the work of nurses may include patient care, relating to other staff members, communicating with relatives, and working with other staff groups, all of these may be considered as potential respondents.

Clearly, the range of respondent groups will vary considerably from setting to setting. It may be impossible to include patients who are extremely ill, but possible to include those who are relatively well. Similarly, in those settings where the work of nurses takes them into contact with medical staff and para-medical groups such as occupational therapists and physiotherapists, it may be appropriate to invite those groups to contribute. In short, you must decide which groups to include on the basis of their knowledge of the work of the nurse, and which groups to exclude because of their lack of contact with, or knowledge of, these matters.

Consider the number of critical incidents required

There is no way of knowing in advance how many incidents need to be collected to answer the question being researched. As a general guide, the less complex the subject being researched, the smaller is the number of incidents required; conversely, the more complex the subject, the greater the number of incidents required. For example, if you are only concerned with the work of the nurse as it relates to student teaching, far fewer will be required than if you are concerned with all work carried out by the nurse. Even so, there is no way of predetermining the number of required incidents.

As a general rule, begin by collecting critical incidents without having any specific number in mind, and collect the minimum number which will provide an answer to the question being asked. This can be achieved by continuing to collect and analyse critical incidents until the last 100 incidents fail to provide new information about the work of the nurse. Only then can you be reasonably sure that the collection of further incidents would add nothing new, and that the incidents already collected contain a reasonably comprehensive description of the subject being researched.

Please recall a time when a nurse did something which you think should be ENCOURAGED because it seemed to be very EFFECTIVE. Please give your answer in five parts as follows:

A. Grade of nurse being reported on. _____

B. What were the events leading up to the activity? _____

_____

_____

_____

C. What did the nurse do that seemed so EFFECTIVE? _____

_____

_____

_____

D. Why was the activity so EFFECTIVE? _____

_____

_____

_____

E. Grade of respondent. _____

Fig. 25.3   Sample form for collecting effective critical incidents.

Design a data collection form

The data collection form is used to give instructions to respondents and to record their responses. It may also be used to contain additional information such as the grade of the respondent, and the grade of nurse being described in the incident. As with all data collection tools, only information which is needed should be collected.

The form on which the critical incident is to be written will, in most instances, be accompanied by written information giving the respondent additional information such as the purpose of the study, the promise of anonymity and confidentiality, or both. An example of a data collection form relating to effective incidents is shown in Fig. 25.3.

In most instances, it is of value to also collect critical incidents which describe activities which are ineffective, that is the behaviours which should be avoided in order to achieve effective functioning. Figure 25.4 presents an example of a form of collecting examples of ineffective critical incidents.

Please recall a time when a nurse did something which you think should be DISCOURAGED because it seemed to be very INEFFECTIVE. Please give your answer in five parts as follows:

A. Grade of nurse being reported on. _____

B. What were the events leading up to the activity? _____

_____

_____

_____

C. What did the nurse do that seemed so INEFFECTIVE? _____

_____

_____

_____

D. Why was the activity so INEFFECTIVE? _____

_____

_____

_____

E. Grade of respondent. _____

Fig. 25.4   Sample form for collecting ineffective critical incidents.

Decide where to collect critical incidents

The setting in which incidents will be collected depends largely on the purpose and scope of the study. If you are concerned only with the work of nurses within a single ward of one hospital, then only incidents from respondents who are familiar with the work of nurses in that particular ward are collected. Alternatively, to describe the work of nurses in six surgical wards within a hospital, the source of critical incidents must be extended accordingly. Finally, if you are interested in describing the work of nurses in the region, you will have to include a sample of respondents who are familiar with the work of nurses in the region.

Decide how to collect critical incidents

Two methods of collecting critical incidents, which resulted in very different response rates, were used by Cormack (1983). First, groups of potential nurse respondents were personally given appropriate forms and instructions and asked to use the internal mailing system to return the completed critical incident to the researcher. The response rate using that method was 2.45%. Second, groups of nurse respondents were given the appropriate form and instructions and asked to complete them in his presence. The response rate using that method was 79%.

It is probably best to begin by gathering potential respondents in small groups and to ask them to participate by giving appropriate information about the study, what is required of them, and to answer questions they might have. Cormack (1983) asked his nurse respondents to provide two effective and two ineffective critical incidents.

Analyse critical incidents

Although all critical incidents will relate to the same general subject, the work of the nurse, for example, they will describe differing aspects of that work. Some incidents may relate to administrative tasks, while others may relate to patient care or teaching, for example.

Analysis of data usually takes the form of inductive classification of incidents. This means that a classification system is constructed as the data are being analysed, rather than before. If the first incident relates to 'Physical nursing care', then one part of the classification will relate to 'Physical nursing care'. If the second incident relates to 'Teaching learners' this clearly does not fit into the only existing part of the classification system, therefore a second part must be created. This process continues until all incidents have been classified within the system which is being created as a result of the classification. The incidents may well be classified using a two- or three-tier system which starts with a fairly general description and progresses to an increasingly more specific one. The classification system may contain a number of general areas, one of which is 'Nursing care', a category of which may be 'Physical nursing care', and which contains a sub-category such as 'Gives bed bath'. In using critical incidents to describe the work of psychiatric nurses, Cormack (1983) created a classification system with four major areas, each with a number of categories, with each of these having a number of sub-categories. An adaptation from that classification system (shown in Fig. 25.5) will demonstrate its structure.

If the critical incidents relate to the work of the nurse, you now have a

AREA A: STAFF INITIATED THERAPEUTIC INTERVENTION
Categories
(1) Uses self as a therapeutic tool
    Sub-categories:
    (i) Makes self available to patients
    (ii) Provides opportunities or encourages patients to talk about their problems,
        etc. etc.
(2) Makes therapeutic use of the environment
    Sub-categories:
    (i) Encourages patient-patient understanding and relationships
    (ii) Encourages or facilitates patients playing an active part in their treatment,
        etc. etc.
Note: AREA A had a total of 5 categories

AREA B: ADMINISTRATIVE ACTIVITY
Categories:
(1) Ensures availability of non clinical patient data
    Sub-categories
    (i) Is aware of identity of patients
    (ii) Is familiar, when necessary, of the location of patients,
        etc. etc.
(2) Protects and secures patients' property
    Sub-categories:
    (i) Arranges for, or offers, security of patients' property
    (ii) Shows respect and concern for patients' property,
        etc. etc.
Note: AREA B had a total of 3 categories

AREA C: PROVIDES, PLANS FOR OR MONITORS PHYSICAL CARE
Categories:
(1) Administers medication
    Sub-categories:
    (i) Administers medications carefully, accurately, and as prescribed
    (ii) Ensures, by observation or assistance, that medications are taken,
        etc. etc.
(2) Gives physical care
    Sub-categories:
    (i) Monitors physical health of patient
    (ii) Selects or initiates appropriate physical care,
        etc. etc.
Note: AREA C had a total of 2 categories

AREA D: PERSONNEL FUNCTION
Categories:
(1) Maximizes staff contribution
    Sub-categories:
    (i) Encourages, accepts, and uses appropriate staff suggestions
    (ii) Arranges work load or routine to maximize staff effectiveness and/or patient
        care,
        etc. etc.
        Note: AREA D had a total of 2 sub-categories

Fig. 25.5 Classification of critical incidents (Example).

description of the work of that group, and can proceed beyond this point according to the purpose of the research. If a description of the work of the nurse is all that is required, the analysis need go no further. If the aim is to establish what nurses require to be taught in order to be effective nurses, the description of the work of that group might be converted into an in-service or continuing education syllabus which will form the basis of the nurse's continuing/in-service education.

A full description of the application of the critical incident technique, and the means of analysing and classifying data, is given in Cormack (1983).

CONCLUSION

As with all data collection techniques, the collection of critical incidents requires careful preparation, planning, and practice. It is heavily dependent on the ability of respondents to provide specific examples of the activity or work being researched, and their ability to distinguish between effective and ineffective practice. These are skills which may not come easily to potential respondents, particularly some nurse respondents who may have little recent experience in examining and describing their work in this way. However, the researcher who chooses this data collection technique can, with sufficient effort, skill, and understanding, minimize the problems which respondents will undoubtedly have.

The provision of ineffective critical incidents, crucial to understanding some aspects of effective nursing, may be difficult for some respondents. Some may be afraid that by describing examples of ineffective nursing, they may be seen as 'telling tales' or 'letting the side down'. Bearing in mind that an understanding of what a work group should not do is as important as the knowledge of what it should do, it is essential that you enable the respondent to provide critical incidents without fear of reprisal or criticism from colleagues or senior staff. In this respect, there is much to be done by you to ensure that the responses are confidential and provided anonymously.

REFERENCES

Clamp C. (1980) Learning through incidents. *Nursing Times* **40**, 1755–8.
Cormack D. (1983) *Psychiatric Nursing Described*. Churchill Livingstone, Edinburgh.
Fivars G. & Gonsell D. (1966) *Nursing Evaluation: The problem and the process.* Macmillan, New York.
Flanagan J.C. (1954) The critical incident technique. *Psychological Bulletin* **51** (4), 327–58.
Jacobs A. *et al.* (1973) *Critical Behaviours in psychiatric mental health nursing.* **Vols. 1, 2 & 3**. American Institutes for Research.
Long T. (1976) Judging and reporting on student nurse clinical performance: some problems for the ward sister. *International Journal of Nursing Studies*, **13**, 115–21.

FURTHER READING

Andersson B. & Nilsson S. (1964) Studies in the reliability and validity of the critical incident technique *Journal of Applied Psychology* **48** (6), 398–403.
Bailey J. (1956) The cirtical incident technique in identifying behavioural criteria of professional nursing effectiveness *Nursing Research*, **5** (2), 52–64.
Dachelet C.J. (1981) The critical incident technique applied to the evaluation of the clinical practicum setting. *Journal Of Nursing Education*, **20**, 15–31.

Grant N.K. & Hrycak N. (1985) How can you find out what patients think about their care. *The Canadian Nurse*, **81** (4), 51.

Rimon D. (1979) Nurses' perception of their psychological role in treating rehabilitation patients: a study employing the Critical Incident Technique. *Journal of Advanced Nursing*, **4**, 403–13.

Ryback D. (1967) A Critical Incident Simulation Technique for Nurse Selection. *International Journal of Nursing Studies*, **4**, 81–90.

Sims A. (1976) The critical incident technique in evaluating student nurse performance. *International Journal of Nursing Studies*, **13**, 123–30.

Woolsey L.K. (1986) The Critical Incident Technique: An Innovative, Qualitative Method of Research. *Canadian Journal of Counselling*, **20** (4), 242–54.

D: Data Handling

The preceding phases of the research process will have taken full account of the need for data to be stored, analysed, presented, and reported and disseminated. Thus, when data are being collected, the researcher should be quite sure as to how they will be handled, rather than be in the unfortunate position of collecting data then asking the question, 'what shall I do with it?'

When planning a study, particularly when considering data collection methods and the quantity and type of data to be collected, the researcher will have taken account of how the collected data will be handled. The handling of data collected during the pilot study will determine whether or not the data can be handled; if there are problems, then the data collection methods can be adjusted in a further pilot study.

Data handling has four distinct elements: storage (see Chapter 26), analysis (see Chapters 27 to 29); presentation (see Chapter 30), and the reporting and dissemination of the research (see Chapter 31).

Chapter 26
Data Storage
Desmond F.S. Cormack

The preceding four chapters have presented a selection of means of collecting research data. As the data are being collected, or at the end of their collection, they will have to be stored and subsequently analysed. Data storage has two basic related purposes: first, to enable information to be contained in a way which makes it reasonably accessible; second, to enable you to analyse the data.

Nurses are no strangers to information collection and storage, much of their time being used to record and store clinical data. Usually, however, it is stored in a way which would make an analysis of large quantities difficult. For example, in relation to each of the 600 patients in a given hospital, information relating to all patients' clinical status will be recorded daily, if not more frequently. However, if a nurse clinician, administrator, or researcher wished to establish how many patients had been incontinent each day during a specific one-week period, this may prove difficult if not impossible to ascertain. The reason for this difficulty is that episodes of incontinence, if they are recorded, are recorded in relation to individual patients and not in a way which would allow easy access, or which would enable overall calculations to be made. Alternatively, a researcher may well collect a large amount of data which, in its original form, is difficult to store and analyse. For example, in relation to the national census, the original data would consist of many millions of census forms. Clearly, it would be difficult, although not impossible, to analyse it by making a manual count of the many millions of forms involved. However, a better approach is to store the data in such a way as to make such analysis easier – for example, in a computer. The purpose of this chapter is to illustrate three commonly used methods of storing data: storage in original form, the Copland-Chatterson card (Cope-Chat card) system, and the computer. As with all phases of the research process, those stages which precede data storage must take account of the proposed data storage method. Similarly, the choice of data storage method will have implications for the next phase of the process, data analysis.

The means and ease by which data can be stored partly depends on whether they are qualitative or quantitative in nature. Qualitative data are not readily transferable into a numerical format; in addition, they are often generated as a result of open questions. An example of an open question is, 'What do you find interesting about nursing?' Responses to this question may include a verbal reply lasting up to five minutes. Such a response is recorded on paper may occupy 2–3 pages and be *relatively* difficult to store in anything other than its original form. By contrast, quantitative data, which are often generated as a result of closed questions, are relatively easily stored in a 'non-original' format. An example of a closed question is, 'Are you a registered nurse?', responses being 'Yes', 'No', or

'Don't know'. The data generated as a result of such a question, answered by 100 respondents, might be:

'Yes'   24
'No'   75
'Don't know'   1

STORAGE IN ORIGINAL FORM

Data are usually recorded initially in writing, occasionally by means such as tape or video recordings. Invariably, but not necessarily, data collected by means other than in writing are transferred into written form. It is appropriate for some forms of data to remain (and to be stored) in writing and subsequently to be analysed directly from that format. For example, if data are qualitative in nature, they might be difficult to store in any format other than the written one. One instance might be when the data were produced as a result of a semi-structured interview in order to determine patients' perceptions of 'being hospitalized', and you feel that analysis is best done by reading and re-reading transcripts of the interviews; maintaining data in their original form might then be the preferred option. Alternatively, the data might be sufficiently compact to require analysis in the original form, for example, a single case study. Finally, data may be of the quantitative type but be of a small enough volume to be handled manually – for example, in the case of 100 questionnaires, each with five questions.

Data, therefore, can be legitimately stored in, and subsequently analysed from, their original format. Storage of data in anything other than their original form is only undertaken if there are advantages in using some other means of storage and subsequent analysis. For example, if the volume of data is such that they cannot be conveniently stored in, and analysed from, their original format, then an alternative must be found.

When storing data in their original format, ensure that each piece of data is clearly recorded. For example, long-hand notes taken hurriedly during an interview might have to be re-written and possibly typed. Secondly, ensure that each answer, or the reply from individual subjects, is discrete and that you can clearly identify and separate each respondent's response generally, and individual questions in particular. Third, ensure that the response from each respondent is clearly labelled, for example, nurse no. 1, 2, 3, etc. Fourth, scan all data immediately after recording and ensure that the record of responses is complete. Finally, seriously consider making a second copy of all data and storing each in a separate location.

Thus, data can, and frequently are, stored in their original form. Many perfectly adequate pieces of research do not require any other means of storage.

The remainder of this chapter will be concerned with the storage of quantitative data. However, bear in mind that qualitative data can be converted into quantitative data by counting the number of occasions that a particular item appears in the qualitative data. For example, you might count the number of times respondents refer to 'working with people' when describing what they find interesting about nursing.

Two further commonly used means of storing data are Cope-Chat cards and on a computer system; each will be discussed using data collected on a four-question

Please place tick (✓) against appropriate reply/replies to each question.

Q.1	Sex:	Male:	✓	1
		Female:	☐	2
Q.2	Qualification/s:	R.M.N	☐	3
		R.G.N	☐	4
		R.M.N.D	✓	5
		R.S.C.N	☐	6
		R.F.N	☐	7
Q.3	Work status:	Full time:	✓	8
		Part time:	☐	9
Q.4	Shift:	Day:	✓	10
		Night:	☐	11

Fig. 26.1 Sample questionnaire (filled in to illustrate data to be stored).

questionnaire as an example. The content of the questionnaire is as shown in Fig. 26.1. For the purpose of illustration, the questionnaire in Fig. 26.1 has been completed in order to demonstrate how the data collected can be stored on Cope-Chat cards.

COPELAND-CHATTERSON (COPE-CHAT) CARDS

The blank Cope-Chat card must first be adapted to suit the data which are to be stored on it. Figure 26.2 demonstrates how the responses to the four questions on the completed questionnaire can be stored on the card. With a short question-naire, you will experience few problems in designing the card to contain the data. With larger questionnaires, make optimum use of the available space on the card in order to contain the data.

Once the first card has been designed to contain the data, it is then typed in preparation for transfer to the printing department for duplication. The number of blank cards sent to the printing department should equate with the number of actual or completed questionnaires. The whereabouts of the printing department will vary depending on circumstances but may include private printers, or those of health authorities or other work places.

As you will note from figure 26.2, holes one to 11 on the Cope-Chat card have been used to contain responses which correspond to boxes one to 11 on the questionnaire. Thus, for question one, sex, two responses were possible; a tick in box 1 indicates the respondent to be male, a tick in box 2 indicates the respondent to be female. Because this particular respondent was male, as indicated by a tick in box 1, the corresponding hole in the Cope-Chat card is used (punched) to record the response made by that individual. An alternative means of entering the data on the card, particularly if a large quantity of data are to be contained on it, is to use the following device which has the effect of optimizing the quantity of data

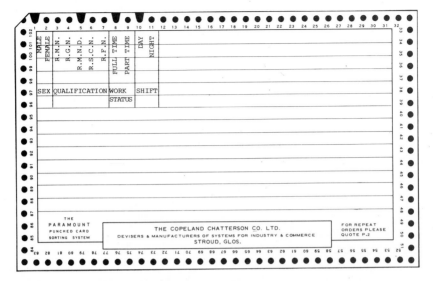

Fig. 26.2 Sample Copeland Chatterson card. (This and Fig. 26.3 are reproduced by kind permission of the Copeland Chatterson Co. Ltd.)

it will contain. When a question has only two possible answers, male or female, for example, only one hole on the card need be used. Thus, the hole may be punched if the respondent is male, and not punched if the respondent is female.

In some instances when the researcher or a research assistant is collecting data, it may be possible to make an entry directly on to the Cope-Chat card. If, instead of asking nurse respondents to complete a questionnaire, you personally interview them and ask the same four questions, you could easily then punch pre-printed cards during the interview.

Retrieval of data from the Cope-Chat system for the purposes of analysis is demonstrated in Fig. 26.3. The stack of cards is taken from their box (one box may hold up to 500 cards). A needle is pushed through the hole relating to the question you wish to answer, the cards are shaken and those which have been punched will fall from the stack. These are then counted and the results subjected to descriptive or inferential statistical analysis. Repeated sorting of the stack of cards can answer more complex questions such as 'How many full-time male staff with RMN, and RGN, qualifications work on day shift?'

The Cope-Chat data storage system comes in various sizes and degrees of complexity; fairly comprehensive systems cost only a small part of even a relatively modest research budget. A basic kit consists of: Copeland-Chatterson cards, storage box, needle, and card punch (a manual tool similar in size to a set of pliers).

This inexpensive and easy-to-use data storage system is ideal for the beginning researcher working on a limited budget. Although Cope-Chat cards represent a manual data storage and data retrieval system, the system can help greatly in relation to both of these aspects of the research process. While it is of little assistance in the application of inferential statistics to the data, it can be of value in relation to reducing the data to a form which is referred to as descriptive statistics (for discussion of inferential and descriptive statistics see Chapters 27 and 28).

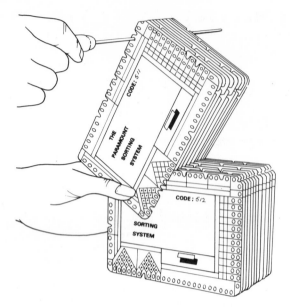

Fig. 26.3 Sorting Copeland Chatterson cards.

For larger quantities of data, perhaps in excess of 1000 questionnaires, and for data which will be analysed using inferential statistics, the use of a computing system becomes rather more necessary although still not absolutely essential.

COMPUTERS

At least two major types of computing systems may be available to you to facilitate storage and analysis of data: the main-frame computer and the micro-computer. Both types may be likened to very sophisticated electronic calculators, with computers having the added ability to store data and accept new programs to enable them to function in a variety of ways.

The physical components of a computer, the parts which can actually be seen and touched, are referred to as hardware. Thus, if you purchase a computer, you are purchasing hardware. The programs which exist within a commercial computer, or are written by a programmer and placed into it, are referred to as software. Computer users can either write their own software (programs), buy them from a company selling specialised software packages, or use the services of a computer programmer. The languages used by computer programmers are many and varied and may only be of passing interest to the researcher. Only if you wish to write your own programs will it be necessary to learn this skill and, therefore, become familiar with one or more computer languages. Examples of commonly used computer languages are COBOL, FORTRAN and BASIC. For a general overview of computing, computer languages and computer applications, see Innes (1982). It is important to remember that it is not necessary to understand how a computer works, or how to write programs, in order to make full use of computers. However, if you do not personally have appropriate computer skills and knowledge, you must have access to someone who does.

Main-frame computers

These are large, extremely expensive machines which may be found at area, district, or regional authority headquarters. At a cost which usually runs into hundreds of thousands of pounds, they will clearly be beyond the budget of all but very large-scale and long-term research projects. However, access to main-frame computers should be considered, even in relation to the most modest piece of research. In principle, researchers employed within the national health service have reasonable access to main-frame computers, as do staff working in universities and other higher education institutions.

In addition to access to the computer, nurse researchers should also negotiate access to computer programming staff, and to NHS-employed statisticians who may be required to give advice regarding data analysis. Thus, the nurse researcher should negotiate, where appropriate, the same access to computing and related facilities as is available to other researchers: medical staff and psychologists, for example.

Micro-computers

An average micro-computing system can now be bought for a relatively modest price, one that is within the range of even the modest research budget. Systems normally consist of:

(1) A micro-computer with visual display unit and typewriter style data input facility;
(2) Printer and supply of printout paper;
(3) Disk drive and supply of disks.

At present, an increasingly large range of micro-computing systems are available, and you will profit by consulting someone experienced in computing systems before buying one.

The advantage of the micro-computer lies in its relatively low cost, its portability, and the ease with which it can be installed and maintained in any domestic-style environment that has an electricity supply. The storage capacity of the system, although smaller and less flexible than a main-frame one, can be extended by the use of additional computer disks which can be used to store and analyse data. Disks, which may be as small as $3\frac{1}{2}$ inches in diameter, can hold considerable quantities of data; they are easily stored and can be marked in order to identify the data which they contain.

As with the main-frame system, commercial software packages are available, and these will enable you to make full use of the micro-computer, even if you have limited programming skills and do not have access to specialist programmers. Such programs include a number which enable descriptive and inferential analysis and specialized data presentation.

USE OF COMPUTERS

Computers have been designed to enable large quantities of data to be stored and quickly analyzed. Not all data, however, are suitable for computer application but most can be converted into a form which is suitable. Data of the quantitative type are most suitable; qualitative data are less suitable but may be converted into a form suitable for computer storage and analysis (see Baker 1988). Figure 26.4 illustrates how a four-question questionnaire might be constructed in order that the resulting data can be stored in a computer.

	Please place tick (✓) against appropriate reply/replies to each question.		Do not write in this margin
Q.1	Sex:	Male: ✓ Female:	1 2 [✓][ ]
Q.2	Qualification/s	R.M.N R.G.N R.M.N.D ✓ R.S.C.N R.F.N	1 2 3 4 5 [ ][ ][✓][ ][ ]
Q.3	Work status:	Full time: ✓ Part time:	1 2 [✓][ ]
Q.4	Shift:	Day: ✓ Night:	1 2 [✓][ ]

Fig. 26.4 Sample questionnaire (prepared for transfer to punch card).

The sequence of events in the collection of data on this questionnaire – which would obviously be accompanied by detailed instructions and a letter of explanation – is as follows:

(1) The respondent places a tick in the boxes which correspond to his answer;
(2) On receipt of the questionnaires, you record each of the four answers in a selected single box located at the right margin of the questionnaire;
(3) Responses are transferred to a means by which the data can be placed into a computer.

In relation to a micro-computer, the data will have to be punched in using a keyboard similar to that on an ordinary typewriter. In relation to a main-frame computer, there are a number of methods used to insert data; these include typing in the data using the typewriter form of keyboard and the visual display unit, entering the data via magnetic tape or punched paper tape, or using punch cards. The latter means of entering data, although now less frequently used than the others, will be discussed in detail in order to demonstrate how you might collect data in a form which is suitable for storage in a main-frame system.

Punch cards

Punch cards are 7 in. × 2 in. with 80 columns of possible hole positions (see Fig. 26.5). A special machine, used by a trained operator, is used to punch a hole at the appropriate point in each column. After the cards are checked, they are then

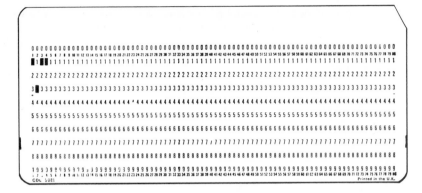

Fig. 26.5 Punch card. (Reproduced by kind permission of Control Dataset Ltd.)

placed into a card reader which enables data from the cards to be transferred into the computer. Cards can be retained by the researcher for use in relation to further data analysis, or as back-up in case of the unlikely event of the computer accidentally losing the data.

Once it has been established that the research data should be stored in a main-frame computer, consult a computer programmer and establish the form the data should take in order to facilitate their transfer to the machine. An example of how data might be coded has already been shown in Fig. 26.4, a similar system being used for storage on Cope-Chat cards, (Fig. 26.2). For example, in relation to question 1 of the questionnaire (sex), the answer is 'male', indicated by a tick in box 1.

The answer to question 1 is subsequently punched into the first column of the card, this being done by punching a hole where 'No. 1' appears (No. 1 equals male; No. 2 equals female). Similarly, the answer to question 2 is recorded in column 2 of the card and a hole would be punched in No. 3 in this case. Each punch card can contain up to 80 coded answers. As an example of how this works, the punch card in Fig. 26.5 has had the answers to the four questions given in Fig. 26.4 punched in.

In collecting data for storage and subsequent analysis in a computer, the important point is to collect the data in a format which is suitable for transfer to a computing system. Providing that this is done – usually with advice from someone with an understanding of computing systems – the data can then be transferred into the computer by someone with the requisite specialist knowledge. Thus, if you ensure that data are in a computer-compatable format, then using the computer to store and analyse them will not present problems. The essential points are:

(1) Give each subject an *individual code number*, e.g. 001, 002, 003, etc.;
(2) Give each question an *individual code number*, e.g. 01, 02, 03, etc.;
(3) Give each potential response an *individual code number*, e.g. Male = 1, Female = 2; Yes = 1, No = 2, Don't know = 3.

Before deciding which method of data storage to use, consider available alternatives and their relative strengths and weaknesses. The advice of researchers who have used data storage techniques, and of those with experience of computing systems, should be obtained during the planning phases of the research.

REFERENCES

Baker C.A. (1988) Computer Applications in Qualitative Research. *Computers in Nursing,* **6** (5), 211–4.
Innes A.E. (1982) *Data Processing for Business Studies.* McDonald and Evans, Plymouth.

Chapter 27
Quantitative Analysis: (Descriptive)
Peter T. Donnan

This chapter and the chapter that follows discuss the quantitative analysis of data. The amount and nature of the data collected in a study will depend on the purpose of the study. A small or large number of cases may have been collected; the study may be either simply descriptive or consist of a comparison of groups, for example. In any case, numerical information on a number of individuals is collected and these form the *data set*.

It would be unwieldy to try to present all of the data every time the study was considered. Instead, descriptive statistics are used to summarize and present the data, extracting the salient points from the results. Descriptive statistics will form the subject matter in this chapter.

Inferential statistics, on the otherhand, are concerned with making judgements; testing hypotheses about the population of interest based upon the information obtained from a sample of that population. This will be explored more fully in Chapter 28. The use of these two approaches depends on whether the purpose of the research is to describe, show differences, predict, or show relationships. In practice both approaches are used as they provide complementary views.

GOOD DESIGN/GOOD STATISTICS

Good statistics start with good design. A study needs to be well designed in order to provide useful results and conclusions. It is thus important to consider all aspects of the statistics at the outset. It is not efficient to consider statistics only after the research has been carried out. Instead, it is necessary to set out the study in such a way that the research is more likely than not to provide the answer sought. The most important part of the design stage is therefore to state clearly the *aims* of the investigation.

If the aims are stated clearly (see Chapter 8), then all other aspects of design will follow, such as:

(1) The nature of the data;
(2) How the data are to be collected (Chapters 22–25);
(3) The appropriate analysis (Chapter 28).

Assuming a well designed study, with adequate data collection, the next step is to consider ways of presenting the results. Communication of the results is a vital aspect of any research. The appropriate use of statistics can provide a systematic means of assessing, summarizing and presenting the findings of such research. As already stated, this can be done in two main ways (not mutually exclusive): using descriptive and/or inferential statistics.

In most research it is not possible to obtain all the possible information from the population of interest because of resource constraints. A *population* is not only a group of people, but, more exactly, is a collection or set of measurements. For example, you might be interested in the proportion of HIV positive patients who develop full-blown AIDS after a certain period of time. The population consists of all patients who are HIV positive. The data acquired (using the methods of Chapter 21) forms a *sample* of this population – one from a single hospital, for example – which it is hoped has characteristics similar to the population from which it was drawn, that is, it is representative of that population. In fact, it is possible to do better than 'hope' that this is so by using simple random sampling (Chapter 21) which means the selection of each member of the population for the sample is equally likely and is independent of any other selected case. Since lack of time and money may not allow the acquisition of data on all patients confirmed as HIV positive the researcher takes a random sample to represent this population.

Importance of sample size

The size of the sample collected may be outside the control of the researcher. For example, the researcher may be interested in a rare disease and so the number of patients with the disease (those whose records are available) will form the sample. However, in most cases, the researcher will have some choice in the size of the sample to be used. If the questions posed by the study involve the comparison of groups, it is especially important to have an adequate sample size. This is estimated at the design stage. It would be wasteful of resources to sample more than is required. However, a more usual error is when the sample is too small, such that the data acquired is useless in fulfilling the aims of the study. Consider also the ethics of the latter case, especially if the research involved includes an intervention trial of a new treatment. The topic of sample size is a factor of major importance, although it will not be pursued further here. Textbook formulae are available for use in the calculation of sample size (see Armitage & Berry 1987), and these should be consulted with the aid of a statistician prior to data collection.

Type of data

It is necessary to consider the type of data being dealt with in your research since the statistical methods used and the presentation of the data will depend on this. For example, sex (male/female) as a piece of data is very different from birthweight measured in kilogrammes. As has been said, the main distinction to be made is that between the two types: *qualitative* (or categorical data), and *quantitative* data. The qualities and quantities measured are known as variables, height, for example, is a continuous variable; degrees of pain is an ordered categorical variable.

Qualitative data arise whenever individuals are classified into groups such as sex (male/female), marital status (married/divorced/separated/single) or bloodgroup (A/B/AB/O). There is no numerical relationship between these categories and hence this type of data is known as nominal (Table 27.1). A special case arises whenever there are only two categories, such as male and female, which form a binary variable. The outcome of a study is often expressed as a binary variable, for example, satisfied/unsatisfied; hypertensive/not hypertensive. On the other hand, there is sometimes a natural order to the groups, for example, degrees of pain in the categories of none/slight/moderate/severe and this is referred to as an ordered, categorical, or ordinal variable.

Quantitative data (Table 27.1) arise from counts such as the number of hospital beds or the number of angina attacks in a specified time period. These can only have discrete values so any intermediate level is not possible: as, for example, half a bed. Finally, quantitative data come in the form of continuous measures such as weight or blood cholesterol level, and these can take any value in a specified range. These values are only limited by the accuracy and precision of the measuring instrument.

As well as being useful for presentation purposes, this classification also moulds the way in which the data can be analysed. Discrete and categorical variables lend themselves to comparisons of proportions in different groups. For example, in comparing the proportions of nurses who consider that more emphasis should be placed on their professional role at two time points, immediately after completing training, and after one year of working.

Continuous data tend to be summarized by some form of average, the mean or median along with a measure of spread, and these terms will be described fully later. If an intervention study intended to reduce blood cholesterol in one group compared to a control group, for example, the comparison might be made in terms of the difference in mean reduction in cholesterol between both groups.

Table 27.1 Types of data.

Type	Description	Examples
Qualitative (categorical)	(1) Nominal: data in separate classes which have no numerical relationship	Types of burn: thermal, chemical, electrical, . . . absence/presence pain (binary)
	(2) Ordinal: data in separate classes with order relationship	Degrees of pain, social class, degrees of satisfaction
Quantitative	(1) Discrete: arise from counts	Number of hospital beds, number of teeth filled
	(2) Continuous measurements: can take any value in range	Height, weight, haemoglobinn level, cholesterol level

The distinction made between qualitative and quantitative, although essential in deciding how to present and analyse data, is not completely clear-cut. It is possible to convert a quantitative variable into a qualitative variable by dividing the range of values into groups. If this is carried further, a variable with two categories can be produced known as a binary variable. For example, let us, initially, consider age as a quantitative variable (Fig. 27.1).

Note that at each step from left to right information is lost, that is, the measure becomes more coarse. All of these age variables may be useful; the form of the variable chosen depends upon the question the study wishes to address. It would

Age (0 to 50) $\longrightarrow$ <20, **20–30**, 30+ $\longrightarrow$ <25, 25+
                                1,   2,   3   1,   2

Continuous   Ordered, categorical

Quantitative   Qualitative   Binary

Fig. 27.1 Age as a quantitative and qualitative variable.

be possible to transform in the reverse direction only if the original data were available.

AIDS TO THE DESCRIPTION OF DATA

Having decided upon the type of data to be collected, and then having collected the data (Chapters 22–25), the initial step in any data analysis is to look at the data themselves. In fact, this may be the main purpose of the study: to provide a description of a situation if this is unknown, for example, the extent of knowledge amongst the nursing profession regarding the condition of AIDS. Even when more sophisticated analyses are planned, looking at the data and the relationships between variables is extremely valuable in deciding what analyses would be appropriate. It is also useful as an aid to interpretation after the analyses have been carried out.

The main ways of describing data are in the form of tables, pie charts, bar charts/histograms, scatter diagrams, and line graphs. Tables and histograms together can convey the same information, with tables emphasizing particular numerical values, while histograms show overall patterns. All of these can be produced using statistics/graphics computer packages, but although the computer will do most of the tedious work, the researcher needs to consider the purpose and format of these visual presentations, and perhaps more importantly, the relevance of the tables to the presentation.

Tables

A simple table is often all that is required to convey information from a study. Thought should be put into the format, the number of tables, and the type of values to go into the body of the table: counts, totals, and percentages. Note that if percentages are to be presented, the number and the total should be stated. Table 27.2 illustrates how a table should be set out, with an informative main title, and column titles. These data come from a survey of health behaviours of 29 adults with cardiovascular disease compared to 29 healthy adults (Laffrey & Crabtree 1988). The number in each category is stated together with the corresponding percentage. Be wary of any table which gives only percentages, especially if small numbers are involved; a 100% increase from an initial value of 1 is 2! Huff (1988) explores in a light-hearted way some of the more common misuses of statistics in tables and plots.

Whenever a survey is reported, the first table presented often shows the characteristics of the sample. Table 27.3, below, shows the characteristics of the two samples in a study to assess differences in severity of morbidity in the first year

Table 27.2   Number and proportion of persons in each group who mentioned health behaviours (n = 58).

Behaviours	Cardiovascular No.	%	Healthy No.	%
Exercise	21	72	22	76
Nutrition	19	66	26	90
Medications	14	48	3	10
Psychological well-being	11	38	20	69
Sleep/rest	11	38	10	34
Relaxation/recreation	5	17	19	66

of life in infants born at term compared to those born moderately premature (Urtis, Clayton & Jay 1988).

Such a table is a formal presentation of a number of descriptive statistics such as the mean with a measure of spread (standard deviation), or counts in groups (which will be described in detail later).

Table 27.3   Demographic data: premature and term infants.

	Premature Mean (s.d.) (n = 20)		Term Mean (s.d.) (n = 20)	
Gestational age (wk)	34.4	(1.2)	39.3	(1.7)
Birth weight (kg)	2.27	(0.41)	3.33	(0.44)
Hospitalization (days)	13.0	(10.1)	3.8	(1.2)
Sex: Male	8		8	
Female	12		12	
Feeding method in hospital: Breast	5		10	
Bottle	11		6	
Both	4		4	

s.d. = standard deviation

Line graphs

The line graph most frequently encountered by nurses is possibly that of the temperature of a patient recorded over time. Figure 27.2 is an illustration of a line graph of the median total length of stay in an acute orthopaedic unit recorded for different age-groups (Whitaker & Currie 1988). The median is the middle value when the observations are placed in order. The plot shows the pattern occurring in the data at a glance, the rising length of stay with age of the patient; in a table, this pattern would not be so immediately obvious.

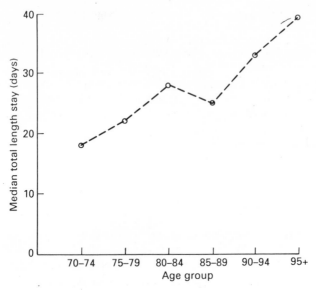

Fig. 27.2   Length of stay in an acute orthopaedic unit (Whitaker & Currie 1988).

Pie charts

A pie chart consists of a circle representing the total data or 100%, with each slice of 'pie' being proportional to the percentage in a particular category. Thus, a pie chart can convey the information in a table at a glance. Figure 27.3 shows the reading rate of the population of Switzerland for an information booklet on AIDS (Lehmann *et al.* 1987) illustrating the slight separation that distinguishes between those who have read the booklet and those who have not.

Beware of 3-dimensional pie charts which, because they show volume, are misleading in that it is the size of the 'slice' in two dimensions which represents the proportion.

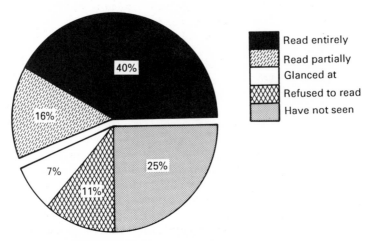

Fig. 27.3   Reading rate of the population of Switzerland for the information booklet on AIDS that was distributed in March 1986 (Lehmann *et al.*, 1987).

Histograms

These are an effective way of presenting the counts of the number of cases in each category of a qualitative variable. The count in each category is known as the *frequency* of that category. Histograms, as well as displaying qualitative data, can also be used to display continuous variables, such as mental ability scores of children, by dividing the range into equal-sized intervals. Table 27.4 divides the distribution of mental ability scores into non-overlapping intervals, and serves to illustrate an investigation of the effect of exposure to lead dust on these scores (Fulton *et al.* 1987).

Table 27.4   Frequency distribution of ability scores.

Interval	Frequency	Relative frequency	Percentage
67.5– 72.5	2	0.004	0.4
72.5– 77.5	0	0.0	0.0
77.5– 82.5	6	0.012	1.2
82.5– 87.5	14	0.028	2.8
87.5– 92.5	22	0.044	4.4
92.5– 97.5	26	0.052	5.2
97.5–102.5	42	0.085	8.5
102.5–107.5	58	0.117	11.7
107.5–112.5	66	0.133	13.3
112.5–117.5	79	0.16	16.0
117.5–122.5	81	0.163	16.3
122.5–127.5	42	0.085	8.5
127.5–132.5	28	0.056	5.6
132.5–137.5	18	0.036	3.6
137.5–142.5	9	0.018	1.8
142.5–147.5	3	0.006	0.6
Total	496	1.0	100

In this form, the data can be plotted as a histogram (Fig. 27.4). This was produced by the computer package SPSSGRAPH. The values of mental ability scores are on the horizontal axis with the mid-point of each interval; the frequencies are placed on the vertical axis. The area of each column represents the absolute count in each category. The frequencies in different categories can be directly compared if the size of each interval is equal. However, the frequency in each category is meaningless by itself; instead the *relative frequency* or proportion in each category is calculated by dividing the number in each group by the total number in the sample (see Table 27.4). If the proportion in each category is calculated, the full set of possibilities is known as a *frequency distribution*.

The histogram of this would be the same as that shown in Fig. 27.4, except that the vertical axis would be the relative frequency or percentage. For this histogram, the total area of the columns must represent 100%, assuming that all possible categories are described, and so the area of each column must represent the

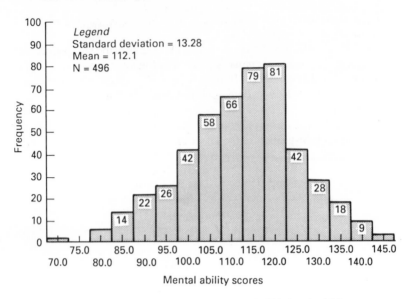

Fig. 27.4 Histogram of mental ability scores for 496 Edinburgh children.

proportion in each category, or the *probability* of being in that category. Since the proportion in the 112.5–117.5 category of mental ability scores is 16% (Table 27.4), the probability of a member of the sample being in that category is 16% or 0.16. This combined set of probabilities is also known as a *probability distribution*.

The actual size of interval is arbitrary; trial and error will show which is most appropriate for a particular dataset, although between 10 and 20 intervals are generally used. Most computer packages will plot histograms with the facility of adjusting the interval width (e.g. MINITAB [Ryan *et al.* 1985]). A histogram can also be compiled by hand for small samples sizes by tallying the data.

NORMAL DISTRIBUTION

As stated above, the set of all probabilities forms a probability distribution. This example was for a sample, so let us assume that we have a complete population. This would also form a probability distribution and if the size of the interval for the histogram were to become smaller and smaller, a curved line would eventually be produced. We would then have the *probability density function* of the population. The probability of lying between any two values can then be calculated as the area under the curve between the two values and, as for the histogram described above, the total area under the curve represents a probability of 1.0. Thus, if you wanted to know the probability of, say, having systolic blood pressure of 130mm Hg or above, you could calculate the area above this value from the frequency distribution of blood pressures. It would, however, be difficult to calculate the area under a curve each time this was required. Expressed mathematically, you would have to know the equation for each distribution and use integration to obtain the probability of lying between two points.

Fortunately, there is one particular probability distribution which approximates to reality in a large number of cases and for this reason the areas under the curve have been tabulated extensively – this is known as *normal* or *Gaussian* distribution.

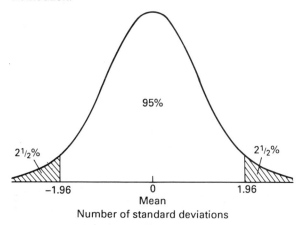

Fig. 27.5   The standard normal distribution.

The normal curve is bell-shaped with most of the values clustered around a central value, with smaller and smaller frequencies moving further and further from the centre. The distribution is symmetric with equal proportions on either side of the centre. The property of symmetry is extremely useful. As noted above, the probability of lying between any two values can be calculated as the area under the probability density curve between these two points and since the normal distribution is symmetric. If the probability of one area in one half is known, the total probability for the two tails is twice this value (Fig. 27.5). The normal distribution is often a useful approximation to reality. Returning to the distribution of the sample of ability scores, a normal curve has been superimposed on the histogram (Fig. 27.6) showing a reasonably close fit.

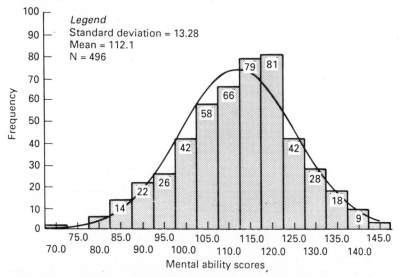

Fig. 27.6   Histogram of mental ability scores for 496 Edinburgh children.

The shape and location of a normal distribution is characterized by two values known as *parameters*, the mean, and the standard deviation. The mean gives the central point of the distribution while the standard deviation determines the shape; the larger the standard deviation, the more spread out will be the distribution. A special case is when the mean is zero and the standard deviation is one, the *standard normal* distribution. Figure 27.5 shows that for this distribution, 95% of the observations will lie between 1.96 standard deviations on either side of the mean.

Skewness

Whenever a greater proportion of cases fall at one end of the tail the distribution is said to be skewed. For example, Fig. 27.7 shows a positively skewed distribution

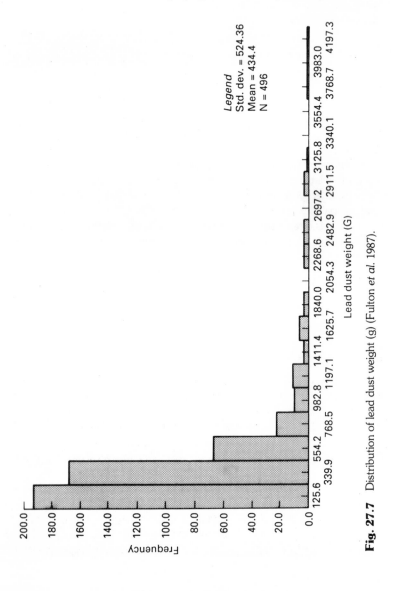

Fig. 27.7 Distribution of lead dust weight (g) (Fulton *et al.* 1987).

of the weight of lead dust in households in Edinburgh (Fulton *et al.* 1987). A negatively skewed distribution is the opposite of this, with most of the data to the right of the centre. The normal distribution is clearly *not* a good approximation to these distributions.

Scatterplots

These are used to represent the relationships between pairs of quantitative variables. They consist of one axis for each variable and usually a point (although any symbol will do) representing each data value; this is placed a distance along each axis corresponding to the values in these two dimensions. The ways in which these relationships can be explored will be discussed in Chapter 28. Figure 27.8 shows the relationship between mental ability scores and standardized height from the lead study (Fulton *et al.* 1987) showing generally higher scores for taller children.

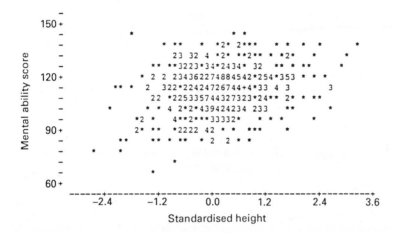

Fig. 27.8   Mental ability score and height in 496 children in Edinburgh (Fulton *et al.* 1987).

SUMMARY STATISTICS

In presenting results, it is unwieldy for the reader to have to consider all the data each time the evidence is examined. It can be more helpful for the reader to be given a few numbers which concisely convey the gist of the results, that is to say, *summary statistics* are calculated. The most common of these are measures of the centre of the distribution of the data, and measures of central tendency, such as the *mean, median,* and *mode.* The case of the common term 'average' is not advised as it is often not clear what is meant. Often these are presented along with measures of spread or variation such as the standard deviation, semi-interquartile range, and range.

The *mean* ($\bar{x}$) is simply the sum of all the observations divided by the number of observations. The mean of the numbers 6, 5, 8, 5 is $(6+5+8+5)/4=6$. The mean is most useful when the histogram of the distribution looks symmetrical. It has useful mathematical properties and is incorporated into many analyses. The formula for the mean is written thus:

$$\bar{x} = \frac{\Sigma x}{n}$$

where n = the total number of observations and the Greek capital letter sigma (Σ) indicates the sum of all the values of x. The mean is a very useful summary statistic. For example, the mean gestational age for the premature babies in Table 27.3 was 34.4 weeks. The mean has the disadvantage that it is very sensitive to extreme values or outliers.

The *median* is the centre of the distribution whenever the observations are placed in order or *ranked* so that 50% of the observations lie above and below it. This measure is most useful whenever the distribution of the data is skewed, but it can also be used with a symmetrical distribution. In fact, it is highly misleading to quote the mean when the data are skewed. Consider a report stating that the mean salary for nurses is £12,000! This is misleading if the population of nurses includes nursing officers, and so the distribution of salaries is therefore skewed; the median salary may be nearer £9,000. The main drawback of the median is that it is not so easily mathematically manipulated as the mean.

If the number in the sample is odd, the median is simply the middle value when they are placed in order. It is the (n + 1)/2th value. If there are 5 values, the median will be the 3rd value when the data are ranked.

If the number in the sample is even, the median is the average of the two middle numbers. It is the (n/2th + (n/2 + 1)th)/2 value. This looks complicated but is actually straightforward in practice. The median of 4 values is the average of the 2nd and 3rd values when the data are ranked, so, for example, the median of 6, 5, 8, 5 is (5 + 6)/2 = 5.5.

The lead dust data (Fig. 27.7) were highly positively skewed. Consequently, the median of 288 g is more representative of the centre of the distribution than the mean of 434 g.

The *mode* is the most common observation and is of limited use. In terms of the normal distribution, it should be noted that the mean, median, and mode all coincide, forming the central point of the distribution. Hence, one way of assessing whether a sample is approximately normal, is to compare these three measures of central tendency.

Percentiles

The median was calculated as the value above and below which 50% of the data lie if placed in order. A percentile is a value below which a percentage of the observations lie. In terms of percentiles, the median is the 50th percentile. The most commonly used percentiles are *quartiles*. There are three quartiles, in other words, three values which divide the data into quarters. The first quartile (Q_1) is the value below which 25% of the data lie, the 2nd quartile is the median, and the 3rd quartile (Q_3) is the value above which 25% of the data lie. For example, if heights were recorded for a sample of nurses, then 25% of these nurses would have heights which are greater than the 3rd or upper quartile. These measures are also useful to assess the shape of the distribution of a sample. One visual method of exploratory data analysis, consists of the representation of the distribution of a variable in the form of a *boxplot*. In a basic boxplot, the median is represented by a plus, the ends of the box are the upper and lower quartiles, while the maximum and minimum are the ends of the hinges if there are no extreme values. Figure 27.9 shows a more complicated boxplot produced by MINITAB (Ryan *et al.* 1985).

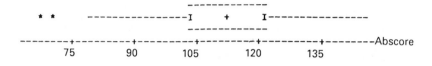

```
                        -------------
  *   *      ----------------I    +    I---------------
                        -------------
  --------+---------+---------+--------+--------+-------Abscore
         75        90        105      120      135
```

    * Extreme values

    + Median

Fig. 27.9 Boxplot of mental ability scores standardized by age of 496 Edinburgh children (Fulton *et al.* 1987).

Measures of variability

As well as these measures of central tendency, some measure of the spread of the data about these points is necessary to fully describe a distribution. The most commonly used measures of variability are the standard deviation, variance, range, and semi-interquartile range.

Standard deviation

This is a measure of the average spread of the data about the mean, assuming that the sample has an approximately normal distribution. One way of measuring the spread would be to subtract each value of the sample from the sample mean, and sum the differences. Unfortunately, the result would be zero! Instead, the standard deviation is calculated by squaring the difference between each data point and the mean, summing these squared differences, and dividing the result by one less than the sample size. This is the sample *variance*, denoted by s^2. Finally, taking the square root of this value gives the standard deviation, s. We divide by one less than the sample size because by calculating the mean we have only $n - 1$ ways left in which the rest of the sample can be chosen. In mathematical notation, this is written:

$$s = \sqrt{\frac{\Sigma (\bar{x} - x)^2}{n - 1}}$$

For the following data, 6, 5, 8, 5, which has a mean of 6, the standard deviation is calculated as the square root of $((6 - 6)^2 + (6 - 5)^2 + (6 - 8)^2 + (6 - 5)^2/3 = 2$. Hence the standard deviation is 1.41.

As already stated, the normal distribution is symmetric so that it is possible to calculate the proportion of cases between any two points. Figure 27.5 shows the most used percentage point of the normal distribution, with 95% of the observations lying between 1.96 (often rounded to 2) standard deviations above

and below the mean. The main drawback of the standard deviation as a measure
of spread, is that, like the mean, it is affected by extreme values.

Standard error (s.e.)

The standard error of the mean is often encountered in the literature in tables and
should not be confused with the standard deviation. They are, however, related,
but while the standard deviation measures the variability of the *observations* about
the mean, the standard error measures the variability of the *mean* of the sample
as an estimate of the true population from which the sample was drawn. They are
both measures of variability, but of two different distributions. If more samples
were taken from the population and the mean calculated for each sample, a
distribution of means would be obtained and the standard error would be the
measure of variability of this distribution of means. The standard error is easily
calculated as:

$$\text{s.e. } (\bar{x}) = s/\sqrt{n}$$

Thus the standard error is smaller than the standard deviation. This is not a good
reason for its use in tables. Whenever the purpose of the table is to compare
means, the standard error should be quoted along with the mean. However, if the
purpose of the table is to compare the spread of the observations, then the
standard deviation should be used. The standard error and the standard deviation,
along with the mean, are used for the purposes of statistical inference and this will
be discussed in the next chapter.

The *range* is simply the difference between the maximum and minimum data
value. As such, the usefulness of the range is rather limited and is unduly affected
by extreme values.

The *semi-interquartile range* is half the difference between the first and third
quartiles. It is calculated as:

$$1/2 \ (Q_3 - Q_1)$$

It has the advantage as a measure of spread that it is not unduly affected by
extreme values.

All of these summary statistics give slightly different information concerning the
characteristics of a distribution. The command DESCRIBE in the statistical
package MINITAB (Ryan *et al.* 1985) gives all of these values (Fig. 27.10). These
values, along with a plot or histogram, are useful initial steps in looking at the data.

SUMMARY

This chapter has described the most commonly encountered ways of describing
and summarizing data. The importance of looking at the data in as many ways as
possible has been stressed, not only as an end in itself, but also as a means of aiding
further analysis.

The chapter that follows moves on to the next step, that of generalizing the
results from the sample to the larger population of interest by the application of
inferential statistics.

N	MEAN	MEDIAN	TRMEAN	STDEV	SEMEAN
496	112.07	113.00	112.24	13.29	0.60

MIN	MAX	Q_1	Q_3
68.00	146.00	103.00	121.00

```
        N  - number in sample
   TRMEAN  - trimmed mean
    STDEV  - sample standard deviation
   SEMEAN  - standard error of the mean
      MIN  - minimum data value
      MAX  - maximum data value
       Q₁  - lower quartile
       Q₃  - upper quartile
```

Fig. 27.10   Output from DESCRIBE command in MINITAB (Ryan *et al.* 1985).

REFERENCES

Armitage P. & Berry G. (1987) *Statistical methods in medical research*. Blackwell Scientific Publications, Oxford.

Fulton M., Raab G., Thomson G., Laxen D., Hunter R. & Hepburn W. (1987) Influence of blood lead on the ability and attainment of children in Edinburgh. *Lancet*, **i** (8544), 1221-6.

Huff D. (1988) *How to lie with statistics*. Penguin, London.

Laffrey S.C. & Crabtree M.K. (1988) Health and health behaviour of persons with chronic cardiovascular disease. *International Journal of Nuring Studies*. **25** (1), 41-52.

Lehmann P., Hausser D., Somaini B. & Gutzwiller F. (1987) Campaign against AIDS in Switzerland: evaluation of a nationwide educational programme. *British Medical Journal*, **295**, 1118-20.

Ryan B.F., Joiner B.L. & Ryan T.A. (1985) *Minitab handbook* Duxbury, Boston.

Urtis J.M., Clayton D. & Jay S.S. (1988) Infant morbidity: A measurement of severity and occurrence of illness in preterm and term infants. *Journal of Pediatric Nursing*, **3** (2), 110-7.

Whitaker J.J. & Currie C.T. (1988) Elderly acute orthopaedic patients - Where they come from and where they go. *Health Bulletin*, **46** (2), 98-105.

Chapter 28
Quantitative Analysis: (Inferential)
Peter T. Donnan

In the previous chapter, various ways of describing the data in a sample were discussed. This is fine as far as it goes, but usually the researcher will wish to say something more general concerning the target population from which the specific sample was drawn. This is achieved through the use of *inferential statistics*.

Consider a survey carried out to discover the satisfaction of mothers with midwifery care in a particular city. The results of this survey will be most useful if the results can be applied to the entire city without the sample and so inform the decision makers of provision of midwifery care in that city. From this sample, one may wish to say something about the population of mothers in the city, that is, inferences are made about the population based on the sample. If the sample is biased, then statistical procedures will not rectify this problem and hence the need for good design in the first place.

As another example, consider a random sample of patients confirmed as being HIV positive. From this sample, a proportion might develop full-blown AIDS, and it would be useful to know for the population of all patients who were HIV positive how likely is it that this proportion will develop AIDS. In addition, the researcher would like to know how precise this estimate of the population proportion in fact is. Statistical inference helps to answer these questions.

The answers to these types of question involve the use of various statistical methods. Before expanding on particular methods, it is worth discussing the use of computer packages. Nowadays it is not essential to know the mechanics of calculations since computers are more efficient at this task, as well as being faster. However, some calculations are presented in this chapter, firstly, as an aid to understanding, secondly, because computers are not always available, and finally, for those who are interested in the mechanics of calculations. Although computers are more efficient, the widespread availability and use of statistical packages creates a danger of using inappropriate methods, coupled with a lack of understanding of the output. Computers follow the maxim 'rubbish in, rubbish out'! What is therefore required is the intelligent use of computers and the knowledge to know when to seek expert advice.

There are many user-friendly packages available for use on micro-computers as well as main-frame computers. Two of the most commonly used are SPSS-X and MINITAB (Ryan *et al.* 1985).

In selecting statistical methods, what is essential is an understanding of when particular methods are appropriate, what assumptions are being made – and whether these assumptions are valid – and how to interpret the output. Often you will have access to a statistician or find that one is a member of the research team; in endeavouring to manage this part of the research process, it is always worth consulting a statistician.

INFERENTIAL STATISTICAL METHODS

There are two main types of inferential statistical methods, known as *parametric* and *non-parametric*. Parametric methods, not surprisingly, centre around estimating parameters of the population – such as the mean – based upon the sample. These methods depend heavily upon making distributional assumptions about the population. On the other hand, there are what are known as non-parametric (or sometimes distribution-free) methods. These synonyms are slightly misleading in that some tests involve parameters and/or distributions. However, these methods are applicable to estimation or hypothesis testing when the population distributions are not rigidly specified, that is, they do not have to belong to specific families such as the normal distribution. The pragmatic difference is that non-parametric methods are based upon the *ranking* of data rather than the actual data itself. For example, the following measurements of haemoglobin levels: 13.3, 10.5, 12.6, 14.1, have ranks 3, 1, 2, and 4 respectively.

Faced with a bewildering array of methods, it is tempting to churn out results from as many programs as possible in a statistical package in the hope that some will be useful. A more systematic approach would be to decide initially between parametric statistical methods and non-parametric methods.

In deciding between parametric and non-parametric methods, the following should be considered:

(1) Distributional shape
Parametric tests often depend upon the assumption of normally distributed data for the population of interest. This is often assessed visually from a histogram of the sample. For example, in Chapter 27, the histogram of ability scores (Fig. 27.4) indicates that the assumption of normality would be reasonable. On the other hand, Fig. 27.7, which is highly positively skewed, suggests that this assumption would be unwarranted and non-parametric methods are indicated. An alternative would be to *transform* the data such that the transformed data are approximately normal. For the data in Fig. 27.7, a log transformation is appropriate and parametric methods could be applied to the transformed data. Sometimes there is no simple transformation which 'normalizes' the data and non-parametric methods should be used.

(2) Power
If the data are in fact normally distributed, the two methods have approximately the same power (the power of a test is the chance of detecting a significant difference if it is present in the population).

For non-normal data, the power of non-parametric tests may actually be superior.

(3) Ease of calculation
For small sample sizes, non-parametric tests can be carried out without the help of calculators or computers. On the other hand, ranking becomes very laborious for large samples.

(4) Very small sample sizes
Non-parametric methods are not very useful when the total sample size is less than 6 since they cannot give significant results even if the test statistics achieve their

most extreme value. As a general rule, any inferences made from very small sample sizes are very weak and should be treated with extreme caution.

Since there are many excellent textbooks devoted to non-parametric methods, I will not describe these here. However, if these methods are indicated, a classic textbook is that of Siegel (1989) which is recommended for the details of any test. For a basic introduction the work by Sprent (1981) is useful.

Since parametric methods are those most commonly encountered, this chapter will concentrate on these methods. Having decided on parametric methods, the choice of method is dependent on the nature of the data.

PARAMETRIC METHODS

As discussed earlier, information is obtained concerning the population of interest from a smaller sample. From this sample you may want to say something about the whole population, that is, inferences are made based on the sample.

Assuming an unbiased study, statistical methods can help you to assess whether the result is spurious or not (hypothesis testing). In other words they evaluate the role of chance as an explanation of the results. In addition, statistical methods also allow calculation of the precision of a given sample estimate such as a proportion (confidence interval). The latter approach is dealt with first. Often this is of more relevance to you than whether an estimate is statistically significant or not. For example, you may be interested in by *how much* anxiety is reduced (measured on a validated scale), and by how much the reduction would vary after the introduction of a self-help package rather than whether the reduction is significant or not. In practice, these two approaches are often presented together since each provides different aspects of inference. For a detailed discussion of the relative merits of these approaches, see Gardner and Altman (1989).

Confidence interval approach

Consider a population parameter of interest, such as a proportion or mean, which is estimated from the sample. A *confidence interval* is defined as a range of values within which it is reasonably certain (often 95%) that the population value lies. For example, if a painkiller was administered to a random sample of female patients and it was recorded that 60% no longer felt any pain after one hour, the researcher would like to know the precision of this estimate if the painkiller were to be applied to the population in general, that is, to all female patients of the same age range with the same condition. If the confidence interval suggests that the population value could be as low as 20% or as high as 100% then the value of 60% is very imprecise and of little use. If, on the other hand, the confidence interval is from 55% to 65%, then this is a more precise estimate and also more meaningful. You could then make a stronger inference about the effect of the painkiller on the population at large than in the former case.

Confidence intervals are concerned with precision, that is, by how much the sample estimate is likely to differ on average from the 'true' population value. Thus we require an interval defined by two values (Fig. 28.1) which has a reasonable chance of containing the 'true' value.

Sample estimate ± Constant × Standard Error of the estimate

(The symbol ± means addition and subtraction to give two values.)

Fig. 28.1   Equation for a confidence interval.

This can be represented pictorially as an interval on a number line.

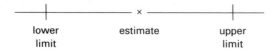

| lower | estimate | upper |
| limit | | limit |

Fig. 28.2   Representation of a confidence interval.

When the constant is appropriately chosen (percentage point from a probability distribution: see Fig. 28.1 and Fig. 28.2), this defines a confidence interval with a specified percentage chance (often 95%) of containing the true value, and the boundaries of the interval are called confidence limits. Hence the terms 95% confidence interval or limits. Note that this does not mean that the 'true' or population value cannot lie outside the limits; it means that this is less likely. The 95% confidence interval is the one most commonly encountered, but any percentage point is possible; others often used are 90% and 99%.

In Chapter 27, the standard error of the mean was introduced. This can be generalized to any parameter estimate so that if the standard error of a parameter estimate is known, then a confidence interval can be calculated using the equation shown in Fig. 28.1.

The size of the confidence interval depends on the size of the standard error and the size of the constant in this equation. In order to emphasize that confidence intervals are concerned with the precision of point estimates, Fig. 28.3 illustrates an estimate with precise and imprecise confidence intervals.

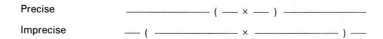

Fig. 28.3   Precision and imprecision.

Confidence interval for a proportion

Consider a random sample of 50 patients who have been confirmed as HIV positive. It would be useful to know what proportion of these patients developed full-blown AIDS in the seven years following confirmation. Suppose 30 (or 60%) developed AIDS. This figure, by itself, does not tell the complete story. We cannot say that, in general, 60% of all patients confirmed as HIV positive will develop AIDS in the following seven years. This is an estimate, based on one sample, and it would be useful to know how precise it is. In terms of proportions $p = 0.6$ and the standard error of a proportion is given by:

$$\sqrt{p(1-p)/n}$$

where n is the size of the sample and, using the 5% point of the normal distribution

Table 28.1   Critical values for the standard normal distribution.

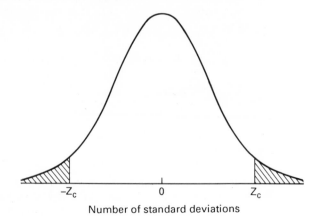

Number of standard deviations

Levels of confidence	90%	95%	98%	99%
Area in two tails (*p*-value)	0.10	0.05	0.02	0.01
Critical values Z_c (number) of standard deviations)	1.64	1.96	2.33	2.58

(Table 28.1), assuming a large enough study, from the equation in Fig. 28.1, the 95% confidence interval for the population proportion is:

$$p \pm 1.96 \times \sqrt{p(1-p)/n}$$
$$= 0.6 \pm 1.96 \times \sqrt{0.6 \times (1-0.6)/50}$$
$$= 0.46 , 0.74$$

In other words, we can be 95% certain that the true proportion could be as low as 46% or as high as 74%. From the standard error of p, $\sqrt{p(1-p)/n}$ it is clear that if n is larger, the standard error will be smaller and the confidence interval narrower. Thus, if this is not precise enough to fulfil the aims of the study, a larger sample should have been taken.

Confidence interval for a mean

In Chapter 27, the standard error (s.e.) of the mean was calculated as $s/\sqrt{n}$ where s is the sample standard deviation, and using this value, a 95% confidence interval can be calculated from the equation in Fig. 28.1 as:

$$\bar{x} \pm 1.96 \times s/\sqrt{n}$$

Here, as for the confidence interval for a proportion, we are using the 5% point of the normal distribution. However, this often gives too narrow a confidence interval, especially whenever the sample size is small, and in this case the percentage points should be taken from the t-distribution.

The t-distribution

For the mean of a small sample ($<$ 50 observations), the approximation using normal percentage points gives too narrow a confidence statement and so wider limits are necessary. This is because the standard error itself is also estimated, and if it happens to be smaller than the true value, the interval will be too narrow. To guard against this possibility, the constant multiplier of the standard error is taken as a percentage point of the t-distribution. These values are larger than those from the normal distribution by an amount that depends on a parameter known as the degrees of freedom (d.f.). This relates to sample size (n), and is taken as (n – 1), denoted by $t_{(n-1)}$, in calculating the confidence limits for a sample mean. Note that in Table 28.2, percentage points of t for large degrees of freedom are only slightly greater than the normal ones, indicating that one may safely use the normal approximation without seriously affecting the confidence statement.

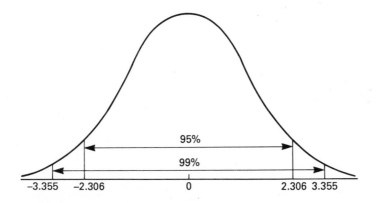

Fig. 28.4   The t-distribution with 8 degrees of freedom.

The shape of the t-distribution is similar to that of the normal distribution, except that it is more spread out (Fig. 28.4). Thus in the calculation of a confidence interval for a mean from a small sample, the 5% point of the t-distribution with (n – 1) degrees of freedom is used for a 95% confidence interval (Table 28.2).

$$\bar{x} \pm t_{(n-1)} \text{ s.e. } (\bar{x})$$

Two sample methods

So far, a single estimate has been considered, a mean or a proportion, for instance. In many studies, the main result may be a comparison of two groups. This could be in terms of comparing two mean outcomes for continuous data, or comparing two proportions for categorical data. For example, a study to assess whether preparation of the parents before hospitalization of their child is effective or not, would involve random allocation of some parents to receive this preparation, while others not receiving the preparation formed the control group. The analysis of this

Table 28.2   Critical values for the t-distribution.

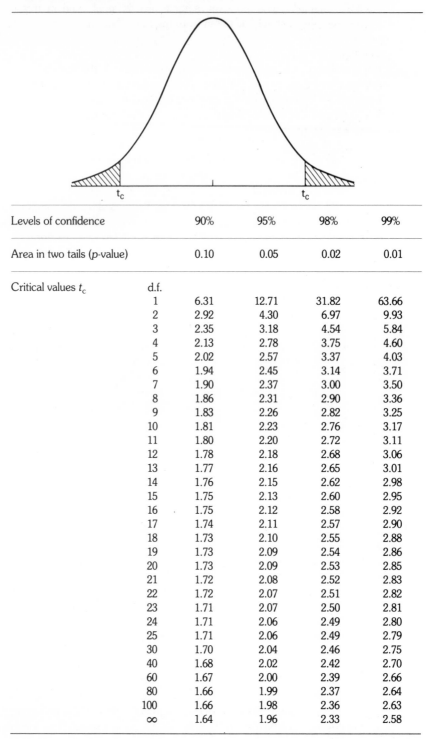

Levels of confidence		90%	95%	98%	99%
Area in two tails (p-value)		0.10	0.05	0.02	0.01
Critical values t_c	d.f.				
	1	6.31	12.71	31.82	63.66
	2	2.92	4.30	6.97	9.93
	3	2.35	3.18	4.54	5.84
	4	2.13	2.78	3.75	4.60
	5	2.02	2.57	3.37	4.03
	6	1.94	2.45	3.14	3.71
	7	1.90	2.37	3.00	3.50
	8	1.86	2.31	2.90	3.36
	9	1.83	2.26	2.82	3.25
	10	1.81	2.23	2.76	3.17
	11	1.80	2.20	2.72	3.11
	12	1.78	2.18	2.68	3.06
	13	1.77	2.16	2.65	3.01
	14	1.76	2.15	2.62	2.98
	15	1.75	2.13	2.60	2.95
	16	1.75	2.12	2.58	2.92
	17	1.74	2.11	2.57	2.90
	18	1.73	2.10	2.55	2.88
	19	1.73	2.09	2.54	2.86
	20	1.73	2.09	2.53	2.85
	21	1.72	2.08	2.52	2.83
	22	1.72	2.07	2.51	2.82
	23	1.71	2.07	2.50	2.81
	24	1.71	2.06	2.49	2.80
	25	1.71	2.06	2.49	2.79
	30	1.70	2.04	2.46	2.75
	40	1.68	2.02	2.42	2.70
	60	1.67	2.00	2.39	2.66
	80	1.66	1.99	2.37	2.64
	100	1.66	1.98	2.36	2.63
	∞	1.64	1.96	2.33	2.58

study might involve comparing mean anxiety levels of the parents in the two groups during the period in hospital.

In comparing two samples, it is important to make the distinction between paired (or matched) groups and unpaired groups, since the statistical methods used differ for these two cases.

Paired and unpaired samples
The calculations of a confidence interval depends on whether the data are paired or unpaired.

Unpaired data implies that the samples are independent of each other, that is, the selection of individuals in one group does not affect the selection of individuals in the other group.

Pairing arises when every individual in one group has a unique match or pair in the other group. This can take two forms:

(1) *Natural pairing*: measurments are made on the same individual at two different time points, or each member of one group has a relative in the other group.
(2) *Artificial pairing*: each member in one group is matched by certain characteristics (age, sex, etc.) to a member in the second group.

Confidence interval for a difference between two unpaired means

For each of the samples, we can calculate the mean and standard deviation, and an obvious way of comparing the two samples is to look at the difference between the two means ($\bar{x}_1 - \bar{x}_2$). In the example discussed in Table 27.3 (Chapter 27), we could compare the mean birthweight of the term infants ($\bar{x}_1 = 3.33$; $s_1 = 0.44$) with the mean birthweight of the premature infants ($\bar{x}_2 = 2.27$; $s_2 = 0.41$). Clearly, the term infants are generally heavier at birth compared to the premature infants, the difference being 1.06 kg. The question arises as to the precision of this estimate. If different samples had been taken, the difference between the means would be different due to biological variation. The answer is to calculate a confidence interval for this difference using the equation given in Fig. 28.1. This is achieved by calculating the standard error of the difference between the means. There will be two standard deviations, and assuming they come from the same population, an average or pooled standard deviation is calculated first. Then the standard error of the difference between the means is calculated and a confidence interval constructed as before using appropriate points of the t-distribution. In the above example, *t*-tables (Table 28.2) would be consulted with $n_1 + n_2 - 2 = 38$ degrees of freedom (since n = 20 in each unmatched group). The formula for the pooled standard deviation and the standard error for a difference between means is given in appendix A.

In the example above, the 95% confidence interval is:

$$1.06 \pm 2.02 \times 0.134$$
$$= 0.79, \ 1.33$$

Thus we can be 95% certain that the true difference between the two means could be as low as 0.79 kg or as high as 1.33 kg. Note that both confidence limits are positive indicating that we can be 95% certain that the term babies are truly heavier than the premature babies.

In the paired case, the difference between each pair is calculated so that the two samples are reduced to a single sample of differences. The confidence interval is then calculated as for a single mean, which in this case is the mean difference.

Similarly, a confidence interval for the difference between two proportions could be calculated. Details are given in Appendix A at the end of this chapter.

Hypothesis testing

The previous sections viewed statistical inference from the idea of estimating a range of values within which we would expect the true population value to lie with a stated probability. Thus a summary statistic was calculated, such as a mean or proportion, and two calculated values defined a confidence interval.

Alternatively, it is possible to test whether or not a particular value of the parameter is consistent with the data, and this is the idea underlying *hypothesis tests*. The outcome of this approach will be a statement to say whether a particular value is *statistically significant* or not.

A hypothesis is a statement about the population; it is made prior to data collection and the validity of this hypothesis or assertion is then tested, based upon the evidence from the sample.

The hypothesis to be tested (denoted by H), for example, whether or not a new drug is better in the treatment of hypertension than the standard one, is couched in neutral terms. In other words, a *null hypothesis* is proposed (the effect of the new drug is the same as that of the standard), and a test is carried out on the sample data. The null hypothesis is analogous to the assumption of innocence of the defendant before a legal trial (Fig. 28.5) and is denoted by H_0. Denote the alternative by H_1. On the basis of this test (examination of the evidence), the null hypothesis is either rejected or not rejected. If rejected, the alternative hypothesis, H_1 is accepted (the new drug is better or worse than the standard). Note that if the null hypothesis is not rejected, this simply means that there is insufficient evidence to reject the hypothesis, analogous to a 'not proven' verdict in Scottish law (Fig. 28.5). This is not the same as 'no difference' or, in terms of the legal analogy, 'innocence'.

LEGAL TRIAL	SIGNIFICANCE TEST
Defendant assumed innocent until proved guilty	Null hypothesis assumes no difference in effect between drug A and drug B
Examine evidence	Calculate test statistic based on evidence from sample
Either:	Either:
(1) Accept evidence proves guilt	(1) Reject null hypothesis and accept significant difference
(2) Accept evidence does not prove guilt 'not proven'	(2) Accept evidence not sufficient to reject null hypothesis; not significant
(*Note*: not same as innocence)	(*Note*: not same as no difference but evidence failed to demonstrate difference)

Fig. 28.5   Legal analogy to hypothesis testing.

All tests are based on a number derived from the sample values; this is the test statistic. The test statistic often consists of a parameter estimate minus the value according to the null hypothesis divided by the standard error of the estimate, thus:

$$\frac{\text{Parameter estimate} - H_0 \text{ value}}{\text{standard error of the estimate}}$$

For example, the test of the null hypothesis that the mean = 0, is carried out by dividing the sample mean by its standard error and comparing the resultant test statistic with percentage points of the normal distribution (assuming a large sample size). In summary, the ordering of this procedure is:

Null $\longrightarrow$ Data collection $\longrightarrow$ Calculate $\longrightarrow$ Accept or
hypothesis   test statistic   reject the
                                                            hypothesis

The details of the test involve calculating a test statistic and comparing the calculated value to theoretical values from a probability distribution such as the normal distribution (Table 28.1). This comparison indicates whether or not the observed value of the test statistic would have been likely to occur if the null hypothesis had been true. If the probability of this happening by chance is sufficiently low (i.e. less than a specified small value called the *significance level*, e.g. 5%), the null hypothesis can be rejected and the sample statistic is said to be significantly different from the hypothetical value.

Significance level

Three significance levels or *p-values* (5%, 1%, 0.1%) are in common use, although this is only a convention because of ease of presenting tables (computers now calculate p-values exactly), reflecting generally agreed cut-off points for strength of evidence against the null hypothesis. It is normal practice to quote the lowest of these levels at which one can reject the null hypothesis; for example, the statement '$p < 0.05$' means that you can reject at the 5% level but not at the 1% level. If you cannot even reject the null hypothesis at the 5% level; the result is not significant (N.S). Since the test of the null hypothesis involves assessment of significance, this procedure is often called a significance test.

Types of error

In making any inference about a population there will always be uncertainty. In setting a significance level for the test of the null hypothesis, we are putting a value on the size of that uncertainty. The significance level is the chance of rejecting the null hypothesis when it is true and so represents the probability of an error – a Type I error. With a significance level of 5%, we are accepting a one in 20 chance of rejecting the null hypothesis when it is in fact true. Obviously, we wish to render the probability of this error as small as possible, so that the lower the significance level, the lower the probability of obtaining a result by chance.

However, there is another type of error, that of not rejecting the null hypothesis when it is in fact false. This is called a Type II error and is related to the Type I error already mentioned. Often this is larger than the Type I error. It is generally assumed that it is more acceptable to have a higher Type II error than a Type I error. In terms of a drug trial, we are saying that it is less acceptable to conclude a drug has an effect when in fact it does not, than to conclude that a drug has no effect when in fact it does. Often, instead of presenting the Type II error the *power* of a test is quoted. The power is simply 100% minus the probability of a Type II error, and so is the probability of rejecting the null hypothesis given that it is false. Hypothesis tests are often carried out at the 5% level with a power of 90% (or 10% Type II error). The power of any test is a function of the size of the sample; small samples will produce tests of low power. Hence the power of any test is decided at the design stage whenever the size of the sample is chosen.

Clinical importance/Statistical significance

In everyday usage the terms importance and significance are synonymous. In statistical jargon, significance refers to the statistical question of whether or not the result could have been obtained by chance; importance relates to the magnitude of the observed effect. Consider a clinical trial in which a new drug reduced blood pressure by, on average, 1mm Hg more than the standard drug and a hypothesis test is statistically significant. However, the result is of no clinical importance, a difference of that magnitude is meaningless. Alternatively, consider a similar trial in which the new drug reduces blood pressure by on average 10 mm Hg more than the standard and a hypothesis test is not significant. In this case, the result is of medical importance. This latter case, in which a clinically important difference is missed because the number in each treatment group is too low to give a statistically significant result, is in fact more common. The way to overcome this is to decide in advance how many patients are necessary for each group to show a clinically important difference at a given statistical significance level. As emphasized in Chapter 27, sample size calculation is very important at the design stage of any study if the results are to be meaningful at the analysis stage.

Comparison of two unpaired means: t-test

We have already calculated the difference between two unpaired means ($\bar{x}_1 - \bar{x}_2$) and the standard error of this difference in the section on confidence intervals. The null hypothesis to be tested in this case is that either there is no difference between the two means, or the difference between the means is zero. As discussed above, a test of this null hypothesis is given by:

$$t = \frac{\text{Estimate} - \text{estimate (if } H_0 \text{ true)}}{\text{standard error (estimate)}}$$

$$= \frac{(\bar{x}_1 - \bar{x}_2) - 0}{s_p \sqrt{(1/n_1 + 1/n_2)}}$$

This value of t is then compared to the theoretical value from t-tables (Table 28.2) with $n_1 + n_2 - 2$ degrees of freedom. Initially, the calculated value of t is compared to the 5% point of the t-tables, and if the value exceeds the tabulated value, the result is said to be significant at the 5% level. The result obtained is unlikely to have occurred by chance and so the difference is statistically significant. If it exceeds the 1% tabulated value the result is significant at the 1% level, and so on. If the value does not exceed the 5% point, it is said to be not significant (N.S.).

The assumptions being made in this test are that both samples come from a normal distribution and hence have the same standard deviation. The assumption of normality can be assessed visually using the methods described in Chapter 27.

In the example above: $t = 1.06/0.13$
$$= 8.15$$

Looking at tables with $20 + 20 - 2 = 38$ degrees of freedom the 5% point is 2.02 (Table 28.2) and the value clearly exceeds the tabulated value. In fact the value of t is significant at the 0.01% level. If we had more extensive tables, the p-value would be even lower. This result is said to be highly significant.

Comparison of two independent proportions

In order to compare two independent proportions, the chi-squared test is used. This is based on the chi-squared (χ^2) probability distribution which is continuous and approaches the normal distribution for large degrees of freedom. However, in comparing two proportions, the χ^2 distribution with 1 degree of freedom is used, which is highly positively skewed.

In order to facilitate the test, the data are laid out in a 2×2 contingency table. The two rows in Table 28.3 represent the two samples, with the row totals being the total number in each sample, and the first column, divided by the row totals, representing the two proportions which are to be compared.

Table 28.3   General form of 2×2 contingency table.

sample 1	a	b	r_1
sample 2	c	d	r_2
	s_1	s_2	n

where r_1 and r_2 are the row totals, and s_1 and s_2 are the column totals.

The test compares the two proportions $p_1 = a/r_1$ and $p_2 = c/r_2$. If the proportions in the two populations are the same, then a/b and c/d should be similar and so $| ad - bc |$ should be small. (The symbols $| \ |$ simply mean that the result of the arithmetic between the vertical bars is given a positive sign.) The table can be rearranged so that the columns become the rows if this is more convenient. The test is one of *association* between the two dimensions which make up the table.

The null hypothesis is that $p_1 - p_2 = 0$ and the test statistic is given by:

$$\chi_2 = \frac{(| ad - bc | - n/2)^2 \, n}{r_1 \, r_2 \, s_1 \, s_2}$$

The value is then compared to the theoretical value from chi-squared tables (Table 28.4) with one degree of freedom and if it is larger the result is significant at that level.

To give an example, it has been found that for babies born at less than 32 weeks gestation, there is a high risk of developing periventricular haemorrhage (PVH). It has been suggested that supplementation of vitamin E for the babies would reduce

Table 28.4   Critical values for the chi-squared distribution with 1 degree of freedom (d.f.).

Significance level (p-value)	0.10	0.05	0.02	0.01
Critical value χ_1^2	2.71	3.84	5.41	6.64

this risk. In order to assess this, one group of babies (n = 102) were randomly chosen to receive the supplement while another randomly chosen group did not receive the supplement, forming the controls (n = 108). The frequency of the outcome, periventricular haemorrhage, was measured and the results could be set out as a 2×2 contingency table (Table 28.5).

Table 28.5   Results of trial using vitamin E supplement.

	Vitamin E supplement		Controls		
No haemorrhage	71	(70%)	50	(46%)	121
Haemorrhage	31	(30%)	58	(54%)	89
	102		108		210

The null hypothesis being tested is that the proportions with haemorrhage in the two groups are the same or $p_1 - p_2 = 0$. The proportion with haemorrhage (p_1) is $31/102 = 30\%$ in the supplemented group, while the proportion (p_2) is $58/108 = 54\%$ in the control group. This suggests that the difference, 24%, is clinically important. To assess the statistical significance of this difference, a chi-squared test is carried out.

$$\chi^2 = \frac{(|\ 71\times58 - 31\times50\ | - 210/2)^2\ 210}{102 \times 108 \times 121 \times 89}$$
$$= 10.74$$

Comparing this value of χ^2 with tabulated values (Table 28.4) shows that the difference of 24% is highly statistically significant. The 95% confidence interval for this difference is (11%; 37%), indicating the size of the effect if the vitamin E supplement were to be applied to the population of ≤ 32 weeks gestation babies.

Note that the chi-squared test for two proportions is one of association and so does not imply that one factor causes the other.

More than two groups

So far, I have only considered one variable and a comparison of this measure in two groups (or samples). There are extensions of the methods described for comparing more than two groups: for example, one way analysis of variance for comparison of more than two means. Lack of space prevents their description here; for details of these methods see Armitage and Berry (1987).

Correlation

The next step is to consider relationships between two quantitative variables. As an initial step, a scatterplot, as described in Chapter 27, will display this relationship. Figure 27.8 showed the relationship between mental ability scores and standardized height (Fulton *et al.* 1987). A single number can be calculated which is a measure of the closeness of this relationship; the *correlation coefficient*, denoted by r.

The correlation coefficient ranges in value from –1 to +1 with a value of ±1 indicating complete correlation, that is, a straight line. A correlation of 0 indicates

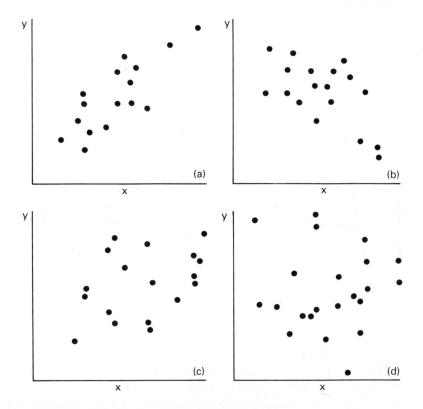

Fig. 28.6 Examples of correlations (a) r = +0.9
(b) r = –0.8
(c) r = +0.6
(d) r = 0.0

(Reproduced from *Statistical Methods in Agriculture and Experimental Biology*, R. Mead and R.N. Curnan (1983), Chapman and Hall)

no correlation or a random scatter of points. The sign of the correlation indicates the direction of the trend, a positive correlation indicates that as one measure increases the other measure also increases; a negative coefficient indicates that as one measure increases the other decreases (Fig. 28.6).

The assumptions made are that there is a linear relationship, that both variables are continuous, and that both variables have an approximately normal distribution. If one or both of the variables are categorical, then non-parametric rank correlation is indicated. The correlation coefficient for mental ability scores and standardized height (Fig. 27.8) was $r = 0.26$, indicating that taller children tend to have greater mental ability (both variables standardized by age.).

As with the other statistics mentioned in this chapter, the correlation coefficient is based on samples, and so the methods of inference can be applied, although this will not be described here. Note that correlation does not imply causation.

Linear regression

The correlation coefficient tells us the strength of the relationship between two quantitative variables. On the other hand, the method of regression tells us about the nature of the relationship between any two quantitative variables and precisely how they change numerically together. In regression, one is interested in by how much one variable increases for a given increase in the other. A linear relationship is assumed to model the data. Figure 28.7 shows the regression line for mental ability scores against standardized height.

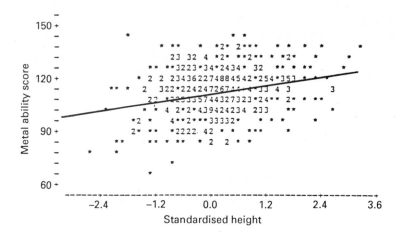

Fig 28.7   Regression of mental ability score on height (both standardized by age) for 496 children in Edinburgh.

In regression, one of the variables is taken as the outcome variable while the other is the predictor variable. For the above example, height would be considered as a predictor of mental ability and not the other way round. Sometimes it is not clear which variable should be the outcome. Although the terms outcome and predictor are used, as with correlation, causality cannot be assumed.

In reality, there will be many possible predictor variables. The method of simple linear regression can be extended for this case and most computer packages contain programmes which will carry out multiple regression. For an explanation of these methods, see Armitage and Berry (1987).

SUMMARY

This chapter has introduced the powerful tool of statistical inference, in terms of estimation and hypothesis testing. These ideas are fundamental, and although more sophisticated methods are not described in this chapter, the outcome from any method will generally involve estimation of parameters, estimation of their confidence intervals, and the testing of hypotheses, followed by an interpretation of these procedures.

REFERENCES

Armitage P. & Berry G. (1987) *Statistical methods in medical research*, Blackwell Scientific Publications, Oxford.
Fulton M. *et al.* (1987) Influence of blood lead on the ability and attainment of children in Edinburgh. *Lancet* **i** (8544), 1221-6.
Gardner M.J. & Altman D.G. (Eds.) (1989) *Statistics with confidence – confidence intervals and statistical guidelines* (Book). *British Medical Journal*, **299**, 690.
Ryan B.F., Joiner B.L. & Ryan T.A. (1985) *Minitab handbook* Duxbury, Boston.
Siegel S. (1989) *Nonparametric statistics for the behavioural sciences*, McGraw-Hill, New York.
Sinha S. *et al.* (1987) Vitamin E supplementation reduces frequency of periventricular haemorrhage in very preterm babies. *Lancet*, **i** (8531), 466-71.
Sprent P. (1981) *Quick Statistics*, Penguin books, London.

APPENDIX A: FORMULAE FOR CONFIDENCE INTERVALS

Confidence interval for a sample mean

The standard error for a sample mean $\bar{x}$ is given by $s/\sqrt{n}$ where s is the sample standard deviation. The confidence interval for a sample mean is:

$$\bar{x} \pm t_{(n-1)} \times s/\sqrt{n}$$

where t is the appropriate value from the t-distribution with $(n-1)$ degrees of freedom.

Confidence interval for a proportion

The standard error for a sample proportion p is $\sqrt{p(1-p)/n}$.
The confidence interval for a sample proportion is

$$p \pm 1.96 \times \sqrt{p(1-p)/n}$$
assuming n is large.

Confidence interval for a difference between two means

Pooled standard deviation is given by:

$$s_p = \sqrt{\frac{(n_1 - 1)\,s_1^2 + (n_2 - 1)\,s_2^2}{(n_1 + n_2 - 2)}}$$

where n_1 and n_2 are the sizes of the two samples. The standard error of the difference $(\bar{x}_1 - \bar{x}_2)$ is

s.e. $(\bar{x}_1 - \bar{x}_2) = s_p \sqrt{(1/n_1 + 1/n_2)}$

and the 95% confidence interval is:

$$(\bar{x}_1 - \bar{x}_2) \pm t_{(n+n-2)}\, s_p \sqrt{1/n_1 + 1/n_2}$$

where the $t_{(n+n-2)}$ is the 5% point of the t-distribution with

$n_1 + n_2 - 2$ degrees of freedom.

Confidence interval for difference between two proportions

For proportions p_1 and p_2 the standard error for their difference $p_1 - p_2$ is:

s.e. $(p_1 - p_2) = \sqrt{p_1(1 - p_1)/n + p_2(1 - p_2)/n}$

and the 95% confidence interval is given by:

$p_1 - p_2 \pm 1.96 \times$ s.e. $(p_1 - p_2)$

(If p is expressed as a percentage, use 100 instead of 1 in the formula for the standard error.)

Chapter 29
Qualitative Analysis
Linda C. Pollock

Chapter 13 focused on the qualitative approach to research design and its application to nursing research. There is a growing interest in qualitative research methods: case study, grounded theory, and phenomenology are but some examples. Each offers a common challenge to the nurse researcher, that of generating results from the qualitative data. The data gathering process is relatively simple: interview schedules, questionnaires, observation logs, journals – whatever enables the researcher to amass, quickly, large volumes of data. Determining what it all means, however, can be less easy, and it is at this stage that you can start to become bogged down. This chapter explores further the data handling aspect of qualitative research. The methods available to facilitate the management of qualitative data are reviewed, and the need for a clear presentation of the data are detailed. Some of the common pitfalls encountered by the novice researcher are outlined, and guidelines are offered to avoid or minimize these difficulties. Writings on qualitative method, ethnographic approaches, fieldwork, and interviewing, are long on discussions of data collection and research experiences, but short on analysis (Miles 1979). Two recent texts redress the balance and fill the gap in the literature: Strauss (1987) and Miles and Huberman (1983). These books will help you see how qualitative analysis can be carried out.

QUALITATIVE AND QUANTITATIVE DATA AND ANALYSIS

Amongst researchers, a distinction is commonly drawn between quantitative and qualitative methods, which produce 'hard' and 'soft' data respectively. Specific disciplines historically prefer particular traditions, for example, sociology has since World War 2 promoted the use of questionnaires and other survey methods of data collection and statistical analysis of findings; social anthropology, in contrast, encouraged the use of field methods which focus on situational and structural contexts and thereby qualitative data was collected and so analysed. Qualitative researchers tend to study one single situation, organization or institution (Glasser & Strauss 1965; Goffman 1961). Quantitative researchers' work, by contrast, tends to be multivariate but relatively weak on context. Analytically, qualitative and quantitative researchers treat their data differently. In quantitative research, statistics or some other form of mathematical operations are used to make sense of the data. In qualitative research, mathematical techniques are eschewed or are of minimal use, although rudimentary counting and measuring may be involved (how many, how often, to what degree).

In daily life everyone engages in some form of qualitative analysis, since no judgements, no decisions, no actions, can be taken in their absence. So in a genuine sense, both commonsense and 'researcher' conclusions are based on 'qualitative data'. Although everyday pragmatic analysis can involve care, self-awareness, and be systematic in character, judgments of researchers are expected to involve all of this and, in addition, to adhere to disciplinary practices associated with the 'good' researcher: that is, researchers must take care to be scrupulously systematic in their treatment of reliable data.

Analysis is synonymous with the interpretation of data. It refers to research activity which involves several different but related tasks. Qualitative analysis occurs at various levels of explicitness, abstraction, and systematization. At the beginning of a research project when the researcher reads a sentence or sees an action, the analysis may be quite implicit; but it is nevertheless analysed as perception, and is selective, mediated by language and experience. Later in the investigation, or even during the first days, when an observed scene, interview, or perused document challenges the researcher's analytic sense, the conclusions will be drawn more explicitly and probably more systematically. Depending on the purposes of the investigator, the final conclusions drawn in the course of research can vary greatly by level of abstraction. At the lowest levels, they can be 'descriptive', and at the highest levels, the researcher may aim for the generation of theory. But description itself can be 'low level': perhaps only reproducing the informants' own words or recording their actions; alternatively, reporting can be at a much more complex, systematic, and interpretative level and result in social theory which may be broad or narrow in scope.

MATERIAL AS DATA

Qualitative research approaches, then, are recommended to bring alive particular situations and people under study, and these approaches are advocated in non-traditional areas where there is little or no technical literature. Researchers using qualitative research methods may come from a variety of disciplines: nursing, medicine, psychology, law, history, education, sociology; different disciplines tend to favour one type of material rather than another. Ethnographers for example have relied mainly on field observations converted into field notes and on interviews for data; historians may use the interview if their work is on contemporary or relatively recent events, but principally they utilize many different kinds of documents, depending on their specific research aims and on the availability and accessibility of materials: records of various types, memoirs, official and personal letters, diaries, newspapers, maps, photographs, and paintings. Researchers in clinical psychology, medicine, or nursing, can base conclusions primarily on clinical observations of patients' non-verbal as well as verbal behaviour and on therapeutic interviews. Many sociologists prefer to analyse written texts rather than engage in field research or interviewing; others generate materials through tape recordings of conversations, transcripts of court trials, and the like. While some materials (data) may be generated by the researchers through interviews, field observations, or videotapes, a great deal already exists, located in settings which can be tapped if the researcher can gain access to study natural environments and working situations.

Systematic approach to qualitative analysis

The introductory paragraph of Barton and Lazarfeld (1969) clearly states the need for researchers to make explicit what they are doing. By making explicit what they do, researchers can then generalize methodological knowledge and transfer from one specific project or subject matter to others, from one researcher, to the scientific community. Becker and Greer (1960) agree and state, 'We need a systematic statement of canons to be applied to individual items of evidence'. The need for a systematic approach to the analysis of qualitative data has been reinforced by the comments of the following authors. Brown (1973) stated that observations can have alternative interpretations. Trend (1978) described this as the 'Roshomon' effect and asserted that the same social field viewed from different perspectives could produce explanations that might as well have been based in two different realities. Bailyn (1977) adds:

'The presentation of data must be sufficiently focused so that the reader can easily assimilate the central research results. At the same time it must be open enough to allow interested readers to make their own inferences and thus to evaluate the cognitive process the analyst went through to reach the presented conclusions.'

Bailyn's article is a landmark, in that she thoughtfully reviews the cognitive processes involved in dealing with survey data. Turner (1981) uses Bailyn's thesis and asserts that for qualitative researchers:

'. . . the practical details of data handling are even more closely associated with central aspects of research cognition, some form of explication seems to be desirable.'

There is a definite need for researchers to make explicit the methods they use to facilitate the management of large amounts of qualitative data. Without this, the advancement of knowledge is impeded within the social sciences, and conclusions will not be considered reliable. Without available tools to manage the data, analysis and presentation of the findings may not even take place. Control of the cognitive complexity of data is perhaps most crucial and most difficult to achieve in the compilation phase, as anyone who has ever been faced with six inches of computer output relating everything to everything else, or mounds of transcribed interviews, can testify. Otherwise, without control, there will be complete cessation of all thought because of overload. In view of the need to clearly detail and present the qualitative information, the techniques available for use are summarized below.

Techniques of qualitative data management

The introductory paragraph of Barton and Lazarfeld (1969) held promise that further reading would lead to a clarification of the research procedure involved in qualitative analysis. The authors indeed comment that their intention is to attempt to answer the question: 'What can a researcher do when confronted with a body of qualitative data?' (p. 163) and present 'a guide through qualitative research' (p. 164). What is offered ultimately, is a presentation (laudable in its scope and variety) of the results of 'about 100' studies, in an attempt to distinguish 'types' of qualitative research. No endeavour is made to focus on what the researcher does to arrive at the analysis.

In general textbooks on qualitative analysis, the content is often aimed at intellectual discussion of the value of a qualitative approach to theory building and development of models (McCall & Simmons 1969; Glaser & Strauss 1967), or on a discussion of the outcomes of qualitative research, with a detailed presentation of the findings and conclusions (Cressey 1932; Whyte 1943; Becker 1961; Becker 1962, Glaser & Strauss 1965). In 1967, the latter authors argued for:

'Theory based on data which can usually not be completely refuted by more data or replaced by another theory. Since it is too intimately linked to data, it is destined to last despite its inevitable modification and reformulation.' (p. 4)

They also emphasise a process of

'Theoretical sampling in which the analyst jointly collects, codes and analyses his data and decides what data to collect next and where to find them in order to develop his theory as it emerges.' (p. 45)

Still later publications are less helpful than might be anticipated. Glaser (1978) deals extensively with some problems faced by the grounded theorist. His style is dense and elliptical and assumes a prior familiarity with the method and does little in the way of offering practical suggestions on data management. He expresses a preference for writing category titles in the margin of carbon copies of field notes, subsequently cutting up those for sorting and also declares index cards a hinderance (pp. 71-2). The description of the procedure of theory generation can be rather nebulous and, as Melia (1982) pointed out, 'at times tended to confuse rather than clarify' (p. 358).

Turner (1981) has cited Sieber (1976) who had analysed seven texts on field method. Sieber found that most of the publications examined paid little attention to the problem of data analysis, rarely devoting more than 5–10% of their pages to the topic. Lofland and Lofland (1984; pp. 127-9) offer practical suggests in relation to qualitative analysis. They comment that: 'At the very least it [the data] should be filed in chronological order and tapes should be labelled and dated'; research workers are also recommended to make copies of field notes and file them under various headings. Vague reference is made to ideas emerging from writing:

'He [the researcher] may begin to find that a section just does not make sense. It will not write. Even and should or must be re-done, re-conceived or re-ordered. . . .
Description and analysis together, without one crushing the other, constitute enlightening and balanced sociological work.'

There seems then, to be a magical aura around the management of observation and qualitative data which assumes a rather mystical and elusive quality. Becker and Greer (1960) provided the seminal work of offering clarification of technique. The authors outlined a model which explained the steps taken (and the assumptions underlying them), to handle data derived from participant observation. Becker and Greer talked about 'coding of data; formulation of the content of the perspective; frequency checks; checks on the range; tabulation of collective character'. The steps outlined were not especially clear but their stepwise model provided the initial impetus and focus for further discussion of what they term 'strategies for a natural sociology'. They also distinguished three types of notes that observers may make: observational, theoretical, and methodological. The first type pertains to observational notes, those based on watching and listening, and these should state what happened and be as accurate as possible. The second, theoretical notes, refers to the researcher's inferences and subjective comments. The final type, methodological, refer to the researcher's comments on the method itself or on himself or the situation. Further writers have detailed in more meaningful ways tips that help new researchers examine the data.

Norris (1981; p. 337) summarized the problems of the analysis of soft data and offered advice on the management of large quantities of descriptive data. She proposes a method of systematic indexing, which facilitates the development of conceptual frameworks from the most frequently recurring topics. She states:

'A useful scheme is to keep an alphabetical index an address book would suffice for a small project in which subjects which constantly recur may be entered. If every page of data is numbered when filed and those page numbers entered in the index ... this makes for easy reference back to similar incidents or

'Stage	Main activity	Comment
(1)	*Develop categories:*	Use the data available to develop labelled categories which fit the data closely
(2)	*Saturate categories:*	Accumulate examples of a given category until it is clear what future instances would be located in this category
(3)	*Abstract definitions:*	Abstract a definition of the category by stating in a general form the criteria for putting further instances into this category.
(4)	*Use the definitions:*	Use the definitions as a guide to emerging features of importance in further fieldwork, and as a stimulus to theoretical reflection
(5)	*Exploit categories fully:*	Be aware of additional categories suggested by those you have produced, their inverse, their opposite, more specific and more general instances
(6)	*Note develop and follow-up links between categories:*	Begin to note relationships and develop hypotheses about the links between the categories
(7)	*Consider the conditions under which the links hold:*	Examine any apparent or hypothesized relationships and try to specify the conditions
(8)	*Make connections where relevant to existing theory:*	Build bridges to existing work at this stage, rather than at the outset of the research
(9)	*Use extreme comparisons to the maximum to test emerging relationships:*	Identify the key variables and dimensions and see whether the relationship holds at the extremes of these variables'

Fig. 29.1   Turner's nine stage framework of qualitative analysis (Turner 1981, p. 244).

statements about the topic as work proceeds . . . and frequent references to particular topics indicate a ready made framework of second order constructs. . . .'

This indexing system has been used by Wheatley (1980) who taped interviews with carers of elderly demented patients, and Dickson (1980), who examined the effects of giving birth on a woman's sexuality.

Turner (1981) elaborated a meticulous and systematic method of handling the practical elements of managing qualitative data (Fig. 29.1). He developed this procedure with a colleague (see Woodward 1970); and it was aimed specifically to be used in the development of grounded theory. Turner (1981) isolated nine stages within his framework and used qualitative data category cards to sort the data into categories. This has been used in a recent piece of nursing research (Pollock 1989) and Figure 29.2 shows an illustration of a data category card used in this study which examined the work of community psychiatric nurses. The first stage is elaborated at length, as the most opaque step in the analysis. From transcription of taped material, Turner (1981; p. 232) labelled the phenomena he was perceiving. He describes the process thus;

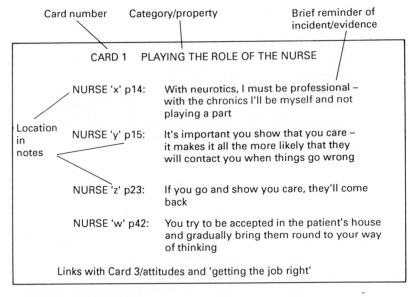

Fig. 29.2 Example of qualitative data category card, showing types of information noted (data from Pollock 1989).

'I deal with the material paragraph by paragraph numbering the paragraphs for reference purposes. Starting with the first paragraph of the transcript I ask "What categories, concepts or labels do we need in order to describe or to account for the phenomenon discussed in this paragraph?" When I think of a label I note it down on a 5" × 8" file card, together with the number of the file and file the card. I then check whether further cards are needed to note significant phenomena referred to in this paragraph. I generate cards with titles of categories, until I am satisfied with my coverage of that paragraph, until I seem to have noted all of those features which are of significance to me, and then move on to the next paragraph. The labels used in this categorisation may be long winded, ungainly or fanciful at this stage and they may be formulated at any conceptual level which seems appropriate, but it is important that they should possess one essential property: as far as the researcher is concerned the label should fit the phenomena described in the data exactly. If the fit is not perfect, the words used should be changed and rechanged and adjusted until the fit is improved, for the value of the whole approach depends upon this goodness of fit as the basis of subsequent operations.'

Transcribing interviews

The transcription of audio-tape recordings of structured interviews is considered a pre-requisite to qualitative analysis (Field & Morse 1985). As detailed earlier, however, this may not be the only material available for analysis. Nevertheless, use of taped interviews is a popular means of obtaining data, and mention is made specifically of analysis of this type of data. Financial resources to meet the heavy cost of professional (secretarial) help have to be assessed when undertaking such an approach to data collection and analysis.

Transcribing is a lengthy process and it can take at least 10 to 12 hours to transcribe a 90-minute tape (see Pollock 1989). This aspect of the analysis, then, involves a considerable investment of time — and this is only a beginning step in the process. Another daunting feature of transcribed tapes is that one 45-minute interview can give you 25 pages of text which then need to be coded, sorted, and analysed. As soon as possible after a taped interview, the researcher will find it helpful to replay the interview carefully noting content and the emotional tone of responses. The typed transcripts should include information of pauses (dashes), gaps and pauses (dots) and comments in brackets detailing laughter, etc. Generous margins on each side of the typescript and double spacing should allow for the researcher's coding and critique of the interview (left margin) and comments regarding content (right margin) to be added. The checking of typed transcripts against the tapes is also necessary.

Options are available for coding interview data. Highlighter pens can be useful, as can cutting and pasting categories into cards for manual sorting (Field & Morse 1985); other researchers have used category numbering to sort the codes (Miles & Huberman 1983); Chenitz and Swanson (1986) show how the use of memos and diagrams can aid coding and analysis. You will find these texts to be an excellent help.

INTERPRETING QUALITATIVE DATA

Emphasizing the use of techniques to handle the analysis of qualitative data tends to underplay the part of the researcher in the understanding of the data. The researcher brings her own theoretical and personal perspective to bear on the analytical process, and the research questions articulated at the beginning of the study will provide an essential structure for guiding the data analysis and interpretation. It is important to emphasize that the analysis does not just involve describing the data. The techniques described above help the researcher focus in on themes and concepts. The researcher thus avoids merely describing the data collected. The results of qualitative studies should not just be idiosyncratic thumbnail sketches of particular human experiences but rather represent concepts that express the meaning of those shared experiences and add to knowledge.

Novice qualitative researchers tend to want to describe and account for *all* the data that have been collected, struggling to fit ever-growing masses of data into precise categories. This can be an overwhelming experience which delays interpretation of the data and formulation of the results. Ammom-Gaberson and Piantanida (1988) provided an account of one such 'submerged' researcher:

> 'I had the image of gathering colorful pebbles from a variety of beaches and then fussing endlessly to sort the pebbles into piles of comparable size, color, texture, beach of origin, etc. Despite the volumes of pebbles I had gathered it seemed terribly superficial and banal to talk about the various piles. Slowly I began to realize that I could use the pebbles in a very different way. I could stop trying to maintain the identity of each separate pebble, and could instead, use them collectively to create a colorful mosaic. Suddenly I realized that the significance of my data did not lie in the individual pieces of data, but rather in using the pieces to create a meaningful picture of hospital education.'

The task at hand then, in qualitative analysis, is not to describe every piece of the jigsaw but rather to stand back and paint a picture of the whole. Interpretation of the meaning arises from the arrangement of data in a way that transcends the significance of individual data bits. The challenge to the researcher is to connect data bits to each other and to a body of literature that yields a meaning that is useful to a professional audience.

Novice qualitative researchers must guard against 'data shuffling' – continually sifting and sorting through the data. This is a necessary part of data management but this stage can become dysfunctional if attempts are not made to piece together the mosaic or jigsaw as described above. One can extend the pebble metaphor. Imagine an artist standing in a studio surrounded by piles of pebbles. Off in a corner stands a large board on which a mosaic is to be created. Instead of bringing the board to the work table and beginning the process of selecting and arranging pebbles to create a picture, the artist spends his time moving the pebbles from pile to pile. No matter how neatly or thoroughly the pebbles are sorted, the mosaic will never be created if the artist does not begin to visualize the picture and start placing pebbles on the board.

Quantitative data lend themselves to classification in clear cut, mutually exclusive categories, whereas qualitative data can potentially fit into several different ones. An indeterminate amount of time can be wasted sorting the data into an ever-increasing number of categories. It is impossible, before making the mosaic, to know which aspects of a particular pebble's characteristics will ultimately be most useful: its colour, shape, texture, or some subtle combination of qualities. By pondering the various possibilities and trying alternative groupings, you become acquainted intimately with the data. This immersion in the data is necessary as a precursor to generating the results, but there is a danger that you become totally preoccupied with the arranging and rearranging of the piles of categories and elaboration of the actual mosaic is delayed. The techniques mentioned above, necessary and helpful though they are, provide temporary storage areas from which the data can be retrieved as they are needed to create the mosaic.

CONCLUSION

Qualitative analysis is not easy and the findings of such studies can be challenged on the grounds of questionable reliability and validity. To counter such accusations, read Hinds *et al.* (1990), and take heart. Try and be as open as possible in your presentation of findings so that your methods and analysis can be critically examined by researcher colleagues. You will find this openness threatening and will be at risk of, like the emperor, being discovered without clothes. If you have taken note of the hints of this chapter, however, you will be at little risk of such embarrassment. The interests of nursing research can only be furthered by the opportunity you have provided for discussion of details of your research process and procedures. Enjoy making and presenting that mosaic, and remember not to get too preoccupied with the pebbles!

REFERENCES

Ammon-Gaberson K.B. & Piantanida M. (1988) Generating results from qualitative data. *Image: Journal of Nursing Scholarship*, **20** (3), 159–61.

Bailyn L. (1977) Research as a cognitive process – implications for data analysis. *Quality and quantity*, **11**, 97–119.

Barton A.E Lazarfeld P.F. (1969) Functions of a qualitative analysis in social research. In McCall G.J. and Simmons J.L. *Issues in participant observation: a text and reader*. (Ed. by G.J. McCall & J.L. Simmons), Addison-Wesley, Wokingham.

Becker H. & Greer B. (1960) The analysis of qualitative field data. Chapter 11 in *Human organisation research*. (Ed. by R.N. Adams & J.J. Preiss) Dorsey Press, Illinois.

Becker H. (1962) *Outsiders*. Free Press, Glencoe.

Becker H. (1961) *Boys in White*. University of Chicago Press.

Brown G.W. (1973) Some thoughts on grounded theory. *Sociology*. **7** 1–16.

Chenitz W.C. & Swanson J.M. (1986) *From Practice to Grounded Theory. Qualitative Research in Nursing*. Addison-Wesley, Chicago.

Cressey P. (1932) *The taxi-hall dance*. University of Chicago Press.

Dickson A. (1980) *An investigation into the effects of the birth of a first child on a woman's sexuality*. MSc thesis, University of Surrey.

Field P.A. & Morse J.M. (1985) *Nursing research. The application of qualitative approaches*. Croom Helm, London.

Glaser B.G. (1978) *Theoretical sensitivity. Advances in the methodology of grounded theory*. Sociology Press, Mill Valley, California.

Glaser B. & Strauss A. (1965) *Awareness of dying*. Aldine Publishing Company, Chicago.

Glaser B. & Strauss A. (1967) *The discovery of grounded theory*. Aldine Publishing Company, Chicago.

Goffman E. (1961) *Asylums: essays on the social situation of mental patients and other patients*. Penguin, London.

Hinds P., Scandrett-Hibden S. & McAulay L.S. (1990) Further assessment of a method to estimate reliability and validity of qualitative research findings. *Journal of Advanced Nursing*. **15**, 430–5.

Lofland J. & Lofland J. (1984) *Analysing social settings. A guide to qualitative observations and analysis.* 2nd edn. Wadsworth, California.

Melia K. (1982) Tell it as it is – qualitative methodology. *Journal of Advanced Nursing,* **7**, 327–35.

McCall G.J. & Simmons J.L. (1969) *Issues in participant observation: a text and reader.* Addison-Wesley, Wokingham.

Miles M. (1979) Qualitative data as an attractive nuisance: the problems of analysis. *Administrative Science Quarterly.* **24**: 590–601.

Miles M. & Huberman M. (1983) *Qualitative data analysis: data source book.* Sage, California.

Norris M. (1981) Problems in the analysis of qualitative data – suggested solutions. *Sociology.* **15** (3), 337–51.

Pollock L.C. (1989) *Community Psychiatric Nursing: myth and reality.* RCN Reseach Series, Scutari Press, London.

Sieber S.D. (1976) *A synopsis and critique of guidelines for qualitative analysis contained in selected textbooks.* Unpublished paper. Project on social architecture in education. Centre for policy research, New York.

Strauss A.L. (1987) *Qualitative analysis for social scientists.* Cambridge University Press.

Trend M.G. (1978) On the reconciliation of qualitative and quantitative analysis – a case study. *Human Behaviour,* **37**, 5–54.

Turner B.A. (1981) Some practical aspects of qualitative data analysis: one way of organising the cognitive processes associated with the generation of grounded theory. *Quality and Quantity* **15**, 225–47.

Wheatley V. (1980) *Supporters of elderly persons with a dementing illness – living in the same household.* MSc thesis, University of Surrey.

Woodward J. (1970) *Industrial Organisation, behaviour and control.* Oxford University Press.

Whyte F.W. (1943) *Street Corner Society.* University of Chicago Press.

Chapter 30
Data Presentation
Desmond F.S. Cormack and David C. Benton

The dissemination of research has long been recognized as being crucial to the development of nursing's research base (Horsley *et al.* 1983; Phillips 1986). However, not only have there been difficulties in gaining access to much of the material produced, but there have also been problems in comprehending some of that material. Data presentation, or to define it more explicitly, getting your results across and understood by your readers, is a critical element of any study.

By examination of the definition given, it is evident that it is not adequate to simply display results since they must also be understood. Unless results are comprehended by your audience, there is no opportunity for you to receive feedback or for readers to consider and reflect on their own practice in the light of new information. It is essential that data are presented in a manner that is clearly understood via an appropriate medium, using an appropriate format, so as to facilitate both individual and our professions' development.

Data can be presented in many ways. The book that you are currently reading is a data source; it has a wealth of information about the research process. Hopefully, this information will be read, reflected upon, integrated into your personal knowledge base, and used at some point in the future.

As you can see from this text, in addition to the written word, you can also find numeric, graphical, and pictorial data, all of which have particular strengths and weaknesses. Before dealing with each of these specific approaches, a number of general issues relating to data presentation are examined.

DATA PRESENTATION TECHNIQUES – GENERAL ISSUES

The method chosen to present data is obviously dependent on a number of factors such as the type of data, the target readership, and the overall design of your study. In today's technological world, there is an ever-increasing number of aids which can be used to assist in the presentation of our material. If communication of results is to be effective, the appropriate use of technological aids must be made.

Whether these aids are used to prepare a scientific paper, a journal article, a book chapter, or simply an overhead transparency, there are a number of fundamental principles which must be considered.

Computer technology has given the researcher, via the word processor and desk top publishing system, access to a wide variety of means of emphasizing data (Powell 1989). Figure 30.1 lists a number of commonly available means of gaining readers' attention.

There are several means of highlighting data so as to enable it to stand out and attract an individual's attention. **Bold** and underlining can easily yet effectively help focus attention on a particular point.

Highlighting
Capitals
Size
markers – Pointers
Colour blocks – Variations in shade
Change of Colour
Differing fonts
Indenting – sub-sections

Fig. 30.1 Approaches to gaining your readers' attention.

Another simple yet effective way of drawing attention to a point, is to use CAPITALS. This can be particularly effective when the rest of the data are presented in lower case.

The ready availability of word processors and desk top publishing systems have given ready access to a number of techniques which were in the past only generally available to printers, graphic artists, and designers.

With new technological assistance, it is easy to produce print in a variety of sizes. This feature is particularly useful if you are using overhead transparencies or a poster presentation format. Unless data are presented in large bold characters, an audience will have great difficulty in seeing and hence interpreting the value of your work.

Pointers in their simplest form may only consist of an asterisk, and are commonly used as a means of highlighting statistically significant associations, see Table 30.1. However, with the introduction of new technology, much more sophisticated characters can be used.

With high technology printers, it is possible to use either colour or variations in shade as a means of enhancing the clarity of data presentation. Colour laser photocopiers can reproduce material (at a cost) such as photographs or other figures which can add significantly to the quality of a presentation. Consider how effective it is to show a photograph of a wound rather than trying to accurately and succinctly describe it. However, great care must be taken when colour print is used on colour back-grounds. If an inappropriate choice is made, the colours may clash or worse still, due to poor contrast, be illegible. As an example, the colour combinations indicted in Fig. 30.2 are acceptable and easy to read.

Table 30.1 Correlation table demonstrating pointers.

	Variable 1	Variable 2	Variable 3	Variable 4
Variable 1	1.000			
Variable 2	0.857**	1.000		
Variable 3	−0.486	−0.771**	1.000	
Variable 4	−0.403	−0.692*	0.820**	1.000

n=17

1-tailed significance level   * = 0.01   ** = 0.001

Text colour	Appropriate background colour
White	Red, Blue, Black
Yellow	Blue, Black
Cyan	Black
Green	Black
Red	White, Yellow
Blue	White, Yellow, Cyan
Black	White, Yellow, Cyan

Fig. 30.2   Legible text and background colour combinations.

Even the most basic word processing systems offer the researcher the use of at least two fonts. A font is the term given to a particular typeface in a particular size of print. Commonly, a font such as '*italics*' is readily available in addition to a basic style. Italics is particularly useful for reporting quoted subject material. By incorporating both italics and indenting, verbal quotes from subjects can be efficiently identified from the main text. For example:

> '*We think new technology offers the researcher a great number of useful and easy to use means of improving the clarity and quality of data presentation.*'

Unfortunately, new techniques can be seductive and there is a danger that they will be overused. The net result is that instead of enhancing clarity, the effect is one of confusion resulting in poor data presentation. A good guide is to try and keep the number of techniques you use in any one table, text, or figure to a minimum. Use highlighting techniques to help get your message across, not just as a means of showing that you have the facility available.

PRESENTING DATA AS TEXT, NUMBERS, GRAPHS, AND PICTURES

Text

The written word is a useful and powerful means of getting views and results across, and is particularly efficient when an individual is attempting to describe a situation or event that is charged with emotion. It also has the potential ability to convey large amounts of data in considerable detail in a relatively compact form. There are times, however, when such an approach is less than ideal. For example, when reporting the results of a survey, it is common to see material presented in the following form: 'A total of 257 questionnaires were distributed of which 203 were returned. Of these, 87, 47, 39 and 30 were received from the Acute, Mental Health, Mental Handicap and Community Services units respectively.' Data presented in this form, despite being accurate and factual, are unattractive from the visual and literary viewpoint. More worrying is the point that such a presentation lacks clarity, for it requires considerable concentration and re-reading to ensure that the correct numbers are associated with the correct unit. Furthermore, the use of text to present numerical data gives the reader little visual

Table 30.2   Skill mix of nursing staff, by grade, in medical unit.

Grade	Numbers of staff (n = 47)	% of staff in each grade
G	3	6
F	6	13
E	16	34
D	6	13
C	4	8
A	12	26
Totals	47	100

All percentages are rounded.

assistance in relation to identifying trends or differences between groups.

It is not always possible to present data in descriptive format; equally, it might be extremely difficult to do so. Consider how difficult it would be to describe the layout of your ward or office compared to the relative ease of drawing a plan.

Numbers, graphs and pictures

By using numbers, graphs, and pictures as an alternate form of data presentation, you can take advantage of the reader's ability to interpret more visually stimulating material. How often have you flicked through a journal stopping momentarily to examine an article which catches your eye, usually as the result of an interesting heading, graph, picture, or table.

Visually dynamic data can not only attract an audience but also can be an efficient method of summarizing large quantities of information in such a way as to illuminate underlying trends. It is not always the case that the researcher takes an either/or decision and quite often will use both textual and graphical data presentation. The use of the two approaches can help clarify the data and also emphasize its importance.

Tabular data presentation

Certain types of data do not lend themselves to textual presentation. Survey data often requires the researcher to summarize findings in tabular form. For example, the skill mix of staff working in a hospital can be effectively and clearly displayed by use of a table (Table 30.2).

Presenting data in tabular form is perhaps one of the most common means of summarizing large quantities of numeric data. Despite the popularity of this approach, it is common for writers to produce tables which are poorly laid out and confusing to the reader. Common mistakes are: inadequately descriptive titles, misaligned columns, use of abbreviations or units within data columns, omission of totals, totals that do not add up correctly, and omission of the number of respondents upon which the data are based, detracting from the quality and clarity of the presentation.

With the aid of new technology, many of these mistakes can be avoided and many of the basic problems of layout can be dealt with automatically. For example, the Statistical Package for the Social Sciences (SPSS) is now available on microcomputer and can present data in tables for you in an adequate and accurate manner, avoiding all the above noted flaws.

Tables are extremely useful and relatively easy to construct but care is needed not to overload them with information. Always remember that the primary objective is to ensure that your reader gets the correct, accurate, and clear information intended. It is far better to use two or more tables that are effective than one that leads to confusion.

Graphic presentation formats

There are several different ways of presenting data in a graphic form. In the past, it has been necessary for writers who wish to present their data graphically to draw their figures by hand and then to physically 'stick' them into their report at the appropriate point. Thankfully for those with access to new technology, all these steps can be automated. Data can be exported from statistical analysis packages into graphics packages and then electronically 'pasted' into the final report.

There are many programs available which will enable you to perform such activity. The specific program you may decide to use will be a personal choice which will inevitably be constrained by the type of computer you have access to and the amount of money you have to spend on the software. In view of the cost of some of these packages, it is recommended that you should attempt to negotiate access to such facilities through your employer. Most health authorities or boards will have these resources and people skilled in their use who can advise you. Generally, the types of package that can be particularly useful when presenting data are integrated software packages. These packages incorporate word processors, spread sheets, data bases, and graphics. In addition, desk top publishing systems that enable you to paste together the output from other programs such as stand-alone word processing, statistical analysis, or graphics packages, are also available.

For those who are less fortunate, and cannot gain access to new technology, do not despair: all the graphical presentation formats that follow can be produced by hand. The end product can be just as effective although it does take a little longer.

There are several types of graphs that can be used for data presentation. Examples of graphs that can be used include those of line, bar, and stacked. Furthermore, it is possible to use either two or three dimensions when plotting data, thus further adding to the repertoire of options available.

Whichever option is selected to present data, it is important that the scales on both axes are chosen appropriately. In most cases it is usual, as in Fig. 30.3, to plot the independent variable, in this case, 'months' along the 'X' (horizontal) axis, and the dependent variable, here, 'shifts lost due to sickness' along the 'Y' (vertical) axis. The scale for the dependent variable is extremely important since the scale can over- or underemphasize any trends present. A small gradual increase in sickness rates can be made to look extremely dramatic if the scale is so sensitive that a single day's sickness is represented by a visually dramatic rise. Great care and common sense is obviously required when selecting scales.

With the advent of new technology, some graphics packages will automatically scale the data for you and will attempt to emphasize differences and trends –

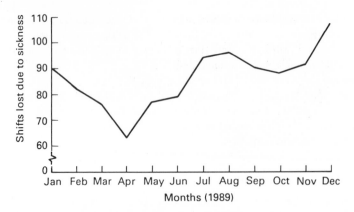

Fig. 30.3 Shift lost due to sickness during 1989.

trends are the tendency for a set of observations to increase, decrease or remain static in relation to time or some other variable. If differences or trends are over emphasized then under such conditions it may be necessary to over-ride the automatic scaling. The omission of the source of the data is also a frequent error and prevents the interested reader from checking your data.

Certain issues are specific to the construction of the various types of graph and these are dealt with in the following paragraphs.

Line graphs

Line graphs are particularly useful for displaying changes and are ideal for showing recurring patterns over time; it is important, however, to ensure that the time intervals along the horizontal axis are equal. A common error seen in graphical data presented in line graph format is the omission of any discontinuities in the scale. That is, if the first scale point is '60' then the discontinuity between '0' and '60' should be indicated, as in Fig. 30.3 (⌇).

There is no real limit as to the number of points that can be shown on a line graph; indeed, the greater the number, the more accurate any interpretation between points. However, for clarity, it is advisable to limit the number of lines (variables displayed) on any one graph to five or six, particularly if the lines frequently cross.

Bar graphs

This type of graph is one of the most commonly used in the presentation of data. The bar graph is particularly useful if you are trying to convey the concept of 'leader' or there are pre-set targets, since such an approach clearly demonstrates those who are meeting the goals and those who are not (see Fig. 30.4).

Unlike line graphs, it is unusual to have dicontinuities in the 'Y' axis since it is then necessary to show the discontinuity in each of the bars.

When drawing a bar chart, it is extremely important to keep the widths of the bars constant since it is in fact the area of the bar which conveys the information.

Bar charts are often 'stacked' when the most important feature is to convey the total magnitude of the dependent variable being measured. However, there may be some interest in the breakdown of the component parts of the variable and it is then that the total magnitude can be shown as the sum of a number of elemental

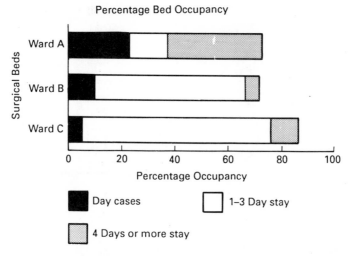

Percentage Bed Occupancy

Fig. 30.4   Surgical unit bed occupancy for April 1990.

parts (see Fig. 30.4). In such a case, it is necessary to illustrate the meaning of the
elements by the inclusion of a legend.

Pie charts

Pie charts, as the name suggests, are circular in format. The overall circular
structure is divided into segments which proportionally represent, by area, the
data to be presented. Many computer packages will generate the pie chart
automatically, but if such a facility is unavailable, a pair of compasses, for drawing
the circle, and a protractor for dividing the circle into proportions determined by
the data to be displayed, are required.

As an example, the data previously presented in Table 30.2 is displayed in the
form of a pie chart in Fig. 30.5. The entire 'pie' represents 100% of the data (47
members of staff). Since it is necessary to rotate compasses through an angle of
360° to fully describe the circumference of a circle, 1% of the data is represented
by a segment with 360/100° at the centre. Therefore every 1% of the data is
multiplied by 3.6° to enable the segment to proportionally represent the
percentage fraction of the data.

When using pie charts to display results, it is important to consider the visual
impact. If there are too many divisions, the pie chart will become cluttered and
small segments will be difficult to interpret. With these points in mind, it is best to
limit the number of segments to less than ten, and also ensuring that no one
segment represents less than 5% of the data.

Since the pie chart is designed to enable data to be presented in percentage
form, it is common to note that some researchers neglect to state the total number
of subjects upon which the data are based.

Pie charts can be labelled in several ways. First, it is possible to label each
segment within the circumference, that is, to superimpose the labelling upon the
specific segments if both the segments and the pie chart are big enough. Second,
it is common to see labelling to be attached to, or placed just outside, the
circumference of the circle. Third, it is possible to use different types of shading

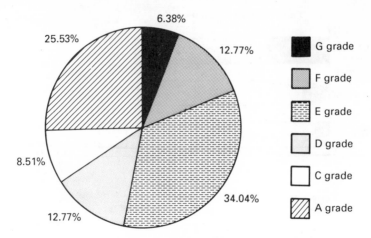

Fig. 30.5 Skill mix of 47 nursing staff by grade, in medical ward.

and then use a suitable legend to define the various areas. Figure 30.5 uses two of these techniques: percentages are placed outside and adjacent to the various segments, but a legend also is used to define the meaning of the shades used.

Sociogram

Sociograms are particularly useful in the display of interactions between a number of individuals. Not only can they visually represent who talks to whom but also they can be used to analyse the types and quantity of each member's contribution over a certain time period.

From the sociogram (Fig. 30.6), it is possible to identify those individuals who dominated group conversation (subject 'L'), those who did not contribute (subject 'H'), and those who form a sub-group (subjects 'E' and 'F').

Problems can arise if researchers use too long a sampling time period, causing the sociogram to become cluttered and extremely difficult to interpret. Similarly, if the technique is being used by an observer to record the interactions of a very vocal group, it can be extremely challenging to ensure that all conversations occurring are noted.

Organizational chart

The purpose of an organizational chart is to demonstrate the (usually formal) managerial relationships and lines of responsibility between individuals or positions in various parts of an organization. Traditionally, health service provision is managed by means of a hierarchical management structure. Figure 30.7 illustrates the use of the organizational chart as a means of succinctly representing the formal lines of communication within a functional unit of a health authority.

Although these charts are frequently used to illustrate lines of communication, it is important to note that these are the 'official' or 'formally' recognized paths. In many cases these will not be the actual paths along which information flows and this can cause problems and mislead naive researchers who take things at face value.

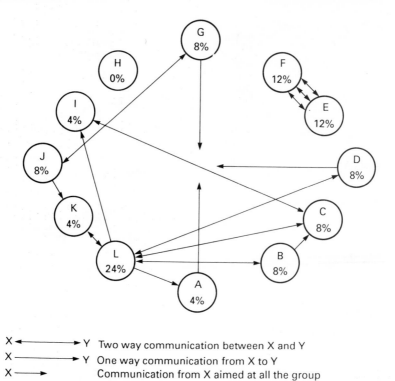

X ◄──────► Y   Two way communication between X and Y
X ──────► Y   One way communication from X to Y
X ──────►   Communication from X aimed at all the group

Fig. 30.6 Number and percentage of interactions between group members over a half-hour period.

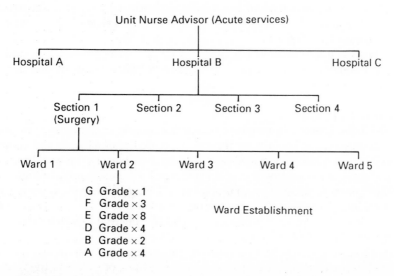

Fig. 30.7 Formal lines of communication in acute unit.

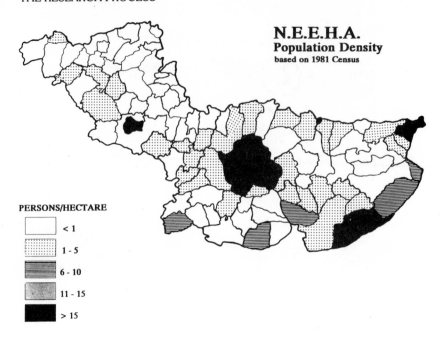

Fig. 30.8 Population density for North East Essex Health Authority District based on 1981 census data. (Reproduced with permission from the North East Essex Health Authority.)

Geographic mapping

This technique is frequently used when a researcher wishes to show the distribution of a variable in relation to a geographic area (Laborde *et al.* 1989). A geograhic area can be an entire country, a county, or even a postal code zone. Figure 30.8 shows the population density of a health authority area, and as can be seen from the legend, increasing population density is represented by increasing darkness of shading.

Such a mapping as in Fig. 30.8 can be produced by hand but with new technology it is possible to translate data directly from data files into this format by means of a suitable software package.

Flow charts

Originally, flow charts were used by systems analysts as a means of interpreting and representing the actions required to guide the development of computer software production. However, many researchers have recognized the utility of this approach in succinctly conveying to readers the relationship and sequential direction of ideas, concepts, or propositions. Although it has a use which is, strictly speaking, often different from actual presentation of data, it remains a very useful and powerful tool for the researcher. The flow chart in Fig. 30.9 presents the phases of the nursing process.

Flow charts should have definite start and end points which are clearly defined, enabling readers to understand how the sequence of events is triggered and completed. The layout of flow charts is also extremely important if clarity of

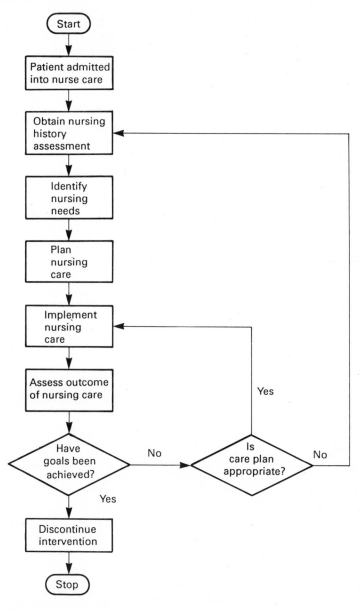

Fig. 30.9 Flow chart of nursing process application.

information flow is to be ensured. The best and most easily understood charts should read from top to bottom, with feedback loops going in the reverse direction. Specific activities or processes should be included in rectangular boxes and decision points in diamond shapes.

Common errors seen in the production of flow charts include: the omission of decision conditions, that is, the requirements that have to be met before the particular path is followed; the omission of arrows to guide the reader through the chart; and the crossover of feedback paths over preceding sections of the chart.

Photographs

Both black and white and colour prints can be used as a means of presenting data which would be extremely difficult to show by other means. For example, photographs are an ideal medium to demonstrate pictorially 'before and after' views of some treatment such as the effects on posture of an intensive exercise programme on a child with multiple physical handicap.

Although the cost of producing the original photograph may be relatively inexpensive, the researcher, if planning to publish the material, should note that not all journals will accept photographic plates; equally, they may require a special size or type of negative. It is therefore essential if you are considering submitting work for publication that you should inquire about such points at an early stage.

One positive point to bear in mind is the fact that most health authorities will have a small medical illustrations department who may be quite willing to help with the production of photographic prints. These departments are usually both small and over-worked so it is important to give sufficient warning if you require assistance.

The reproduction of monochrome or colour prints can be achieved by means of suitable photocopying machines but, although colour is perhaps more striking, it is also far more expensive. You therefore should assess the benefits versus the costs of using colour.

Blueprints – scale drawings

Blueprints or scale drawings are used to portray the size, contents, position, and spatial relationships of an item or area such as a hospital, ward, or room. Figure 30.10 is an example of such a blueprint.

If the blueprint requires to be drawn to scale, each of its parts must be carefully calculated, measured, and drawn. While a scale drawing may be essential in some instances, it may not always be needed. The reader, however, must be informed

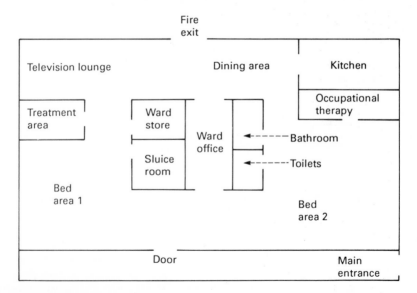

Fig. 30.10   Blueprint of ward 1 layout (not to scale).

whether it is or is not a scale drawing.

Only items which are necessary should be included in the blue-print. If the major point of the presentation is to indicate the position of each of the rooms in the ward, it would obviously be inappropriate to include individual beds, wash-hand basins, and windows.

Scatter diagram

Before the development and ready availability of computers, researchers who wished to examine data for correlations used the initial technique of plotting a scatter diagram. By plotting the value of the independent variable against the dependent variable, it is possible to visually determine whether there is likely to be a statistically significant correlation between the two variables. The decision can then be taken as to whether a statistical calculation should be performed.

Examination of the overall shape of the data distribution pattern can reveal such information as positive, negative, or no correlation between the variables. The closer the data pattern resembles a straight line, the greater the degree of correlation between the variables. It is common practice to encompass the data points so as to highlight the overall data pattern (Fig. 30.11).

Due to the increased availability of computers and statistical analysis packages, there is now less need to use scatter diagrams, but they are nevertheless a useful way of demonstrating to an audience who have limited understanding of statistical techniques the correlation between two variables under examination.

Contour plots

Perhaps the most readily recognized contour plot in the United Kingdom, is that of the air pressure over the British Isles displayed by the weather forecasting service on television. In the plot, points of equal air pressure are connected, thus displaying a series of contour lines.

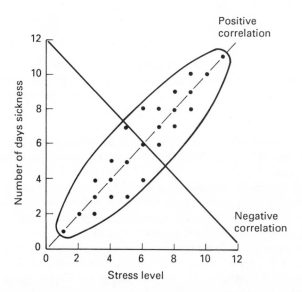

Fig. 30.11 Correlation between stress and days lost due to sickness.

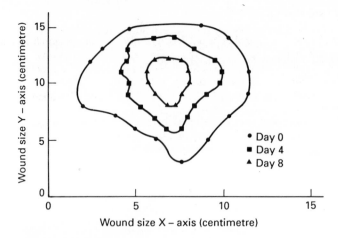

Fig. 30.12   Contour plot of outline of granulating wound.

Contour plots are frequently used in diagnostic medical physics departments where the emissions of radioactive isotopes are recorded as a means of identifying, for example, vascular lesions. However, researchers can put the technique to use for far less technology-based applications. For example, if you are interested in the effect of a new treatment on the granulation of a *decubitus ulcer*, it might be useful to plot the outline of the wound at specified time intervals. It then would be possible to calculate the rate of wound granulation for that patient. The technique would provide an objective accurate visual record, overtime, of the healing process. Figure 30.12 illustrates the technique.

CONCLUSIONS

Many techniques are available for the presentation of data and if results are to have optimum impact, great care must be taken to ensure that an appropriate method is selected. Unless results are presented in a clear and visually dynamic format, readers may have difficulty in interpreting findings, or worse still they may not be read.

New technology offers a wide variety of aids which can enhance the standard of data presentation and reduce the time taken to prepare material. Nevertheless, remember that the purpose of the presentation will affect many of the choices you make in deciding the most appropriate format. Do not use inappropriate approaches just because they happen to be readily available to you.

Finally, throughout this chapter, specific specialized methods of data presentation have been illustrated but, perhaps more importantly, a number of general points have been emphasized. These points can be easily remembered by use of the acronym VACUME. That is, is the format **V**isually stimulating? Are the results **A**ccurate, **C**learly **U**nderstandable and **M**eaningful? Is the format chosen the most **E**fficient means of getting the message across? If the answer to all these question is 'Yes' then it is likely that you have made the correct choices.

REFERENCES

Horsley J.A., Crane J., Crabtree M.K. & Wood D.J. (1983) *Using Research To Improve Nursing Practice: A Guide CURN Project.* Grune & Stratton, Orlando.

Laborde J.M., Dando W.A. & Hemmasi M. (1989) Computer Graphics a tool for decision making in nursing. *Computers in Nursing.* **7**: 1, 15–20.

Phillips L.R.F. (1986) *A Clinician's Guide to the Critique and Utilization of Nursing Research.* Appleton-Century-Crofts, Norwalk.

Powell D. (1989) How to get your message across with maximum effect. *Business Graphics Review.* **1**: 1, 8, 10–11; 13.

Chapter 31
Reporting and Disseminating Research
Alison J. Tierney

The research process is not complete until a written report of the study which has been undertaken is prepared and disseminated. Through the activities of reporting and dissemination, the 'doer' of the research communicates with the potential 'users' and, of course, without this there is little point in having done the research in the first place.

This chapter looks at what is involved in writing a research report, preparing research papers for publication, and, more generally, at research dissemination. The guidance given should be particularly useful for nurses who are embarking on research for the first time. But, equally, the chapter may be helpful for others who are not doing research but who simply wish to learn about the research process. An understanding of how research reports and papers are structured helps one to read this kind of literature and, importantly, to evaluate it critically.

WRITING A RESEARCH REPORT

Preparing a research report on completion of a study is a researcher's responsibility even when there is no obligation to do so. Often there is this obligation. If the study has been supported financially, it is usual for the funding body to make the submission of a written research report one of the conditions of the grant contract. Many nursing research studies are not grant-supported but are carried out in an educational context. In such circumstances the requirement would be in the form of a dissertation or thesis. Even if there is no formal requirement to produce a written report – for example, in the case of a small, unfunded study carried out in the context of a nurse's work – there is still the need for some form of research report. This need applies to small-scale studies as much as to large-scale research, and to studies which produce inconclusive findings as well as research which generates new insights and knowledge. It is from the written research report that others can be made aware of the work, be able to critically appraise its relevance, and, as appropriate, make use of its findings.

The format of a research report

Obviously, depending on the nature of the study and the circumstances, there are variations in the way research reports are written and in their length. A pilot study or small-scale project report may be quite short, containing only brief details of the background and method and with main findings succinctly presented. In contrast, a complex large-scale study is likely to merit a full report in order to provide a comprehensive account and discussion of all steps of the research process. If the research is being written up in the form of a thesis to be presented for a higher degree, there are specific requirements laid down by the educational establishment concerned which govern the format and length of the report. In other cases, it may be that the grant-giving body specifies how the report is to be presented and in what amount of detail.

Although the style and length of presentation may vary, there is, in all cases, a basic format for a research report. This format is simply a logical reflection of the research process and, following the sequence of the steps, the report is usually structured into the following sections:

(1) Introduction;
(2) Literature review;
(3) Method;
(4) Findings;
(5) Discussion;
(6) Conclusions and recommendations.

Some basic comment is made below on each of these sections in turn. First, it may be helpful to suggest that much of the ground-work for the final report can be done long before the study itself is completed. As each stage of the research is completed, notes for the relevant section of the report can be made and even some first draft writing up attempted, for example, in the case of the literature review and method sections. By doing this, time will be saved (not to mention panic!) when work on the final report has to be got down to in earnest; the danger of forgetting details or mislaying vital information will be avoided; and, perhaps most important of all for the newcomer to this exercise, some valuable practice at writing will have been obtained.

Introduction

The very beginning of a research report needs to be especially clear and engaging if the reader is to be persuaded to venture further. First of all, there should be a clear statement of what the research was all about. It has been emphasized earlier in the book that the business of identifying and formulating the research problem/ question is a vital, but difficult, first stage of the research process (see Chapter 8). Assuming the task was accomplished properly, then it will not be difficult to provide a clear statement of the research task in the introduction to the report.

It is also interesting, and often helpful, to outline the thinking which was involved in translating the original idea into the researchable question or hypothesis which the study was designed to explore, answer, or test. It is useful, too, if the boundaries of the research are explained; in other words, what was not being studied as well as what was included. In explaining the focus and scope of the study, some background is often both interesting and informative; for example, the reader might be told what prompted the researcher's interest in the study, particularly if its origins lay in direct practice experiences or problems.

After reading the introductory section of the report, the reader should be clear about the precise nature of the research being reported and know something about its background and context.

Literature review

The task of 'searching the literature' has already been described and, in the final report, an account of this early step in the research process is given (see Chapter 9). This is not simply a case of listing a string of references which were found and looked up; nor is it an endless discourse on the literature. The aim is to present a distilled and critical *analysis* of the relevant literature, showing how the study being reported was based on previous research and existing knowledge, and how the new work was intended to take that forward. This is no easy task, even for experienced researchers. If a decent job is made of it, however, the reader will benefit from the literature review in its own right as well as being able to judge the extent to which the present study was properly grounded. The reader is, of course, entitled to be informed about all relevant literature and all perspectives on the subject. This includes references to theories and studies which conflict with, as well as support, the perspective and approach adopted in the research.

Writing the literature review section of the report will be made easier if, as suggested earlier, some work has been done towards this already. Even if a draft was not prepared, it will be helpful if the outline is ready. A literature review of any length needs to be divided into sections, each covering an area of the literature. It is, of course, imperative that references have been documented in full, and helpful if summaries and/or copies of material consulted were filed away carefully. At the stage of writing up, there will be little time available to waste on hunting for lost references, checking incomplete ones, or, even worse, scouring the library for that crucial chapter in the book by Anderson (. . . or was it Henderson? . . .), the one with the purple cover! Organization and diligence at the time of the original review of the literature will pay off when the final report has to be written up. All that remains to be done is a last check on more recently published work, noting any important new research which impinges on the present study.

Method

Information about how the study was planned and conducted is a vital part of a research report. Without this, the reader cannot judge the validity of the findings and conclusions presented by the researcher. Details of method are certainly needed for anyone who might wish to replicate the study.

A re-cap of the research problem/question(s) and a statement of the aims of the study should be given at the start of the method section. Thereafter, how this section is structured and presented needs to take account of the nature of the study and the method(s) employed. It may be, for example, that use of qualitative research approaches to investigate a question hitherto only tackled by standard quantitative methods will need not only to be explained, but defended as well.

With a more conventional research design, description of the method is usually written up under a series of fairly standard sub-headings. After the *research questions or hypothesis* have been stated, the *study setting* is described and then *the sample*; this in terms of size, mode of selection, assignment to groups (if relevant), and consent procedure adopted. Any *intervention* must be detailed and *data collection methods and instruments* described, including any piloting and reliability testing undertaken. (Copies of instruments can be put in an Appendix to the report or offered as available on request to the researcher.) Finally, methods of *data analysis* require to be reported.

Most of this information will be in written form already, in the research proposal.

The proposal, however, will have been written in the future tense in terms of intentions, whereas, in the final report, the account is given in the past tense and is a description of how the study was carried out. Any significant changes, made in the event, should be explained, as should any major difficulties which were confronted. This information is important since it might suggest changes needed should the study be replicated.

Findings

Unless described in the method section (under 'sample'), the characteristics of the sample are presented at the beginning of 'findings'. Specific characteristics such as age and sex, socio-economic status, and health history, along with a description of the sample as a whole, provide background to the findings and their relevance. Response rates, for example, to a questionnaire, are also reported at this stage.

Beyond that, how findings are presented really depends on their nature and the type of analysis undertaken. But, in all cases, this section of the report needs to be well organized so that the reader is taken through what was found in relation to the questions which the study set out to explore or answer.

In a qualitative study, findings are usually presented in terms of themes which emerged from the data and, by way of substantiation and illustration, examples of raw data will be given (e.g. direct quotes from an interview transcription, or accounts of observation). In contrast, quantitative analysis produces findings of a numerical type and much of the presentation will be in the form of tables. Each table must be numbered, given a legend, and referenced in the text with explanation of statistical tests employed. The reader should not be expected to work out what all these tables show and what relationships were found. Such explanation is the responsibility of the researcher, as is comment on any inconclusive or contradictory findings or on results which were incidental (but interesting) or different from those which could have been reasonably expected.

Discussion

While some discussion may have been entered into in the course of presenting the various findings, the final discussion should provide a broader and deeper interpretation of the results of the study. This section of the report can be thought of as attempting to answer the question 'So what?'. The aim is to draw together the findings of the study and to discuss these in the light of what the research was set up to do and in the context of previous research and the current state of knowledge of the subject.

For the reader, the results of this task should be illuminating and so should it be for the researcher. Preparing the discussion involves more thinking than any other part of the research process except perhaps the very beginning stage of teasing out the research idea in the first place. What is being sought here is an explanation of the *meaning* of the research findings – their inherent limitations as well as their value.

Conclusions and recommendations

From the discussion, the conclusions should follow fairly obviously and these require to be stated clearly and succinctly. On the basis of the conclusions, recommendations can be made as to how the findings of the study might be picked up in practice, education, management, and future research. By doing this, the researcher will stimulate and assist the reader to consider the relevance of the recommendations in relation to their own circumstances as well as appreciating the more general relevance of the study to nursing knowledge. This, after all, is the point of research in nursing.

PUBLISHING RESEARCH

In the course of describing how a research report is written, numerous references were made to 'the reader' because, obviously, the only reason for producing a written research report is for others to read it. As such, however, research reports seldom have a wide readership. Reports in the form of a thesis or dissertation will be stored in a university or college library and borrowed only by students and the occasional outsider who finds out about the work and has a particular interest in it. Research reports submitted to a grant-giving body or steering committee, or close colleagues, will be scrutinized with interest by those groups but are unlikely to be disseminated more widely. Thus, for the most part, written research reports are not made widely accessible and, indeed, may be too detailed in that form for the needs of a wider readership. If the researcher is to make the work known more widely and easily available, then the research needs to be published.

There are many reasons why publication of research is especially important in the case of nursing. Research is a relatively recent development in nursing and much of the work is in the form of small-scale, one-off studies. Further research will be all the more useful if it builds on studies previously undertaken and, for this to be done, there needs to be access to earlier work in published form. It is not only intending researchers who need access to this material. Students and teachers need it too if research is to be incorporated into nurse education. And, clearly, for nursing practice to be developed and changed on the basis of research, then those members of the profession who are in a position to bring this about – the practitioners and the managers – must also be kept informed through publication of the findings of recent research. The potential readership of nursing research is both large and varied and not confined only to members of the nursing profession.

Preparing research for publication

A number of decisions must be taken before any actual work begins on the preparation of research material for publication. The researcher has to decide *what* would be most useful to have published; *how many* publications are merited; *who* each of these is intended for; *where* publication would be most suitable in order to reach the targeted readership; and the *form* of presentation which would be most appropriate.

If it seems that the written research report merits publication more or less in full, then length dictates that this will be in the form of a book or monograph. Few publishers will be interested in a research publication of this type unless it is of sufficiently wide interest to be commercially viable. It has been invaluable, therefore, for British nursing to have had a publishing outlet for monographs (The Nursing Research Series), initially through the Royal College of Nursing, and more recently its publishing house (Scutari Press).

Publishing research material in the form of journal articles is much more common and, indeed, has a number of advantages over publication in book form.

An article is usually in print much more quickly than a book, an important consideration when the subject is research. Journal articles are also much more likely to be read by many more nurses than a research monograph and, depending upon the journal selected, an article can be targeted at a particular section of the profession. Journal articles differ from monographs in two main respects; they are shorter, and they are selective in the aspects of the research reported.

What the researcher should not do is write an article and then look around for a journal willing to publish it. This sounds rather obvious but it is something that is often done by first-time researchers. As has been pointed out above, before putting pen to paper, there are various decisions to be made. From the outset, it must be clear *what* is to be covered in the article. If it is considered that general rather than detailed information about the study would be most useful, the article could take the form of a resumé of the total research study (really an abridged form of the written research report). In another case it might be the findings of the study which merit concentration, particularly if these appear to be potentially influential on nursing practice. Alternatively, the focus of an article might be the research method employed, or perhaps even more specifically, the particular data collection instruments used or developed in the study. Or it may be that the most useful type of publication is the literature review undertaken. Usually there is sufficient material of interest and importance in any one research study to merit several articles rather than just one.

Once the topic for the article is clarified, it is important to turn attention to another issue; *who* the publication is intended for. Being clear about this is vitally important. Every journal has a quite distinct readership and so identifying the intended readership is essentially synonymous with selecting the right journal. If the article being planned is aimed at a large and varied readership, then the researcher should seek publication in a nursing journal which has a large circulation among nurses representing various levels and branches of the profession – *Nursing Times* would be the likely choice in this case. If the article is of special relevance to nursing practice, a journal which caters especially for practising nurses may be most suitable: *Nursing*, the *Journal of Gerontological Nursing*, or *Cancer Nursing*, to mention some examples. However, if the research is concerned with an aspect of nursing education, and the article planned is aimed at nurse educators, then *Nurse Education Today* would be a suitable choice. If the article is to be longer, and intended for readers with knowledge of research methods, the *Journal of Advanced Nursing* might be selected. For an article of interest to an international readership, the researcher might seek publication in the *International Journal of Nursing Studies*. The journals named above are simply mentioned to illustrate the point that selection of the journal is dependent on having clearly identified the targeted readership. In some cases, the researcher may consider it appropriate to seek publication in a non-nursing journal if the research has particular relevance for other health care professions or academic disciplines. If the choice of journal does not immediately seem obvious, then a helpful step is to spend time in a library which is well-stocked with a wide range of current periodicals. Browsing through many different journals, even quite quickly, is a good way of getting to know their various readerships and assessing likely interest in the research material you have available.

The decision about which journal to write for to a great extent pre-determines the length, format, and style of the article. Careful scrutiny of back issues of the selected journal will provide a good idea of how the article should be presented. Most journals have quite specific guidelines concerning length, format, and style of presentation, including illustrations and references. If the journal does not carry notice of these, the editor will provide guidelines for authors on request. It may also be a good idea to send an outline of the proposed article to the editor in order to obtain an indication of whether or not there is likely to be interest in the material. In most, if not all instances, editors insist that prospective authors submit a particular article to only one journal at a time.

With all this planning accomplished, there is only one job left to do – to sit down and write the article for publication!

WRITING FOR PUBLICATION

The actual prospect of writing for publication often seems daunting to those with no experience and a self-consciousness about writing. Nurses seem particularly prone to thinking that writing for publication is something which only the exceptionally talented can accomplish! Writing well is, of course, a very skilled activity and there is no simple formula to follow. There is no quick and easy way to write and it is perhaps reassuring for the rest of us to realize that people who do have a flair for self-expression and a good command of language and grammar are the exception rather than the rule. Mostly, writing is a slow, laborious and often frustrating business but, when done, it gives a great sense of satisfaction and accomplishment.

The key is to allow plenty of time for writing (and, even more important, for *rewriting*), and not to become discouraged by the slow progress or the seemingly disproportionate number of drafts consigned to the wastepaper basket! Some of the hints about writing for publication which are given below may be helpful. These, of course, are equally pertinent to the business of writing a research report. In that case, however, the readership is likely to be more limited and probably less critical of presentation than readers of published material.

Planning the writing

The drafting of an article for publication becomes instantly easier if sufficient time is spent on planning it out. This involves making an outline, which consists of headings and sub-headings, with brief notes of the main points to be included under each. This exercise helps to organize ideas and material logically and into a sequence. It also divides the writing task into manageable portions, so making it all less daunting. Most journals restrict the length of particular kinds of articles so, bearing this in mind, each section can be allocated an approximate number of words so that, from the start, there is a clear sense of how much detail can be afforded.

Early drafting

Once a satisfactory outline has emerged, and thought given to the content, a first draft of the article can be attempted. It may be helpful to start at the beginning but it is often encouraging to work first on the parts which seem the easiest to write. Knowing how important it is for the introduction to be clear and engaging, starting here can often result in your getting quickly bogged down in pursuit of inspiration and perfection. Better just to get writing. The putting together of all the sections of the article, each linking logically with the next, is a job which can be done later.

Once an initial draft is done, the next step is to re-read it carefully and review it critically and objectively. Revision and rearrangement are usually needed. If you are using a word processor, this is a relatively easy and rather enjoyable job. If working with pen and paper, the same process of rearrangement can be done by 'cutting and pasting' with revisions marked up alongside.

The goal at this stage is to produce a paper which is organized in a sensible way, which deals with the points to be covered in the various sections, and which, overall and in its parts, is balanced and approximately of the right length.

Final touches

However tedious, a final stage of work still remains. This involves one last, but detailed, check of the finished research paper. What is being looked for now is that each sentence conveys what was intended; every detail is correct (check especially the accuracy of data, quotations, references, and cross-references); language and grammar are as good as possible; spelling and punctuation are correct; and that the style is readable, even if not remarkable. Improving and refining writing takes a lifetime of practice, but many of the features of poor writing can be avoided if adequate time and concentration are invested on this final stage of the process.

A frequent criticism of research publications is that they are too full of technical language and jargon. Avoiding unnecessary technical terms greatly extends the readership but, if such terms need to be used, their meaning should be explained. Nursing, like other disciplines, runs the risk of becoming jargon-laden. The goal should be concise and natural language, and this is especially important if nursing research is to be read and appreciated by all members of the profession.

Preparing tables, references, appendices

A research report or article normally involves a combination of text and visual forms of presentation of material. Tables, graphs and charts can be valuable for presenting complex information in a concise and ordered way. But, if poorly presented or too complicated, they can confuse the reader. Each table must be numbered, accompanied by an explicit legend, and placed in the report or article following the reference to it. Any necessary explanation of the table or figure should be provided in the text (see Chapter 30 for a full discussion of data presentation).

It is essential for one standard style of referencing to be used consistently throughout the report or article; in this book, the Harvard system is adopted. This particular style involves reference to the surname of the author(s) and year of publication in the text, with the full reference provided in the reference list at the end, ordered alphabetically by authors' surnames. Details of references should be checked and double checked.

A written research report (although not usually a journal paper) is likely to contain appendices for the inclusion of material which is too lengthy or too detailed to include in the body of the report – for example, a copy of a questionnaire used. Appendices are placed at the end of the report and referred to at the appropriate point in the text.

Appendices, tables, and figures, and a list of contents, should be contained in the 'prelims' at the front of the report. The full range of the items which may precede the text of the report, are:

(1) Title page;
(2) Contents page;
(3) List of tables and figures;
(4) Preface (if the report is published in book form);
(5) Acknowledgements;
(6) Abstract.

In a research paper intended for publication in a journal, any acknowledgements would normally be inserted at the end. The inclusion of an abstract (at the beginning) is usually a requirement.

Preparing an abstract

An abstract (a concise summary) is a useful feature of a reserch report or article; it is usually a requirement in a thesis. It is also possible to have an abstract of a research report published in its own right. Abstracts of nursing studies are printed, for example, in *Nursing Research Abstracts* published by the Department of Health in London (see Chapter 9 for further details).

Titling the report or article

Although the title is the first thing a reader looks at, it is very often the last thing the author of a research report or article attends to. It is extremely important for a research publication to have a meaningful and unambiguous title. Nurse authors (and, dare it be said, editors of some nursing journals) sometimes show a preference for titles which are intriguing and anecdotal, but which are not always informative and are sometimes downright misleading.

It is the title which clarifies the topic of the research being described and gives the potential reader an indication of the content and scope of the report or article. More importantly, the title is reproduced in references, bibliographies, indexes, and abstracts. As literature retrieval through on-line computer systems uses 'key words', it is vital for the title to contain the most relevant words. Nurse researchers should not be tempted to dream up clever but totally useless titles for their reports and publications – these can be reserved for that bestselling novel, yet to be written!

Preparing the report or article for typing

Little needs to be said about this here, except to point out that a research report or article must be produced in typed form. This requires adequate time allowance for the task. The typist must be given full details of any particular typing requirements laid down by the educational establishment (in the case of a thesis), publisher, or journal in question. Most experienced typists can interpret these requirements more successfully than can the amateur. Although typing the manuscript oneself may seem easier and cheaper, the services of a proficient professional are not to be underrated.

Only one job – careful proofreading – remains to be done before the hard work is over and the report or article is at last ready to be submitted.

DISSEMINATING RESEARCH

The completion of a written report and the preparation of articles for publication are really only the starting point of research dissemination and not, as is sometimes assumed, the complete job. Making available the information in written form cannot automatically ensure that the research becomes known about and appreciated, or that the maximum use will be made of its findings. In nursing, there is particular reason for realizing this because those who do the research are seldom in a position within the professional structure to influence its uptake.

If writing about research is only one way of publicizing a study, what else can the nurse researcher do to disseminate the research? One widely used and very useful approach is for the researcher to accept and seek opportunities to talk about the research to members of the nursing profession. Talks can be given at anything from large conferences and international meetings to small-scale study days and in-service education activities. Giving talks is a particularly effective way for the researcher to communicate research findings to others. In particular, talks can be targeted at practising nurses who may well be in the best position to consider the implications of research for nursing practice, at least initially.

For the researcher, a talk is not only a means of information-giving but also of stimulating questioning and discussion. However, preparing and giving talks and engaging in face-to-face discussion is a time-consuming business and there is seldom any allowance of time made for researchers to concentrate solely on this dissemination phase. Increasingly, nurse researchers are making more use of modern audio-visual technology to disseminate research findings in an appealing way to a wider audience.

Whichever novel ways of publicizing research might be tried, the written word is likely to remain *the* communication vehicle. There remains the question of how we can ensure that what is written is read. As is so often the case in nursing, Florence Nightingale's example is worth following. No apology should be necessary for referring to her considerable influence on any aspect of nursing, and certainly not when discussing the subject of writing and publishing a research report. Nurses know so much about her work, and about her as a person, because she wrote and published. Much of her writing was in the form of research reports, and display her passion for statistics. Her writings are distinguished not only by the astuteness of her observation, and her farsightedness, but also by their clarity and eloquence. But Florence Nightingale was only too aware that simply to write, even to publish, was not enough. She expended considerable energy to ensure that her reports were read by those she wanted them to influence. Of course, in this she had the advantages of royal patronage and influence in high places. However, even without these advantages, it is likely that she would have found ways of disseminating her work because of her awareness of the necessity of doing this. A margin note on her draft of the Report of the Sanitary Commission on the Health of the Army (July 1857), noted: 'Reports are not self-executive'.

Although this Nightingale comment has been often quoted, efforts to improve research dissemination in nursing have been neither widespread nor determined. There are signs, however, that researchers and others in the profession are beginning to attach a higher priority to dissemination. This, at least, is a step in the right direction towards ensuring that the best possible use is made of research which has not only been undertaken, but adequately reported.

FURTHER READING

Tornquist E.M. (1986) *From proposal to publication: An informal guide to writing about nursing research.* Addison-Wesley, California.

Watson G. (1987) *Writing a thesis: A guide to long essays and dissertations.* Longman Group, Harlow, Essex.

Part III
The Use of Nursing Research

The main reason for undertaking research is that it is used by nurse practitioners, educators, and managers. The three chapters in the final part of this book are specific to those who make use of nursing research as it applies to nursing practice (see Chapter 32), nursing education (see Chapter 33), and nursing management (see Chapter 34). These chapters also apply to potential researchers in those areas who are considering a possible focus for their own research. Although each of these topics is dealt with individually, it is recognized that considerable overlap and similarity exists.

The ability to make use of completed studies, and to initiate or facilitate new ones, depends on a firm understanding of the research process generally. For this reason, this section, which deals with the use of nursing research, is placed at the end of this text.

Chapter 32
Research in Nursing Practice
Alison J. Tierney

'Applying research findings in nursing practice is perhaps the biggest challenge facing nursing research.' (Sheehan, 1986)

The preceding chapter stressed the importance of effective dissemination of research findings. Dissemination which is targeted at those who are in a position to use research in practice, and in a form which encourages its use, is especially important if research is to make its proper impact on patient care. The *raison d'être* of research in nursing is, after all, to improve the quality of patient care and to increase the effectiveness and efficiency of the nursing service. The mere existence of research cannot in itself alter nursing practice; research has to be *used*.

Using research is a complex task; this is true for all applied disciplines, not just nursing. In nursing, however, we have been slow to appreciate the complexities of 'research utilization'. It tends to have been assumed that use of research in practice would somehow 'just happen' if only researchers reported their findings and practising nurses read their reports.

The apparent lack of research use in nursing practice is discussed in the first part of this chapter. The need to understand the notion of 'research utilization' is then addressed. Finally, the challenge of improving research utilization in nursing practice is explored. This chapter does not provide simple guidelines for the use of research in nursing practice. Rather, it seeks to stimulate readers into thinking more deeply about an issue which tends to have been oversimplified and neglected in nursing research to date.

RESEARCH USE

As the amount of research in nursing has grown, so too has concern about what is seen to be its *apparent* lack of impact on, and use in, practice. In a hard-hitting analysis of current-day clinical nursing, Walsh and Ford (1989) draw attention to numerous examples of regular practice which appear to ignore research evidence. They argue that much of nursing practice remains rooted in myth and traditional ritual, with nurses acting in these ways because 'this is the way it has always been done'. Questions are asked about why, for example, nurses spend time drying out a pressure sore with piped oxygen when research has shown that the best environment for wound-healing is a moist one; about why patients continue to be subjected to unnecessarily long pre-operative fasting times in the face of all the evidence of its adverse effects; about why pre-operative skin preparation has failed to change in the light of all the research; and so on. Perhaps the most catching of their examples is 'the myth of the salt bath'. Walsh and Ford refer to studies which suggest, on the one hand, that there is no evidence to support the notion of the salt bath as therapeutic for infected wounds and, on the other hand, surveys which indicate regular continuation of this practice. While it may not be dangerous, it is at the very least a waste of nurses' time . . . not to mention the good salt!

'Why don't we use the findings?' was the question asked by Hunt (1984) in an article on the issue of lack of use of research in practice. Hunt suggested several reasons. Some of these are what could be regarded as deficiencies in nurses themselves: for example, their lack of knowledge of research and disinclination to 'believe' the findings. Other reasons given reflect deficiencies in the system; for example, the lack of encouragement and incentive for nurses to use research in practice. Greenwood (1984) concurred with this analysis but, in explaining why 'the impact of research findings on the clinical nurse and her work is minimal', he ventured to suggest that:

'Clinical nurses do not perceive research findings as relevant to their practice because frequently they are *not* relevant . . ..' [emphasis added].

It certainly is true that practising nurses have expressed criticism of nursing research as an essentially academic exercise which can seem remote from, and largely irrelevant to, their practice. But, clearly, there are many examples of research which are very obviously relevant to practice but, even then, appear not to be being used. There can be no better example of this than the case of research relating to the prevention and management of pressure sores. Much of that research has very directly relevant implications for practice and yet, as Gould (1986) discussed, the findings are not being applied.

What can be concluded from all of this? Does the problem lie with researchers failing to effectively disseminate research findings? Or is it that practising nurses and nurse managers do not keep up to date with research or, if they do, are simply failing to apreciate its relevance for practice? Or do they possess this knowledge and appreciation but, for whatever reason, find themselves unable to make use of it in practice?

The answer is that we really do not know because there has been so little investigation of research utilization in nursing. The few studies which have been undertaken are, therefore, interesting. In the United States, Ketefian (1975) investigated nurses' use of research findings related to temperature-taking. She chose this topic because it represented a commonplace nursing activity and further, because the research findings had been disseminated widely, and had been available for some time; and, importantly, had been reported with the implications for practice clearly stated. Despite this, Ketefian found that only one of the 87 registered nurses studied knew the correct way to take oral temperature and, indeed, many used this site while believing it to be less accurate than rectal temperature assessment. She concluded that 'the practitioner was either totally unaware of the research literature . . . or, if she was aware of it, was unable to relate to it or utilize it'.

A rather more optimistic picture emerged from a study by Brett (1987). She identified 14 nursing research findings and, from data collected from 216 practising nurses in hospitals of varying size, assessed their awareness of, persuasion about, and use of, the findings. The majority reported awareness of most of the findings and, for seven of the innovations, felt persuaded about use in practice. Actual use of the various findings varied greatly but at least one (relating to closed sterile urinary drainage) was in routine use. Brett concluded that 'at least for the group of nurses and innovations studied and reported here, the findings suggest that research dissemination and use is occurring'.

If little is known about the extent of research utilization in nursing, even less is understood about what effects or inhibits it. An attempt to explore this was made by Champion and Leach (1989) in relation to the variables of (1) support from the work environment, (2) availability of research findings, and (3) nurses' attitudes. From data on self-reported use of research findings in practice from a sample of 59 nurses, both perceived availability of research findings and a positive attitude towards research were strongly related to research utilization. Although only a small-scale study, these findings serve to reinforce the importance of a positive attitude towards research being encouraged in the process of nurse education as well as the need for effective dissemination of research findings to practising nurses.

But even if nurses were to feel positive towards research and be informed about research, the *use* of research in practice would not automatically follow. There is also the need for nurses to understand the nature of research utilization and how to act on this knowledge.

UNDERSTANDING 'RESEARCH UTILIZATION'

Fawcett (1984) has pointed out:

'In the past, many nurses expected all nursing research to have immediate applicability for practice. This expectation probably was based on a misunderstanding of knowledge utilization . . .'

Research rarely produces new knowledge which is instantly usable. Certainly, any single nursing study is unlikely to result in a straightforward and immediate prescription for practice. To expect this is to misunderstand the processes of knowledge building and utilization of knowledge and, as a result, to devalue research.

In nursing especially, where much of the research is necessarily small-scale and both exploratory and descriptive in nature, it is unrealistic to expect results which are immediately applicable. The production of explanatory and predictive knowledge for practice can only be obtained through larger-scale and longer-term investigation and, importantly, the replication of studies to test applicability and generalizability.

But even if research studies do not have any obvious or legitimate direct application to nursing practice, it is seldom the case that there is no potential for utilization. Appreciating that 'utilization of research' and 'implementation of research findings' are not synonymous is a helpful starting point in thinking through this argument. It is also useful to distinguish between 'direct' and 'indirect' uses of research.

Direct uses of research

The most obvious direct use of research is when findings do have potential for application in practice. Here, we are talking about 'implementation of findings'.

Many nursing research studies have not produced findings which are suitable for implementation because of their limited scale and/or specificity to one setting. But there are many examples of findings which have been made available and are suitable for implementation on a wider scale.

Take, for example, the research which has been conducted in relation to the long-standing practice in midwifery of perineovulval shaving before childbirth. The suspicion that this served no real purpose, coupled with mothers' increasing objections to the procedure, prompted research investigation. Finding that this procedure served no real purpose, recommendations have been put forward that this routine practice be discontinued (Romney 1980; Bond 1980). That a survey of 220 maternity units in England found a 'no shave' policy to be operating in as many as 42% of locations (Garcia et al. 1986), shows that this research has been directly used. Many other examples of this kind of specific change in nursing practice could be given to illustrate direct uses of research.

Horsley (1985) draws attention to a very helpful but rarely made distinction between using the *products* of research (i.e. the findings), and using the *methods*. Although the findings of a study may have no direct application, the methods employed may well be directly useful in practice. For example, Brooking's (1989) methodological paper describes her development and testing of a scale to measure use of the nursing process. The suggestion is offered that 'it could be used by nurse managers as an auditing tool and by clinical nurses concerned to examine their own practices in relation to the nursing process'.

Whether or not – in Horsley's analysis (1985) – such instruments are 'products' or 'methods' of research, the transfer of research tools into nursing practice is an important area of direct research utilization.

Indirect uses of research

Seeing the usefulness of research only in terms of its potential for direct use, is to ignore its contribution to 'enlightenment'. The concept of 'an enlightenment model' of social research is contrasted with 'the technological approach' of natural science in Robinson's (1987) discussion of the relationship of knowledge to action.

A similar idea was conveyed by Stetler and Marram (1976) in their use of the term 'cognitive applications' of research. By this they mean using research findings to enhance one's understanding of a situation. Almost by definition, all research and certainly all descriptive studies, encourage reflection and extend understanding of nursing practice. Endless examples from the British nursing research literature alone come to mind in support of this suggestion.

Thinking back further, one obvious example is contained in the work which Stockwell (1972) published under the title *The Unpopular Patient*. That study set out to establish whether there were some patients who nursing staff enjoyed caring for more than others and, if so, why were some patients more or less 'popular' and did the 'unpopular' patients receive 'less good' nursing care? While a great deal was 'found out' by this study, it did not really produce findings with potential for direct use. Nevertheless, it was enlightening. Surely that study could not have failed to stimulate nurses who read it to reflect on their own relationships with patients and, thereafter, to be more sensitive to factors and circumstances which might influence how they regarded and treated various patients.

Similarly, research by Simsen (1986) which explored patients' spiritual resources and needs, produced no particular findings with potential for direct application in practice. What that research provides for practising nurses, however, is provocation to reflect on the idea that the 'search for meaning' may well be much more engrossing for patients than is generally appreciated.

Perhaps, if the indirect benefits of research were more explicitly recognized, and particularly so among practising nurses, then research in general would become more valued. The personal benefit to be gained from reading research reports would also become more obvious. For individual nurses, the feeling of being powerless to implement research findings in practice would then be offset by the knowledge that at least their own thinking had been extended, and become more enlightened.

IMPROVING RESEARCH UTILIZATION

Improving nurses' knowledge of research and their understanding of the complexities of research utilization are crucial, but not, in themselves, sufficient to ensure that research will be better used in nursing practice. The potential for research use in practice needs to be more clearly articulated by researchers and more systematically assessed by practitioners and managers. And once the potential for use of research is recognized, the process of research utilization can begin. This requires planning, management, and conditions which are conducive for change; and, of course, all of that requires resources – both human and material.

Assessing potential for the use of research

The first step, then, towards improving research use in practice is for *potential* use to be better recognized. Researchers in general tend to be hesitant about pointing out how their research might be used. Quite reasonably, academic researchers may have no real interest or necessary concern with 'what gets done' with their research. Their concern is to contribute to the generation of knowledge and to stimulate further research. And so, reasonably, they concentrate on reporting the theoretical and methodological aspects of a research study and discuss the findings in that context.

There are good reasons why nurse-researchers should go beyond that, attempting to delineate the consequences of their work in terms of its potential for application in practice. Tornquist *et al.* (1989), in an article on 'Writing research reports for clinical audiences', make just that point. What practising nurses need is a readable research report which provides adequate information about the study method, and a clear presentation of the findings; but, most of all, they need a full and helpful discussion of the relevance and potential usefulness of the research for nursing practice.

Given that start, practising nurses are more likely to see the potential for use of research in practice. The researcher's recommendations should not be unconditionally accepted, of course. The importance of critical appraisal of research has been emphasized elsewhere in this book (see Chapter 10), with the skills which that requires discussed in some detail.

In judging the relevance of research to practice, whatever the field, a number of issues are being considered. According to Robinson (1987) these are:

(1) the relevance of the research findings to actual day-to-day work;
(2) the quality, objectivity, and cogency of the study itself;
(3) the plausibility of the research given prior knowledge, values, and experience;
(4) the explicit guidance which is given for the feasible implementation of the research;
(5) the challenge presented to existing assumptions, practice, and arrangements.

Along the same lines, although expressed a little differently, Ropka (1983) writes about what is involved in making a decision to use research in nursing practice. She considers that the first step is to evaluate the scientific merit of the study and that the key questions to be asked on reading a research report which recommends adoption of a particular form of nursing intervention are:

(1) Is there adequate support in the literature for a decision to implement the findings?
(2) Are the results clinicially significant in addition to being statistically significant?
(3) Are the results generalizable?
(4) Is the proposed intervention relevant to your practice and feasible in your practice setting?

A great deal then is involved in decision-making about research utilization in practice. The potential user is not only challenging the robustness of the research, but is also being challenged by its findings. Even if the findings are judged to be relevant, the feasibility of their application cannot be taken for granted. There is a need to assess the readiness and receptiveness of the practice setting for the changes which will have to be made if the findings are to be implemented.

Viewing research utilization as organizational change

While it is certainly within the powers of an individual nurse to identify the *potential* for use of research findings in practice, it is rarely possible for one individual alone to act on that, except in the most limited of circumstances where personal control can be exercised. Indeed, Hunt (1987), on the basis of experience gained in the course of an innovative project concerned with the process of translating research findings into nursing practice, concluded that the task of research utilization is 'generally beyond the capacity of any one individual'. She also concluded that it has been simplistic to hope that if individual nurses could be educated to read research, they could then be enabled to change their practice.

Whose responsibility is it, then, to tackle research utilization in practice? Fawcett (1980) described nurse administrators as the 'key to making research an integral part of nursing practice', and suggested:

'They alone hold the power and authority to effect the requisite changes and to provide the necessary incentives and rewards.'

While this view of research utilization as organizational change has become well established in North America, it has been slow to develop in the UK. Some individuals have highlighted the need for managers to become more responsible in this regard. For example, Melia (1984) challenged managers to 'grasp the real nettle of research'. Objecting to the idea that researchers should be responsible for getting research used, Melia bluntly suggested that while 'researchers make the bullets, it is up to the managers to fire them'.

The argument for research utilization being accepted as an aspect of the management of change within organizations is put forward forcibly in a recent publication by MacGuire (1990). Based on a presentation to a 1989 colloquium for senior nurse managers and educators in Wales, MacGuire's paper begins as follows:

'The problem of utilization of research findings in nursing is usually characterized in terms of why nurses in clinical areas do not modify their practice in response to the new knowledge that has been generated . . . I feel that the position has been oversimplified in much of the writing on this subject.'

She takes up the whole question of research utilization as an aspect of the management of change, and comments that:

'The process of *intentional* change in large-scale organisations is complex and involves a great deal more than bringing about modifications in attitudes and behaviours of individual people.'

In concluding, she says:

'What is clear [is] that the whole process is . . . more difficult than any of us imagine when we blithely talk about a wholescale change to research-based practice.'

Research utilization has to come to be viewed, then, as an organizational process, and resources need to be directed towards finding ways of understanding that process and translating it into practice. The flagship of North American efforts in this direction is CURN – The Conduct and Utilization of Research in Nursing Study (Horsley *et al.* 1983). This was a major collaborative study conducted in the late 1970s with the purpose of developing and testing a model 'to facilitate the use of scientific nursing knowledge in clinical practice settings'.

The CURN Project has also been influential in the preparation of some of the next generation's nurses. Larson (1989) describes its use in an undergraduate nursing curriculum, and, although not without difficulties, the experiment was shown to have a positive impact on students' attitudes to carry out research. Perhaps the most important lesson here for us is not what was achieved, but what was being attempted; namely, to change the emphasis in nurse education from teaching the skills of research to encouraging acquisition of the skills required for research *use* in practice.

While education of individual nurses will continue to be important, various approaches are needed in tackling the challenge of research utilization in practice. An innovative approach described by Wilson-Barnett *et al.* (1989) is the introduction of individuals with a researcher-teacher role amid the practitioners. Two studies (one relating to nursing care of patients with a tracheal stoma, the other concerned with nurses' knowledge and attitudes to cancer), are used to demonstrate how the researcher can work with practising nurses to improve patient care on the basis of research. In this 'experiment', both the researchers and the nurses appeared to be persuaded of the benefits of this type of ward-based research and teaching by the researcher.

CONCLUSION

Clearly, this is an era in which such innovative approaches to improving research use in nursing practice are needed. For its survival, and certainly to justify its growth, nursing research will have to begin to be able to demonstrate that it does make a difference in terms of positively influencing nursing care. It may well be that its apparent lack of impact has resulted more from a lack of understanding of the complexities of research utilization – and misplacement of responsibility on individual nurses – than from a lack of desire to see research used in practice. Whatever the reasons, the time has come for us to stop thinking that use of research in practice will somehow 'just happen'; we need to make it happen and all of us – researchers, managers, educators, and practitioners – have a part to play in that.

REFERENCES

Bond S. (1980) Shave it . . . or save it? *Nursing Times*, **76**, (9), 362–3.

Brett J.L. (1987) Use of nursing practice research findings. *Nursing Research*, **36**, (6), 344–9.

Brooking J.I. (1989) A scale to measure use of the nursing process. *Nursing Times*, **85**, (15), 44–9.

Champion V.L. & Leach A. (1989) Variables related to research utilization in nursing. *Journal of Advanced Nursing*, **14**, 705–10.

Fawcett J. (1980) A declaration of nursing independence: The relation of theory and research to practice. *Journal of Nursing Administration*, **10**, 36–9.

Fawcett J. (1984) Hallmarks of success in nursing research. *Advances in Nursing Science*, **7**, (1), 1–11.

Garcia J., Garforth S. & Ayres S. (1986) The policy and practice in midwifery study – progress report. *MIDIRS Information Pack No. 2* (July).

Gould D. (1986) Pressure sore prevention and treatment: An example of nurses' failure to implement research findings. *Journal of Advanced Nursing*, **11**, 388–94.

Greenwood J. (1984) Nursing research: A position paper. *Journal of Advanced Nursing*, **9**, 77–82.

Horsley J. (1985) Using research in practice: The current context. *Western Journal of Nursing Research*, **7**, (1), 135–9.

Horsley J. et al. (1983) *Using research to improve nursing practice: A guide.* Conduct and Utilization of Reserch in Nursing Practice (CURN). Grune & Stratton, New York.

Hunt J. (1984) Why don't we use these findings? *Nursing Mirror*, **158**, (8), 29.

Hunt M. (1987) The process of translating research findings into nursing practice. *Journal of Advanced Nursing*, **12**, 101–10.

Ketefian S. (1975) Application of selected nursing research findings into nursing practice: A pilot study. *Nursing Research*, **24**, (2), 89–92.

Larson E. (1989) Using the CURN Project to teach research utilization in a baccalaureate program. *Western Journal of Nursing Research*, **11**, (5), 593–9.

MacGuire J.M. (1990) Putting research findings into practice: Research utilization as an aspect of the management of change. *Journal of Advanced Nursing*, **15**, 614–20.

Melia K.M. (1984) Using research (letter). *Nursing Times*, **80**, (49), 14.

Robinson J. (1987) The relevance of research to the ward sister. *Journal of Advanced Nursing*, **12**, 421–9.

Romney M.L. (1980) Predelivery shaving: An unjustified assault? *Journal of Obstetrics and Gynaecology*, **1**, 33–5.

Ropka M.E. (1983) Research questions and answers: Utilization of research in nursing practice. *Oncology Nursing Forum*, **10**, (1), 92–4.

Sheehan J. (1986) Nursing research in Britain: The state of the art. *Nurse Education Today*, **6**, 3–10.

Simsen B. (1986) The spiritual dimension. *Nursing Times*, **82**, (48), 41–2.

Stetler C. & Marram G. (1976) Evaluating research findings for applicability in practice. *Nursing Outlook*, **124**, 559–63.

Stockwell F. (1972) *The Unpopular Patient*. The Study of Nursing Care, Series 1, No. 2. Royal College of Nursing and National Council of Nurses of the UK, London.

Tornquist E.M., Funk S.G. & Champagne M.T. (1989) Writing research reports for clinical audiences. *Western Journal of Nursing Research*, **11**, (5), 576–82.

Walsh M. & Ford P. (1989) Rituals in nursing: 'We always do it this way'. *Nursing Times*, **85**, (41), 26–35.

Wilson-Barnett J. *et al.* (1989) Integrating research and practice – the role of researcher as teacher. *Journal of Advanced Nursing*, **15**, 621–5.

Chapter 33
Research in Nursing Education
Patricia Osborne

Many advances have been made in nursing education as a result of educational research in general and nurse education research in particular. Rogers (1985) identified four priority areas for research in relation to nurse education, namely: methods of teaching and learning, assessment of students, curriculum content, and the preparation of nurse teachers.

When considering the literature, it would appear that these aspects have indeed been developed in recent years and it is prudent to consider some key developments more closely.

TEACHING AND LEARNING METHODS

Over the last half of this century, educational philosophy has moved away from a didactic style of teaching towards a more humanistic approach, largely based on the works of Maslow (1954), and Rogers (1969; 1983). This philosophy recognizes the differing developmental needs of individuals and the notion that the subject matter should not be imposed, but rather sought after by the student; the teacher then acts as a facilitator to assist the student in his search.

Nurse education has been somewhat slow in recognizing the advantages of adopting the concepts of androgogy as a theory of adult education as opposed to pedagogy, the theory of child education (Knowles 1973). The findings of Gott (1982) and Alexander (1984) remain applicable in many cases today in that nurse teachers instruct and 'spoonfeed' their students and, in so doing, believe that their obligation to the student is fulfilled once information has been imparted.

Student-centred learning

If follows that if teaching styles can be different so too can learning. Learning occurs in a variety of ways according to the situation, subject, and purpose. It can also be affected by many factors, but if the learning situation is incompatible with the objective that the student is trying to reach, the learning will be ineffective. In response to this, alternative methods of learning have been explored in recent years and these deserve consideration.

Experiential learning
Nursing is a practice discipline and therefore learning by experience is an integral part of nurse education; however, the adoption of experiential learning as a legitimate educational method is still a fairly novel idea in nursing. Rai chura (1987) highlights the different principles and learning methods involved when utilizing this learning style, particularly in relation to the acquisition of interpersonal skills. She

cites role play, simulation, gaming, and sculpting as just some examples and concludes that these methods enhance the development of communication skills in nurses. Other research by Tomlinson (1985) and Miles (1987) has also demonstrated the importance of experiential learning as a useful learning method in nursing.

Merchant (1989) argues that experiential methods change the role of the teacher to that of facilitator as students retain control of their learning. In addition, a pilot study by Burnard (1989), which explored nurse educators' views of experiential learning, concluded that educators are not always clear about the definition and use of this form of learning and this may help to explain why many teachers remain uncomfortable with this educational approach.

Reflection in action

A development of experiential learning is that of learning by reflection described by Kolb (1974). Schon (1983) suggests that thinking adds theory to the action whilst it is occurring and therefore theory and practice are inseparable. Clarke (1986) elaborates on this by discussing reflection in action as a method of addressing the separation of theory and practice in nursing. She suggests that education should be considered the action and that theory and knowledge provide the explanation. Verbalizing this would then constitute the reflection and encourage an ability to see the action from a different perspective, thus creating a positive feedback mechanism which allows for continual appraisal and refinement of both. When researching the use of reflection in action, Powell (1989) found, however, that while it was demonstrated in planning the actions, there was little evidence of it occurring when the action took place.

This form of learning style needs to be considered further by nurse educationalists. The planning of student experiences should be considered in relation to the why, how, and what, regarding that experience. In addition, both teacher and student must take the opportunity to learn and reflect together, and then discuss a basis for action.

Contract learning

Bouchard and Steels (1980) define contract learning as:

> 'a document drawn up by a student and his instructor or advisor, which specifies what the student will learn, how this will be accomplished, within what period of time and what the criteria for evaluation will be'.

This definition underlines the principle that adults are individuals and self directing and are therefore able to take responsibility for the learning process. In turn, the teacher takes on the mantle of a facilitator and is able to witness the development and progress of the student. The basis for the contract is one of negotiation although if the written contract is too rigid, negotiation may be problematic (Allman 1985). Contract learning is still relatively new in British nurse education but nevertheless it can offer a valuable approach to learning. Richardson (1987) found that this method is most successfully used by those students who value independence and this was corroborated by Gibbon (1989) who noted that the successful preparation of the contract was largely due to the high motivation of the student. Burnard (1987) reports that contract learning is particularly useful in continuing education and professional development. Gibbon (1989) suggests that in view of this it could have strong implications for mandatory updating as it may be one way of identifying individual needs.

Learning style inventories

Recently, education has become aware of the different learning styles preferred by individual students. Ostmoe, Van Hoozer, Scheffel, and Crowell (1984) defined this as the student's own preferred method of perceiving and processing information. Remington and Kroll (1990) addressed this topic while considering learning style preferences in 'high risk' students and noted that their strengths lay in reflective observation and concrete experience. This is an important observation as, given that nursing requires to broaden entry gates and consider afresh retention and recruitment in light of demographic changes, it is likely that attraction of 'high risk' students will increase. Consideration of appropriate learning style preferences could be one method of reducing that 'risk.'

Further research by Dux (1989) found, however, that students did not show any one learning style preference. She suggests the need to examine further the reasons why teachers choose one method in preference to another and when, and if, they adapt these.

ASSESSMENT

The discussion above has demonstrated a definite move away from didactic, one-dimensional education. Whatever approach is adopted, however, education demands that learning be measured in some way and this usually occurs as some form of feedback by assessment. Quinn (1985) states that:

> 'if it is accepted that the teacher's role is that of creating the conditions for learning, then regular assessment of those conditions and their outcomes would seem to be necessary'.

Continual assessment

As nursing has moved towards a problem-solving approach to care, it has embraced the development of student-centred learning where the student is responsible for his own educational needs and how he achieves these. This phasing out of uniformity has required the consideration of alternative assessment methods (Cunningham 1983). As the student accepts responsibility for his learning needs, so he has the ability to set his own criteria for checking progress (Knowles 1980).

This has encouraged the development of continual assessment and there are a number of tools that have been designed to assist with this evaluation. Armitage and Rees (1988), in discussing the use of projects as one such tool, note that their use encourages personal development by the student and requires that the teacher or supervisor has the experience to foster these skills in the student. They comment, however, that many of the teachers involved in this manner do not possess such skills as they themselves have not experienced undertaking such a project.

By definition, many of the student-centred learning and teaching methods discussed above require and encourage the student to self evaluate. Reflection in action is identified as a form of assessment by Burnard (1988) when discussing the use of journals and diaries. This occurs when the student reflects prior to writing, converts thoughts into words as he writes, and then evaluates when discussing with tutors or peers. Cunningham (1983) believes that collaborative assessment of this nature has a place in nurse education because it considers the student as an individual. Unfortunately, to date, this approach has not been adopted and clearly this situation requires some thought.

Examinations

Until relatively recently, written examination was the only method of assessment adopted by nurse education. The number of examinations throughout training currently vary but they are usually few and the ultimate aim is to succeed in the final examination (the inclusion of which remains a United Kingdom Central Council (UKCC) requirement).

A large study undertaken by Altschul and Sinclair (1989) considered the problems encountered by Scottish nursing students when curricular changes created an increase in the number of written examinations. The authors commented that increase in stress was experienced by both the teachers and the students, the former with paper-setting and the latter with the examination itself. They concluded, however, that some form of external examination of students should be required to provide standards and that a final course examination is useful to assess the cumulative outcome of modular training.

Examination as a form of assessment is an appropriate method of measuring recall of knowledge but is an unreliable method of assessing the varied and complex sequence of skills attributed to nursing. In addition to this, it is well-known that marking of essay style assessments is fraught with problems due to poor inter-marker reliability (Hartog & Rhodes 1936).

Peters (1966) suggests that:

'Education itself is not the destination but rather it is the experience of travelling along the road which constitutes an individual's education'.

The trend towards continual assessment and the adoption of alternative methods of assessment as outlined above, would seem to support these sentiments. As a result, the student and her teacher will gain a more useful insight into the quality and success of the learning.

THE CURRICULUM

Nursing knowledge

The recognition of a more holistic approach to care, coupled with striving towards professionalism and accountability, has required the theoretical framework for nursing practice to change. This in turn has created a positive feedback system where the nature of nursing has evolved further and become more identifiable.

These changes have created many challenges for the profession. As the knowledge base of nursing has and is continuing to broaden, so nurses are being encouraged to question their practice; this is, however, easier said than done. One of the most pressing problems of all is that of the marriage between theory and practice (Weatherstone 1981; Melia 1983; Bond 1985). Nurse educators have had to deal with this issue and the result is that the curriculum is now being challenged.

Content

The content of a curriculum derives from a developing basis of nursing knowledge and theory and the last 10–15 years has seen an increase in this theoretical base for nursing practice. Initially this has focused on a systematic approach to care, but as this evolved so too have a variety of models, providing a framework upon which to hang the nursing process.

It is now accepted that for nursing to develop on a firm foundation, it must be supported by nursing theory (Dickoff & James 1968; McFarlane 1977). It is suggested by Draper (1990), however, that in order to do this successfully, the theory must reflect realistic nursing practice. It is at this point that the edges become somewhat blurred as this requires that nursing be defined, a task that is not that easy. Indeed, McFarlane and Castledine (1982) state that nursing is such a complex human activity that it defies a simple definition.

This complexity is reflected by the variety of sources from which nursing knowledge derives and there are implications here for educationalists as often these sources influence both the content and delivery of the curriculum.

Tradition

By far the greatest source of all is that of tradition. As Henderson (1986) states:

> 'Most aspects of basic nursing, including the nurse's approach to the patient, are steeped in tradition and passed on from one generation of nurse to another. Too often they are without rhyme or reason. They are learned by imitation and taught with little if any reference to the underlying science'.

Today, this situation is still strongly reflected in the curriculum. Gilling (1989) believes that the introduction of behavioural objectives into the registered nurse training syllabus in 1977 in Britain, has actually hampered the move away from the medically orientated curriculum, creating instead further entrenchment as a subject-bound, medically orientated profession. Janhonen (1989) confirmed this when evaluating written curricula, finding that they were characterized by traditional nursing, while systematic nursing featured only in a minor capacity.

Authority

Other subjective sources of knowledge contribute to this firm hold on traditional educational practice. Many nurse educators have not had much experience in curriculum planning and have by necessity had to rely on colleagues to supply this expertise. Torres and Stanton (1982) discuss the importance of educational expertise when considering the curriculum by stating that if the expertise is not present it should be sought. Indeed Ouellet and Rush (1989) found that lack of procedural knowledge was a barrier to curriculum review.

Intuition

Benner and Tanner (1987) have described in detail the powers of intuition that nurses are noted for and how best this can be utilized. The authors express concern over the devaluing of this skill because of apparent lack of concrete evidence, and suggest that education has rationalized nursing to the exclusion of the skills required for intuitive judgment. They further suggest that pattern recognition can be taught by reflective judgement using the educational approaches discussed earlier. Carroll (1988) seconds this by stating that nurse education must recognize the importance of this source of knowledge by considering reflective judgement skills within curricula.

Science

The development of nursing theory and the acknowledgement of the differing sources of knowledge has brought to a head the argument that nursing theory and nursing practice must be founded on a scientific base (Akinsanya 1985). This involves quality planning when designing or revising existing curricula. Current changes in nurse education in the form of the New Preparation for Practice (Project 2000) (UKCC 1986) and the Post Registration Education and Practice Project (PREPP) (UKCC 1990) are providing ideal opportunities to introduce some of the developments and approaches discussed above. Never again will there be such an opportunity to move away from unsound traditional curricula and teaching methods and towards new, innovative ideas that have a foundation in science.

WARD-BASED LEARNING

A great deal of research has occurred in relation to ward-based learning. Discussion still exists concerning who is in the best position to facilitate this learning experience for students, particularly concerning the role of the ward sister and nurse teacher.

The ward sister

A large part of the student experience is rightly gained from the clinical component of the training programme. McCabe (1985) described clinical learning experience as the 'heart' of professional education. This has resulted in research focusing on the ward sisters' role in creating an environment for student learning (LeLean 1973: Orton 1981: Ogier 1982, 1989; Fretwell 1982). LeLean (1973) indicated in her study of ward sisters, that whilst the teaching element of the role is vital, it was, in reality, sadly lacking. Long (1976) and Reid (1983) found that sister/student contact time was minimal, and therefore (misleadingly) implied that student teaching is considered an unimportant aspect of the sister's role.

The 'hidden' curriculum

Despite these findings, there remains the issue that most of the student's learning originates from the ward. Ogier (1989) has attributed this to the identification of the sister as a role model for the student and thus it becomes evidence of a 'hidden curriculum'. Bevis (1989) described this 'hidden' curriculum as one of:

'subtle socialisation; of teaching students how to think and feel like nurses.'

This, in turn, is measured by rules of performance and the student's ability to conform to the requirements of the ward as seen by the permanent ward staff. In identifying the ward sister as the key person responsible for creating a learning environment on the ward, Orton (1981) suggested that the selection of new ward sisters should consider attitudes and behaviour in relation to student-orientated climates. More recently, a study by Brown (1989) noted that the sister who was 'patient' rather than 'task' orientated, recognized the importance of her own influence on the ward climate and was more in tune with the needs of student nurses.

Clinical instructors

Alexander (1983) discusses the potential of the ward as a learning environment but also identifies a 'hidden' curriculum, believing that ward teaching will be unplanned, poorly executed, and with little relevance to the total curriculum. She further asks if nurse teachers would wish to join a ward team where such roles (the ward sister as the clinical teacher) already exist. In answering this question, it is necessary to consider the current status of the educationalist on the ward.

Traditionally, teaching in the clinical area has been seen as part of the role of the clinical teacher and nurse tutor. Shuldham (1988) suggests, however, that clinical teaching of this nature is not very successful as, despite efforts, teachers often find it difficult to keep up with current ward practices. She continues by stating that those who teach predominantly in the classroom may be seen to have rejected clinical work and to be divorced from it. Wong and Wong (1987) support this by saying that clinical teaching is considered secondary to classroom teaching and thus has been delegated to inexperienced instructors or 'reluctant' educationalists.

Nurse teachers

If the role of the educationalist on the ward is as a reluctant clinical teacher, how can she be better utilized? Studies by Runciman (1983), Stapleton (1983) and Bryant (1985) have all identified lack of preparation as a key issue in considering ward sisters as the provider of learning climates. The strengths of the nurse educationalist therefore must lie in the expertise that can be brought to the ward staff and the support that can be offered in assisting them to recognize the importance of the teaching and learning aspect of their role in relation to student nurses. Wong, Wong and Mensah (1985), in their discussion concerning student unrest, state that incongruity between students' expectations and educational philosophy is one major factor of student stress and unrest. When analysing nurse teacher accountability, Wood (1987) believes that the teacher has the ultimate responsibility of the learning climate in her hands. By offering support and educational expertise to clinical staff, educationalists can remain in touch with clinical reality and assist qualified staff to enhance the quality of the learning experience for the student.

Joint appointments

The continued scrutiny of ward-based teaching has prompted the development of alternative approaches to this important aspect of nurse education. Pembrey (1980) suggests that it is the teaching agent rather than method that is the key to successful ward learning. This has culminated in the development of joint appointments and the advent of lecturer/practitioners.

Orr (1984) argues for the promotion of the concept of joint appointments stating that it is an error to separate those who teach from those who practice. In view of this, he suggests that the only way forward is to provide a situation where the teacher is immersed in practice and the practitioner develops her educational role. Balogh and Bond (1984), when evaluating one such joint clinical teaching–service appointment, noted that the two appointees became more and more identified with nursing and teaching respectively; thus the school–service split, rather than being bridged, was further emphasized.

Mentorship

A further development in the effort to create a better learning environment for students and to ease the transition from student to staff nurse, is that of mentorship. The scheme originated in America in the 1970s but more recently it has been advocated by the National Boards as desirable for students and course participants. Morle (1990) expresses some surprise that the idea of mentorship has caught on so rapidly but suggests that this may be due to a partial understanding only of the meaning of mentor. She further advocates that this must be clarified prior to preparation of the mentor in the clinical setting. She also suggests that the term 'mentor' is too broad, offering the term 'preceptor' as an alternative. Allanach and Jennings (1990), in evaluating nurse preceptorship programmes, conclude that they are important in facilitating the transition and integration of newly qualified nurses. Nyatanga and Bamford (1990), by developing a model for use based on experiential taxonomy, recognize the potential of mentorship schemes, claiming the 'opening of an educational arena'.

INTEGRATING RESEARCH AND TEACHING

It has been demonstrated in this chapter that educational research has infiltrated into many aspects of teaching and learning styles and by doing so has acknowledged individuality of both student and teacher. It has also recognized the development of nursing as a profession and the move towards holistic care. This has in turn required that the knowledge base be broadened and deepened, and that the sources of this knowledge be exploited to the full. These developments have directly affected and influenced the curriculum. Thus the content has changed, and the presentation of it in the form of curriculum design, the range of teaching strategies, and student learning experiences, have been, and still are being considered from an educational perspective.

There is, however, another aspect of research integration to be considered. When demanding that nursing become a research-based profession, the Report of The Committee on Nursing, chaired by Briggs (Department of Health and Social Security 1972), stated that 'research mindedness' should be encouraged during training. Why is it then, that the profession still bemoans the much documented theory – practice gap mentioned earlier in this text?

The task of cultivating research-mindedness must fall largely on the shoulders of nurse educators and this should be done from the commencement of a nurse's education by fostering critical skills and research awareness. Hockey (1981) sees this as 'cultivating the problem-solving mind'. Birch (1979), however, noted with disappointment that, 'tutorial staff in schools of nursing do little to encourage the reading of research material – neither do they use research findings to illustrate their teaching to a significant degree'. Indeed, Myco (1980) found that few educational staff read academic nursing journals regularly, demonstrating that the majority are not using research as a basis for teaching. These discoveries are also confirmed by Gott (1982) who also found that tutors seldom referred to research when teaching. With these serious implications in mind, it is little wonder that Thomas (1985), in considering why research findings were not implemented, found that the fault lay with the reading habits, or lack of them, of students during their training. This absence at the very start meant that the habit was less likely to be cultivated once a nurse qualified due to pressures and responsibilities of work.

A further obstacle for integration of research is that it is still taught as a separate subject. Research is about discovery and identifying questions that require exploration and then critically appraising these efforts. This can be done with every aspect of learning without being taught as an isolated component within a curriculum. Boore (1984) believes that a major element in relation to this is that teachers lack the skills with which to do this. It is clearly not feasible to expect integration of research and education if those concerned do not possess the expertise with which to do so. A study by Norberg and Wickstrom (1990) stressed the need for integrating practice and educational research by stating that the understanding of nursing theory presupposes an understanding of the elements of research.

THE FUTURE

Change

There is little doubt that nurse education is undergoing tremendous change in response to the development of the profession as a whole.

In examining current educational change, Field (1989) identifies this as part of wider changes in patterns of society. She considers Mannheim's (1943) framework for analysing cultural transformation through social change to be relevant when considering change in nurse education, stating:

'change in nursing education can only succeed if the values inherent in the health care system match those values predicted in the educational system.'

Field continues by suggesting that long-range plans for practice must parallel long-range plans for education.

The concept of organizational culture as a starting point for change, has also been considered by Webster (1990). By identifying the school of nursing as a culture, she considers how progression and implementation of change can be achieved using a cultural model. From producing culture profiles, her study identified positive and negative aspects of culture and suggests that these findings are useful as a basis for highlighting areas for development in the change process.

That change is occurring, is a positive situation as it reflects the dynamism of nursing and education; however, it is vital that those involved in the education of nurses meet these changes in a constructive, planned manner and not as a reaction to perceived inevitability. Orr (1990) states that simple introduction of a new Preparation for Practice Curriculum (Project 2000) will increase conflict and create a defensive stance by 'traditionalists' when faced by the new problem-solving nurse student. He believes that it is important for those people to have available every opportunity to enable involvement concerning decisions about how the change should develop.

It has been suggested that change in nursing education has been held back by failure to understand the change process rather than by a lack of innovative ideas. In response to these concerns, the English National Board for Nursing. Midwifery and Health Visiting (1987), produced their learning package to assist nurse educators to understand and embrace the changes that are offered. As Field (1989) says, 'the greatest stumbling block to educational change may be nurses themselves', and she expresses concern that in the past change has been thrust upon education without first educating the educators.

It is clear, therefore, that for the current changes in nurse education to be greeted in a positive, proactive manner, nurse teachers must understand both the origins of that change and the process of change. Achieving this will ensure that education does not become entrenched, as it has been accused of in the past, and that educational needs will be met in the future.

THE WAY FORWARD

Throughout this chapter, discussion has related to the influence of research in nursing education. It is encouraging to note the advances that have been made, particularly concerning learning and teaching strategies, and the developments concerning the curriculum. It is also important to note that research has influenced many other educational issues. These include evaluation of the curriculum, clinical experiences, and evaluation of philosophies of schools and colleges of nursing. Teaching and learning methods have only been touched upon in this chapter, and it is worth noting the development of distance learning, particularly in continuing education.

The challenge of research is that it often creates more new questions than it answers. Outlined below, are just some ideas for consideration in the future.

The role of the nurse teacher has, and is still, changing and more research is needed into aspects of the role in order to facilitate effectiveness in the future, particularly in relation to clinical input and responsibilities.

Further research is also called for concerning various learning styles, for example, reflection in action with reference to the planning of student experiences and the encouragement of mature entrants (who may well be equipped to use this learning style) to nursing. The use of contracts in learning undoubtedly needs to be developed further too, perhaps in relation to those second level nurses opting for conversion to first level and whose needs and experiences will be very diverse. Similarly, further development of the use of learning style inventories would be useful in view of current discussion concerning widening the 'entry gate' for nursing and the enrolment of 'at risk' students previously mentioned by Remington and Kroll (1990).

There is also a great need for evaluation of the curriculum and further development concerning the possible merger of nursing models and educational models as a mode of content presentation.

Further research and evaluation is required concerning the role of the clinical mentor and the use of preceptorship schemes. Once again it appears that models for use have a part to play and there is need for further development.

Davis (1983; 1987) advocates a process approach to nursing education which focuses on the needs of the learner in relation to curriculum content, teaching strategies, and learning environments and evaluation of the student, curriculum and school. It is encouraging to note that research is demonstrating consideration of these aspects of nurse education.

Finally, this chapter has highlighted many of the changes in nursing education that reflect its dynamism today. This has been due to the influences of educational research within and beyond the realm of nursing. Many issues and initiatives have been, and are currently being considered and dealt with, and it is clear that research and development in nurse education today is alive and growing.

REFERENCES

Akinsanya J. (1985) Learning about life. *Senior Nurse*, **2** (5), 24–5.

Alexander M.F. (1983) *Learning To Nurse Integrating Theory and Practice*. Churchill Livingstone, Edinburgh.

Alexander M.F. (1984) Learning to nurse: Beginning has implications for continuing. *Nurse Education Today*, **4** (1), 4–7.

Allanach B.C. & Jennings B.M. (1990) Evaluating the effects of a nurse preceptorship programme. *Journal of Advanced Nursing*, **15** (1), 22–8.

Allman P. (1985) *Towards a Developmental Theory of Androgogy*. Unpublished PhD Thesis, University of Nottingham.

Altschul A.T. & Sinclair H.C. (1989) Student assessment in basic nursing education. *Nurse Education Today*, **9** (1), 3–12.

Armitage S. & Rees C. (1988) Project supervision. *Nurse Education Today* **8** (2), 99–104.

Balagh R. & Bond S. (1984) An analytical study of a joint clinical teaching/service appointment on a hospital ward. *International Journal of Nursing Studies*, **21** (2), 81–91.

Benner P. & Tanner C. (1987) How expert nurses use intuition. *American Journal of Nursing*, **87** (1), 23–31.

Bevis E. O. (1989) New directions for a new age In *Curriculum Revolution: Mandate For Change*. National League of Nursing, New York.

Birch J. (1979) Nursing should be a research based profession. *Nursing Times* Occasional paper, **75** (51), 135–6.

Bond S. (1985) Part of the Union. *Senior Nurse*, **2** (4), 12–13.

Boore J. (1984) Nursing research – nursing education. *Journal of Advanced Nursing*, **9** (2), 93–5.

Bouchard J. & Steels M. (1980) Contract learning: the experience of two nursing schools. *The Canadian Nurse*, **76** (1), 44–8.

Brown R.A. (1989) *Individualised Care. The Role of The Ward Sister* Scutari Press, London.

Bryant R.J. (1985) *The Role and Preparation of The Ward Sister Involved in Nurse Training* Unpublished MSc. thesis, University of Surrey.

Burnard P. (1987) Teaching the teachers. *Nuring Time*, **83** (49), 63–5.

Burnard P. (1988) The journal as an assessment and evaluation tool in nurse education. *Nurse Education Today*, **8** (2), 105–7.

Burnard P. (1989) Exploring nurse educators views of experiential learning: a pilot study. *Nurse Education Today*, **9** (1), 39–45.

Carroll E. (1988) The role of tacit knowledge in problem solving in the clinical setting. *Nurse Education Today*, **8** (3), 140–7.

Clarke M. (1986) Action and reflection: practice and theory in nursing. *Journal of Advanced Nursing*, **11** (1), 3–11.

Cunningham I. (1983) Assessment and experiential learning. In *Learning And Experience In Formal Education* (Ed. by R. Boot & M. Reynolds) Manchester Monographs, Manchester.

Davis B.D. (1983) (Ed.) *Research Into Nurse Education*. Croom Helm, London.

Davis B.D. (1987) (Ed.) *Nursing Education: Research And Developments* Croom Helm, London.

Department of Health and Social Security (1972) *Report Of The Committee On Nursing* HMSO, London.

Dickoff J. & James P. (1968) A theory of theories: a position paper. *Nursing Research*, **17** (3), 197–203.

Draper P. (1990) The development of theory in British nursing: current position and future prospects. *Journal of Advanced Nursing*, **15** (1), 12–15.

Dux C.M. (1989) An investigation into whether nurse teachers take into account the individual learning styles of their students when formulating teaching strategies. *Nurse Education Today*, **9** (5), 186–91.

English National Board For Nursing. Midwifery and Health Visiting (1987) *Preparing For Change*, ENB, London.

Field P.A. (1989) Implementing change in nursing education. *Nurse Education Today*, **9** (5), 290–9.

Fretwell J.E. (1982) *Word Teaching And Learning*. Royal College of Nursing, London.

Gibbon C. (1989) Contract learning in a clinical context: report of a case study. *Nurse Education Today*, **9** (4), 264–70.

Gilling C.M. (1989) A common core curriculum for nurses, midwives and health visitors. *Nurse Education Today*, **9** (2), 82–92.

Gott M. (1982) Theories of learning and the teaching of nursing. *Nursing Times* Occasional paper, **78** (11), 41–4.

Hartog P. & Rhodes E.C. (1936) *The Marks of Examiners*. Macmillan, London.

Henderson V. (1966) *The Nature of Nursing*. Macmillan, New York.

Hockey L. (1981) Research – relevance for reality. *Nurse Education Today*, **1** (5), 5.

Janhonen S. (1989) Traditional or systematic nursing? An evaluation of the written curricula of registered and enrolled nurses in Finland. *Nurse Education Today*, **9** (1), 31–8.

Knowles M.S (1973) *The Adult Learner: A Neglected Species*. Gulf, Houston, Texas.

Knowles M.S. (1980) *The Modern Practice Of Adult Education* 2nd Edn. Follett, Chicago.

Kolb D.A. (1974) On Management and the Learning Process. In *Organisational Psychology: A Book of Readings*. Prentice-Hall, Englewood Cliffs, New Jersey.

LeLean S. (1973) *Ready To Report Nurse*. Royal College of Nursing, London.

Long P. (1976) Student nurse assessment *Nursing Times*, **72** (2), 522–55.

Mannheim W. (1943) *Diagnosis of Our Time: Wartime Essays of a Sociologist* Routledge and Paul, London.

Maslow A.H. (1954) *Motivation and Personality* Harper and Row, New York.

McCabe B.W. (1985) The improvement of instruction in the clinical area: a challenge waiting to be met. *Journal of Nursing Education*, **24**, 255–7.

McFarlane J. (1977) Developing a theory of nursing: the relation of theory to practice, education and research. *Journal of Advanced Nursing*, **2** (3), 261–70.

McFarlane J. & Castledine G. (1982) *The Practice of Nursing* C.V. Mosby, London.

Melia K. (1983) Students' views of nursing. *Nursing Times*, **79** (20), 26–7.

Merchant J. (1989) The challenge of experiential methods in nursing education. *Nurse Education Today*, **9** (5), 307–13.

Miles R. (1987) Experiential learning in the curriculum. In *The Curriculum In Nurse*

Education, (Ed. by P. Allan & H. Joley). Croom Helm, London.

Morle K.M.F. (1990) Mentorship – is it a case of the emperors new clothes or a rose by any other name? *Nurse Education Today*, **10** (1), 66–9.

Myco F. (1980) Nursing research information: are nurse educationers and practitioners seeking it out? *Journal of Advanced Nursing*, **5** (6), 637–46.

Norberg A. & Wickstrom E. (1990) The perception of Swedish nurses and nurse teachers of the integration of theory with nursing practice. An explorative study. *Nurse Education Today*, **10** (1), 38–43.

Nyatanga L. & Bamford M. (1990) Mentorship Scheme using the experiential taxonomy (ET), *Senior Nurse*, **10** (5), 14–15.

Ogier M. (1982) *An Ideal Sister?* Royal College of Nursing, London.

Ogier M. (1989) *Working and Learning: Creating A Learning Environment In The Clinical Nursing Area*. Scutari Press, London.

Orr J. (1984) Joint appointments – the way forward. *Nurse Education Today* **4** (6), 132–4.

Orr J. (1990) Tradition Project 2000 – something old, something new. *Nurse Education Today*, **10** (1), 58–62.

Orton H.D. (1981) *Ward Learning Climate* Royal College of Nursing, London.

Ostmoe P.M. *et al.* (1984) Learning style preferences and selection of learning strategies: consideration and implication for nurse educators. *Journal Of Nurse Education*, **23** (1), 243–8.

Ouellet L.L. & Rush K.L. (1989) Forces influencing curriculum evaluation. *Nurse Education Today*, **9** (4), 219–26.

Pembrey S. (1980) *The Ward Sister – Key To Nursing* Royal College of Nursing, London.

Peters R.S. (1966) *Ethics and Education*. Allen & Unwin, London.

Powell J. (1989) The reflective practitioner in nursing. *Journal of Advanced Nursing*, **14** (10), 824–32.

Quinn F.M. (1985) *The Principles and Practice of Nurse Education* 2nd Edn. Croom Helm, London.

Rai chura L. (1987) Learning by doing. *Nursing Times*, **83** (13), 59–61.

Reid N.G. (1983) *Aspects of nursing training in Northern Ireland*. New University of Ulster, Coleraine.

Remington M.A. & Kroll C. (1990) The 'high risk' Nursing Student: identifying the characteristics and learning style preferences. *Nurse Education Today*, **10** (5), 31–7.

Richardson S. (1987) Implementing Contract learning in a Senior nursing Practicum. *Journal of Advanced Nursing*, **12** (2), 201–6.

Rogers C. (1969) *Freedom to Learn*. Merrill, Columbus, Ohio.

Rogers C.R. (1983) *Freedom to Learn For The Eighties*. Merrill, Columbus, Ohio.

Rogers J.M. (1985) An examination of research priorities in nurse education. *Journal of Advanced Nursing*, **10** (3), 233–6.

Runciman P.J. (1983) *Ward Sister at Work*. Churchill Livingstone, Edinburgh.

Schon D. (1983) *The Reflective practitioner*. Temple Smith, New York.

Shuldham C. (1988) The new nurse teacher: myth or reality? *Senior Nurse*, **8** (2), 6–8.

Stapleton M.E. (1983) *Ward Sisters – Another Perspective* Royal College of Nursing, London.

Thomas E. (1985) Attitudes towards nursing research among trained nurses. *Nurse Education Today*, **5** (1), 18–21.

Tomlinson A. (1985) The use of experiential methods in teaching interpersonal skills to nurses. In *Interpersonal Skills in Nursing: Research and Applications*. (Ed. by C. Kagen) Kogan Page, London.

Torres G. & Stanton M. (1982) *Curriculum Process in Nursing*. Prentice-Hall, Englewood Cliffs, New Jersey.

United Kingdom Central Council for Nursing, Midwifery and Health Visiting (1986). *Project 2000: A New Preparation for Practice*. UKCC, London.

United Kingdom Central Council for Nursing, Midwifery and Health Visiting (1990) *Discussion Paper on Post Registration Education and Practice* UKCC, London.

Weatherstone L.A. (1981) Bridging the Gap: Liaison between nursing education and nursing services. *Journal of Advanced Nursing*, **6** (2), 505–13.

Webster R. (1990) From threat to challenge: a cultural approach to change in nurse education. *Senior Nurse*, **10** (5), 20–21.

Wong J. & Wong S. (1987) Towards effective clinical teaching. *Journal of Advanced Nursing*, **12** (4), 505–13.

Wong J. Wong S. & Mensah L. L. (1985) Student unrest; A challenge for nurse educators *Journal of Advanced Nursing*, **10** (3), 237–44.

Wood V. (1987) The nursing instructor and the teaching climate. *Nurse Education Today*, **7** (5), 228–34.

Chapter 34
Research in Nursing Management
James Connechen

Hunter (1985) makes the point that research on health service organization and management in Britain began to develop in earnest following the 1974 National Health Service reorganization. There are, however, he argues, real difficulties in researching human service organizations like the NHS, often because of lack of precise definitions as to what is management and who are the managers, as well as problems in measuring output and impact on health status. Although the 1980s saw a series of research reports into the preparation and role of the ward sister (Fretwell 1980; Ogier 1982; Pembrey 1980), there has been a paucity of studies into nursing management in general. The reasons for this are probably complex but may be related to what follows.

Firstly, nurse managers, in common with most other managers, are not a particularly reflective or introspective species. If management is about 'doing things' and achieving results, then there is little time to consider the how or indeed the why of what they are doing. Mintzberg (1975) found that managers work at an unrelenting pace and their tasks are characterized by discontinuity, brevity, and variety. They tend to be action-orientated rather than reflective. Stewart (1967) demonstrated how the manager's day is typically fragmented, with constant switches in attention caused by endless interruptions. When asked to keep a diary of their activities, managers are often surprised by how they actually spend their time as opposed to how they think they spend it.

Secondly, problems exist that relate to the definition, nature, and purpose of nurse management. Many nurses equate management with administration and conceptualize the activity in terms of paperwork such as preparing duty rotas or ordering ward supplies. Pembrey's (1980) study showed that many ward sisters experienced difficulty in exercising their management roles. This may be due, in part, to their lack of management training or the organizational expectation that they effectively manage care, while according them minimal management authority and control.

Thirdly, lack of research awareness is another possible reason. An editorial by Ash (1985) lamented the fact that few nurses seem to read or review research reports. Nurse managers seem to share this, in common with their practitioner colleagues. A study by O'Brien and Heyman (1989) looked at a sample of nurses, including 35 Assistant Directors of Nursing Service, and assessed attitudes and knowledge of nursing research and their perception of research priorities. As many as 40% of the sample were unable to indicate one piece of nursing research or to correctly match two authors to their research reports.

Finally, there may be a reluctance on the part of nurse managers to participate or collaborate in research, not only because it is time consuming but as Withams and Knibbs (1988) argue, the end result may be perceived as threatening or potentially disturbing as it may reveal shortcomings in their work.

NURSE OR NURSING MANAGEMENT?

An important distinction that should be clear in the minds of any potential researcher is the difference between *nurse* management and *nursing* management. De Geyndt (1990) argues that management is not an end in itself and that it does not have a function in itself. It is in effect a means to an end and therefore must be defined in terms of what it is supposed to be doing rather than in terms of what it is. This suggests that the function of nursing management is to facilitate the practice of nursing. The introduction of general management into the health service has meant that the NHS tradition of the management of nurses by nurses was broken. Shaw (1989) states that while nurses can be accountable to non nurses for the provision of services, they can only be accountable to themselves for standards of professional practice and quality of nursing care. Rye (1988) sees the differentiation as critical since it underpins the need for a clearer understanding of the development opportunities in nursing that are now on the research agenda.

If the focus of attention (and research) in the past has been on issues relating to the management of nurses, the new agenda for the future must be related to the interface between management and the delivery of patient care, that is the contribution nurse management can make to the effects of nursing care on patient outcomes. Leadership and nursing input at health authority level will continue to be crucial, but professional advice in the future will have to be backed by hard evidence derived from systematic analysis of the nursing function at the bedside.

NURSING MANAGEMENT – THE CHALLENGES

There are probably few professions within the NHS that have been subjected to as much change over the past three decades as that of the nursing profession. The current crisis of confidence in nurse management can perhaps be understood in terms of the fact that nurse managers seem to have suffered more than most since the introduction of general management. In many Health Authorities, the operational level of management is now firmly based at ward level, with the subsequent disappearance of many nursing officer posts. At the planning and policy levels, meanwhile, senior nurses have found themselves stripped of their line management roles while retaining their professional advisory function. The introduction of resource management with its implication of new organizational structures and relationships such as clinical directorates, is seen by many nurse managers as a further threat.

The reasons why nurse management seems to have faired so badly recently can be seen as a consequence of organizational changes in the past. The implementation of the Committee on Senior Nursing Staff structure recommendations (Ministry of Health and Scottish Home and Health Department 1966) created a nursing line management function and career pathway for nurses, while subsequent reorganizations in the 1970s left nursing with a hierarchical management structure that stretched up to the highest levels of health care planning and policy formulation. Unfortunately, it also managed to alienate most nurse practitioners who felt the system did not provide them with enough support or understanding at ward level. Nurses were promoted into middle management posts on the basis of their clinical competence and were ill prepared for their new management roles. Tension was created between the management function of the newly created nursing officer and that of the ward sister. The rigid hierarchical structure ensured that accountability and decision-making were pushed upwards, and communcation downwards. Too much emphasis was given to roles and reporting relationships, with insufficient attention being given to the management process, the jobs, and the people who work in them.

The nursing officer role was originally envisaged as that of an expert nursing adviser who would participate in clinical work. This rarely ever happened and nurse managers often became nothing more than the administrators of the bureaucracy rather than the managers of the service. The low status accorded to nurse managers by their clinical (and medical) colleagues, coupled with the fragmentation and routine nature of much of their work, left many managers feeling disillusioned and stressed. Smith (1977) prophesied that unless the nursing officer role developed into a clinical one, that is one pertaining to or dealing with nursing practice, then it would become a role which would be taken over by a non nurse in the future.

The 'new managerialism' currently sweeping the health service mirrors to some extent the changes in organizational and management structures and practices which are being adopted by successful businesses and industrial concerns. Faced with unstable environments and fierce competition, organizations are adapting themselves to ensure survival. Hierarchy has receded in favour of looser, more 'organic' structures that ensure maximum decentralization and delegation. The 'scientific management' approach, which guided much management thinking for so long, laid great emphasis on an orderly sequence of activity which encompassed planning, organizing, motivating, and controlling as the key functions of management. Now interest is focused upon 'humanistic' forms of management, which attempt to harness people's own motivation and energies to that of the organization's goals. The carrot has replaced the stick. The 'customer is king' concept has meant that the planning and managing of the enterprise must become customer-led, rather than service- or provider-led.

Within the health service there is also the realization that managers will not

---

Where the system is designed to support the manager:

(1) Division of authority/responsibility into self contained tasks
(2) Division of resources closely controlled
(3) Conservation of information
(4) Networks closely guarded
(5) Upward delegation encouraged
(6) Task forces led by the most senior member
(7) Roles tend to be fixed
(8) Mistakes are remembered/recorded
(9) Working environment invokes fear, or comfort, or paradoxically both together.
(10) Manager sees himself as a controller

MANAGERIAL ROLE MODEL = GOD

Fig. 34.1   Controlling power.

achieve the goals of promoting the health of their local populations, while providing good quality, cost effective care to those who require it, without the total commitment and hard work of their staff. General management sought to achieve this by enhancing accountability at the level which the service was being provided and by involving clinicians and other practitioners in the management process. The new clinical grading structure for nurses has created a strong management role, with continuing responsibility for the ward sister; the middle manager's role – where it still exists – is being re-defined in terms of a facilitating and enabling role. Figure 34.1 illustrates the characteristics of the management role in terms of how managers use power to control. An alternative model of how nurse managers can exercise power is shown in Fig. 34.2.

Where the system is designed to support the subordinate:

(1) Extensive delegation of authority across broad tasks
(2) Resources available on request
(3) Openness of information
(4) Networks available for subordinates to use and extend
(5) Upward delegation discouraged (if you bring me a problem bring suggested solutions as well)
(6) Task forces led by most relevant/capable person regardless of seniority
(7) Roles tend to change frequently
(8) Mistakes are used as learning opportunities
(9) Working environment evokes challenge/excitement
(10) Manager sees himself as guide/counsellor/enabler

MANAGER ROLE MODEL = JESUS

Fig. 34.2   Enabling power.

The great challenge facing nurse managers today is whether they can now seize hold of the opportunities to create the kind of climate and culture that will empower their staff to take responsibility, solve problems, and take decisions. Much more research is needed to identify the personal qualities and characteristics of nurses who would feel comfortable working in this type of management culture. Further work is also needed into exploring the most effective ways in which they can be prepared for the role.

RESEARCH IN NURSING MANAGEMENT

Much of the existing research into management and nursing has been focused on inputs and activity (structure and process) into the health care system, for example manpower planning, recruitment and retention, management styles and roles (Fig. 34.3).

This may reflect, as discussed earlier, the prevalent views amongst nurses about the nature and purpose of management, or because nursing has lacked any readily available measures by which nursing performance can be assessed against outcomes. A Delphi survey of priorities for nursing research in Scotland by Macmillan et al. (1989), conducted amongst first level nurses and ranked in order of importance, identified the top three items as understaffing, low morale, and

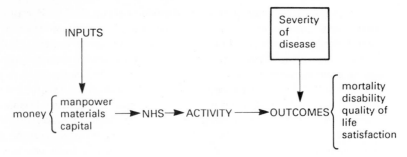

Measurement and Management in the NHS. Office of Health Economics (Teeling Smith 1989)

Fig. 34.3   Model of the NHS.

support of staff. While these items probably reflected the way the nurse practitioners may have felt about the pressures they were working under, it is interesting to note that a North American study by Henry *et al.* (1987), conducted amongst nurse and health administrators, found that the most commonly supported research items included issues related to nursing management such as the relationship between nursing services and patient care.

Nurse turnover studies

Of particular interest to researchers has been the factors that have influenced recruitment and retention in the profession. A survey conducted by the management consultants Price Waterhouse (1988), of 7600 nurses and midwives, found that pay, workload, and management approach were the main factors to influence retention. The report went on to suggest that retention problems can be improved by, amongst other things, making cultural and structural changes in management approaches. The notion that management culture can influence nurse wastage rates appears in many studies. Bamber (1988) looked at why staff nurses left a psychiatric hospital, using a questionnaire to elicit the responses. Of the 162 nurses, the 41% who responded, cited poor management or staff relationships as the main reason for leaving. That author suggests that the real reasons why people leave can only usefully be discovered by having someone – preferably outside the mainstream of nursing management – to conduct exit interviews.

Cavanagh (1989) would seem to support this approach when he took a critical look at nursing turnover studies and concluded that the results are often conflicting and inconclusive. He argued that difficulties arise when different definitions of turnover are used and when measurement techniques fail to take account of the complex and complicated reasons why people leave jobs. This is particularly true when simple bivariate correlation studies are used, for example, job satisfaction being a prominent variable to correlate with turnover. He makes a plea for less reliance to be placed upon quantitative approaches to this kind of problem, while arguing the case for more smaller scale qualitative studies.

Tutton (1989) did conduct a small-scale study, using quantitative methods, to see whether expressed levels of dissatisfaction amongst leavers varied according to different methods of data collection. He was also interested in testing the reliability of data obtained from exit interviews conducted by a 'management' department (personnel) and a 'non-management' department (occupational health). Staff from two district health authorities participated in the study and all received an exit interview from one of the two departments as well as a questionnaire some time later.

The results did seem to indicate that exit interviews and questionnaires produced qualitatively different information on staff's reasons for leaving. Staff interviewed by the personnel department were less likely to give 'management problems' as the main reason for leaving, while staff interviewed by occupational health staff were less likely to give work-related stress as the main reason. Tutton discusses several reasons for the discrepancies but suggests that the question-naire is probably more reliable than the interview in obtaining data on why nurses leave.

Another interesting approach to studying this problem was presented by Barry *et al.* (1989) when he used a computer-assisted analysis of personnel records containing nurses' work histories to identify turnover rate in one health authority. Of interest to the researchers, were variables that might be linked to wastage rates, such as gender, age, first or second level nurses, and time spent in service. This sample of recent studies illustrates how different methodologies can be used to examine the same phenomena, while highlighting the complexities of an apparently straightforward problem. It is also worth mentioning the value of using comprehensive literature reviews such as the one on turnover by Cavanagh (1989).

Nurses and stress

Stress in management is another area that has attracted the interest of researchers – and with some justification since it features so prominently in the literature on nurse management. A seminal piece of work in this area is the study of stress on 515 nurse managers by Hingley and Cooper (1986). One interesting finding, among many contained in that study, was the lack of support in their work that was experienced by so many managers. The kind of support that was missing was of two main types:

(1) Emotional support, that is someone to talk to and share experiences with;
(2) Professional support, that is involving someone who can listen, and who can give advice and direction when necessary, while giving honest feedback on job performance when required.

Individual performance review/appraisal of performance

Although the study of appraisal of performance is well reported in general management literature, little work seems to have been done to assess the impact of such schemes in nursing management. One study, however, Barnett and Anderson (1987), did attempt to look at the effect on the performance of nurses following appraisal. Data analysis included preparation for the interview, the appraisal interview itself, and post interview outcomes. The main finding to emerge was that nurses did not see the appraisal as being related to their present job, perceiving it as being more concerned with preparing them for promotion. Given the importance that appraisal of performance schemes play in allowing managers to set clear objectives with their boss and to receive feedback on their current performance, as well as being coached on ways to improve future performance, research such as Barnett and Anderson's provides valuable information in identifying the inadequacies of existing schemes.

The preparation and role of the ward sister

This area is probably one of the best researched in nursing management and undoubtedly reflects the importance accorded to the role. Researchers in this area have already been mentioned earlier, but attention must be drawn especially to the work of Pembrey (1980) whose study subsequently influenced the King's Fund to set up its experimental ward-based training scheme for sisters. Pembrey demonstrated that using a plethora of research tools, including checklists, semi-structured interviews, questionnaires, and observation, it was possible to identify 'manager' sisters who organized care on an individual basis and 'non-manager' sisters whose form of work organization actively prevented patients from being nursed effectively. Significantly, the 'manager' sisters were the most professionally and academically qualified and had learnt their management skills from working with and observing other more experienced sisters. Farnish's (1983) study on the preparation of the ward sister looked at a sample of 166 ward sisters by questionnaire and demonstrated that few had been adequately trained for their role as ward managers. She discusses in the conclusion of her work the real difficulties in developing appropriate training programmes.

The implications from these and other studies in how we select and prepare ward sisters for their role are profound and are not always realized in practice. It would be interesting now to see whether we have learned from this work by looking at the preparation and role of the 'G' grade ward sister.

RESEARCH IN NURSE MANAGEMENT – AGENDA FOR THE FUTURE

Managing information

Nurse managers have always used information to assist them in day to day decision-making and planning. Monthly staffing returns, sickness levels, bed occupancy rates, theatre throughput, out-patient attendance, and staff wastage rates, have allowed managers to identify potential or actual problem areas and to at least relate resources (inputs) to activity. It is often said that while the health service has been rich in data, it has been poor in information. However abundant the data, it has not always been easily accessible, reliable, up-to-date, or complete enough to have strong utility value for nurses.

The introduction of information technology in the form of clinical and management information systems, has now completely opened up the range and quality of information available to nurse managers. It is difficult to visualize an aspect of the manager's role that will not be affected by new forms of organization and new ways of working that the technology can bring. Managers will have to acquire skills in accessing, using, and managing information, as well as articulating their own information needs.

They could, for example, seek the answers to questions such as:

What decisions am I making?

What information do I need?
Am I monitoring the right things or just the easy things?
Is activity or achievement my key focus?
What measures of achievement do I need?

which in turn would assist in the development of systems that actually work because they have been based on the user's requirements.

The ideal nurse management system is one that can create ward or unit rosters, provide comparison on planned versus actual rotas, link with pay-roll and personnel systems, and relate patient workload and dependency levels to staff deployment and skill mix, while providing financial information and individual patient costs.

The resource management initiative, while relying to a large extent on information systems, is really more about involving doctors and nurses in managing the resources they use and control, supported by essential, timely, and accurate information. This should allow them to review clinical and management practice against agreed standards of care and budgets. Decisions about how resources (staff, budgets, equipment) are used, will lie at the level where the information is generated, that is ward and department level. Research will be required to evaluate the impact that these information systems will have on the management and delivery of patient care. How will managers turn all that information into action and how efficiently will the systems match deployment and skill mix with patient needs? What are the best ways of helping ward managers identify their information needs and what are the most effective ways of developing the new competencies they will require? Resource management will allow nurses to take on new roles and responsibilities, but how effective will they be? Can ward managers contain costs while continuing to deliver good quality care? How difficult will it be to change established routines and practices? The investigation of these and other issues related to information management ought to provide a rich source of material that will lend itself to some valuable research studies.

Managing quality

The development of standards of nursing care within a quality assurance framework is very much a live issue for nurses from most specialities. The development of profiles of care, with built-in minimum standards, for individual patients, will provide benchmarks against which care and treatment can be measured. How can managers nurture quality in their wards or teams and how can practitioners be best supported when developing and using tools to measure nursing performance? What influence do managers have in creating the kind of culture where quality becomes integrated into every nurse's actions? Managers must demonstrate their belief in the primacy of the practitioner to regulate her own practice and determine standards of care. How can this best be done when the manager also needs to ensure that corporate objectives are achieved?

The role of the nurse manager in research

There are probably three main ways that managers can engage in the research process.

Research awareness

Managers need to manage their time so that they leave room to keep abreast of published research in their own field of interest. Even more fundamental to that, however, is the self awareness that comes from critical self examination of their own performance. Managers must question what they are doing by addressing basic questions such as what is my job, and how well am I doing it, and what measures do I have to assess my performance?

Facilitating research

This is perhaps the most important function that managers can perform within the research arena – by highlighting areas of practice where research is required. How can managers create the climate where practitioners are supported and encouraged to carry out research?

Participation in research

A Scottish Home and Health Department report (1988), commenting on the difficulties health service managers have in participating in research, concluded that there was little point in encouraging them to do so. The report goes on to say, however, that they might be persuaded to participate in 'mini-projects', particularly if they could collaborate with research workers. The advantages of participating in inter-disciplinary studies should also be kept in mind.

Areas of possible research interest have already been discussed but a description of the language used to describe management skills, identified by Hirsh (1989), could serve as a model against which managers could usefully view areas of potential research interest.

Management skills

What the job involves: activities, tasks, roles
What the manager can do: skills, competences
What the manager achieves: output, performance
What the manager is: intellect, personality, attitudes
What the manager knows: knowledge experience

The role of the manager in nursing has changed dramatically over recent years. Managers can no longer control what a professional practitioner does. They must instead seek to provide the supportive framework within which nursing practice can be carried out, and this must be underpinned by research. However, the provision of new information is in itself not enough to change practice. There may be resource implications or changes in policy or other organizational issues that will require consideration as well.

Managers need to understand the processes involved in managing change and to network extensively with educationalists, quality assurance staff, information managers, and others, to ensure an appropriate climate for practitioners to put change into practice.

REFERENCES

Ash C.R. (1985) Why Nursing Research *Cancer Nursing*, **8** (4), 17.
Bamber M. (1988) Quitting. *Nursing Times* **84** (22), 33–4.

Barnett J. & Anderson G. (1987) Performance Appraisal Reviewed *Senior Nurse*, **7** (6), 20–2.

Barry J.T., Soothill K.L. & Francis B.J. (1989) Nursing the Statistics: a Demonstration Study of Nurse Turnover and Retention *Journal of Advanced Nursing*, **14** (7), 528–35.

Cavanagh S.J. (1989) Nursing Turnover: Literature review and Methodological Critique *Journal of Advanced Nursing*, **14** (7) 587–96.

De Geyndt W. (1990) Towards a Common Vocabulary for Identifying Management Issues in Health Projects *Health Services Management Research*, **3** (2), 115–26.

Farnish E.G.S. (1983) *Ward Sister Preparation: A Survey in Three Districts*, University of London, Chelsea College Nursing Education Research Unit, London.

Fretwell J.E. (1980) An Inquiry into the Ward Learning Environment *Nursing Times*, 76 (16), Occasional Papers, 69–75.

Henry B., Moody L.E., Pendergast J.F., O'Donnell J., Hutchinson S.A. & Scully G. (1987) Delineation of Nursing Administration Research Priorities *Nursing Research*, **36** (5), 309–14.

Hingley P. & Cooper C.L. (1986) *Stress and The Nurse Manager*, John Wiley, Chichester.

Hirsh W. (1989) Defining Managerial Skills, *Institute of Manpower Studies*, Brighton. IMS Report 185.

Hunter D.J. (1985) Managing the NHS in Scotland: an Agenda for Research and Development *Hospital and Health Services Review*, **81** (3), 114–6.

Macmillan M.S., Atkinson F.I., Prophit P. & Clark M.O. (1989) *A Delphi Survey of Priorities for Nursing Research in Scotland* University of Edinburgh, Department of Nursing Studies, Nursing Research Unit, Edinburgh.

Ministry of Health and Scottish Home and Health Department (1966) *Senior Nurse Staff Structure:* Report of the Committee (Chairman: B. Salmon), HMSO, London.

Mintzberg H. (1975) The Manager's Job: Folklore and Fact *Harvard Business Review*, **53** (4), 49–61.

O'Brien D. & Heyman B. (1989) Changes in Nurse Education and the Facilitation of Nursing Research: an Exploratory Study *Nurse Education Today*, **9** (6), 392–6.

Ogier M.E. (1982) An Ideal Sister? *A Study of Leadership Style and Verbal Interactions of Ward Sisters with Nurse Learners in General Hospitals*, Royal College of Nursing, London.

Pembrey S.E.M. (1980) *The Ward Sister – Key to Nursing: A Study of the Organisation of Individualised Nursing*, Royal College of Nursing, London.

Price Waterhouse. (1988) *Nurse Retention and Recruitment: a Matter of Priority* Price Waterhouse, Bristol.

Rye D. (1988) Managing Nurses or Nursing? *Nursing Standard*, **2** (22), 22.

Scottish Home and Health Department. (1988) *Priorities for Health Research* SHHD Chief Scientist Office, Edinburgh (BGM (P) (88) 15).

Shaw S. (1989) Nurses in Management, New Challenges, New Opportunities *International Nursing Review*, **36** (6), 179–84.

Smith J.P. (1977) The Unit Nursing Officer: Manager of Nursing Care. *Journal of Advanced Nursing*, **2** (6), 571–88.

Stewart R. (1967) *Managers and Their Jobs*, Macmillan, London.

Teeling Smith G. (1989) *Measurement and Management in the NHS*, Office of Health Economics, London.

Tutton J. (1989) Evaluating Exit Interviews *Nursing Times*, **85** (49), 46–8.

Withams S. & Knibbs J. (1988) The Study of Nurse Managers – Seeking co-operation *Senior Nurse*, **8**, (8), 7–8.

Epilogue

As nursing becomes a profession in the fullest meaning of the term, there can be no doubt that it is developing a firm research base. Without such a base, nursing would undoubtedly lack the support, academic and clinical credibility, and professionalism which it deserves and requires. Although there continues to be a place for some intuition, opinion, and untested theory in the art of nursing, this is being tempered with a much stronger research input than has been the case in the past. Although the change of emphasis in nursing which will result in a greater research-mindedness is perceived by some as threatening, it need not be so. The nursing profession is not being criticized for the approaches to care which it has developed thus far; indeed it is to be applauded for the developments which have been achieved. Rather, the profession is embarking on a process of self-analysis and self-criticism which is making full use of a scientific tool not previously available to all its members – nursing research.

Now that the research process is becoming better understood by increasing numbers of nurses, the possibility of making it acceptable to all professional nurses is becoming much more real. Thus far, the majority of nurses who have developed research skills have been based in academic establishments such as colleges and universities, a historical fact which is easy to understand in the context of research having a strong academic component. However, now that a number of academically based nurses have taken the first tentative steps towards making nursing a research-based profession, the time is now right for introducing a greater degree of research-mindedness into the thinking of all professional nurses.

Nursing is a clinically based profession. It is composed largely of clinicians who are supported by a number of sub-groups such as managers and educators. As clinicians, the *raison d'être* for all nurses and nurse groups, is to more fully understand and make use of the research process, so that nursing will become increasingly research-based. This book has been prepared with all nurses in mind, particularly those who are concerned with the delivery of direct patient care, and who wish to do so with a full appreciation of the value of *The Research Process In Nursing*.

Desmond F.S. Cormack

Index

3M, 28

Abstracts, 83, 90, 326
Abstracting journals, 83
Access *see* Research site, gaining access to
Accountability, 37
Action research, 4–5, 125, 155–65
Activity analysis, 139
Advances in Nursing Science, 78
Agencies supportive to nursing research, 23–9
Agreement–disagreement scales, 223
Aims and objectives of research, 100
American Nurses' Association, guidelines on
 ethical values, 34
Appendices, preparing, 325–6
Appraisal of performance *see* Performance
 review
Assessment, continual, 342–3
Audio tape, 131
Author index, library, 82
Author, of research report, 90
Automated observation, 234
Average *see* Mean

Bar graph, 300–9
Baseline conditions, 153
BASIC, 256
Behaviour sampling, 237–8
Bias, 222
Bibliographies, 84
Bibliography of Nursing Literature, 84
Blind assessment, 150
Blind procedure, 150
Blueprint, 314–15
Boxplot, 273
British Lending Library, 79
British Medical Association, 37
British Society of Gerontology, 25
Budget *see* Finance

Canadian Nurses' Association, ethics of
 nursing research, 34
Cancer Nursing, 323

Case study, 178
Categorical data *see* Qualitative data
Categories, 132–3
Category rating scales, 235
Causal relationships, 43
Census, 197
Central tendency, measurement of, 271–2
Checklists, 141, 219
Chief Scientist's Organizations, U.K., 26
Chi-squared test, 287
Citation Indexes, 84
Classification catalogue, library, 82
Clinical instructors, 346
Closed questions, 141, 218–20
COBOL, 256
Code of Professional Conduct (U.K.C.C.), 8
Commissioned research, 33
Comparative descriptive design, 182
Computer(s), 256–60
 data-bases, 80, 84–5
 languages, 256
 in literature search, 84–5
 main frame, 257
 micro, 257
 punch card, 258–9
 statistical packages, 276
Concepts *see* Terms, research
Conceptual definition, 179
Conclusions, 93, 321–2
Conditions, constancy of, 144
Conferences, 20, 69
 proceedings of, 79
Confidence
 in results, 46
 intervals, 278–9
 for mean, 280–1
 for proportion, 279–80
 levels, 202
Confidentiality, 34
Consent, 34
Constant comparative method, 134–5
Continual assessment, 342–3
Contour plot, 315–16